Physical Medicine
and Rehabilitation
Pocket Companion

Physical Medicine and Rehabilitation Pocket Companion

Marlís González-Fernández, MD, PhD
*Department of Physical Medicine
and Rehabilitation
The Johns Hopkins University School of Medicine
Baltimore, Maryland*

Jarrod David Friedman, MD
*Pain Management Physician
Boca Raton, Florida*

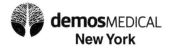

demosMEDICAL
New York

Acquisitions Editor: Beth Barry
Cover Design: Gary Regalia
Compositor: S4Carlisle Publishing Services
Printer: Hamilton Printing

Visit our website at www.demosmedpub.com

Medicine is an ever-changing science. Research and clinical experience are continually expanding our knowledge, in particular our understanding of proper treatment and drug therapy. The authors, editors, and publisher have made every effort to ensure that all information in this book is in accordance with the state of knowledge at the time of production of the book. Nevertheless, the authors, editors, and publisher are not responsible for errors or omissions or for any consequences from application of the information in this book and make no warranty, express or implied, with respect to the contents of the publication. Every reader should examine carefully the package inserts accompanying each drug and should carefully check whether the dosage schedules mentioned therein or the contraindications stated by the manufacturer differ from the statements made in this book. Such examination is particularly important with drugs that are either rarely used or have been newly released on the market.

Library of Congress Cataloging-in-Publication Data

Physical medicine and rehabilitation pocket companion/[edited by] Marlis Gonzalez-Fernandez, Jarrod David Friedman.
    p. ; cm.
  Includes bibliographical references and index.
  ISBN 978-1-933864-53-2
  1. Medicine, Physical—Handbooks, manuals, etc.   2. Medical rehabilitation—Handbooks, manuals, etc.   I. Gonzalez-Fernandez, Marlis.   II. Friedman, Jarrod David.
  [DNLM: 1. Physical Medicine—methods—Handbooks.   2. Rehabilitation—methods—Handbooks. WB 39]
  RM700.P469 2011
  615.8′2—dc22

                                                                          2010047034

Special discounts on bulk quantities of Demos Medical Publishing books are available to corporations, professional associations, pharmaceutical companies, health care organizations, and other qualifying groups. For details, please contact:
Special Sales Department
Demos Medical Publishing
11 W. 42nd Street, 15th Floor
New York, NY 10036
Phone: 800–532–8663 or 212–683–0072
Fax: 212–941–7842
E-mail: rsantana@demosmedpub.com

Made in the United States of America
11 12 13 14 15   5 4 3 2 1

For wisdom will enter your heart,
and knowledge will be pleasant to your soul.
Proverbs 2:10

To Justin B. because a project like this wouldn't be possible
if you were not there for me every day when I get home.
—MGF

This book started as an idea during my residency,
while I watched my paternal-grand-father a dedicated doctor,
editor, teacher and leader in the medical community die.
I dedicate this book to him, Marion Friedman, M.D.
Thank you to the love of my life, my wife, Heidi, for her love and support
during this journey. Thank you to my entire family and my parents: Marsha
and Barry, for all they have done for me. Also special thanks
to my co-editor and friend, Marlis Gonzalez-Fernandez M.D. Ph.D.
Thank you additionally to everyone who has contributed
and helped in the creation of this book.
—JDF

Contents

Appendices

Preface

Finding small (but crucial) information is important in clinical practice particularly for residents who are required to learn, incorporate, and utilize vast amounts of information on a daily basis. Physical medicine and rehabilitation residents also have the unique challenge of mastering a field that covers multiple medical and nonmedical disciplines that are not normally taught in great detail during medical school. There are many excellent and comprehensive books on physical medicine and rehabilitation (PM&R); even books devoted to single rehabilitation topics, but finding the right information at the right time can be elusive for trainees and practitioners alike.

For those at an early stage in their career (students or residents), this book will provide an introduction to the PM&R patient care approach and a bird's eye view of critical topics. For those at later stages of their career, it should provide easy access to facts and core information on areas of rehabilitation medicine that have not been recently visited.

To that end, we chose to divide the book into four sections. The first section introduces the reader to the spectrum of rehabilitation practice. The second section provides an overview on the scope of practice of allied health professionals who are part of the rehabilitation team. Rehabilitation topics and practice areas are discussed in section three. The last section of the book is an extensive Appendix with tables, scales, figures, algorithms, and other facts useful in daily practice.

We are optimistic that this book will be a useful tool for medical students, residents, and the seasoned practitioner.

Marlís González-Fernádez, MD, PhD
Jarrod David Friedman, MD

Contributors

Lisa S. Barrett, MD
Medical Director
Inpatient Rehabilitation Medicine
Marietta Memorial Hospital
Marietta, Ohio

Katherine E. Binder
Staff Prosthetist
Dankmeyer, Inc.
Linthicum, Maryland

Erik Stanton Brand, MD, MSc
Chief Resident
Department of Physical Medicine
  and Rehabilitation
The Johns Hopkins University
  School of Medicine
Baltimore, Maryland

Martin B. Brodsky, PhD
Assistant Professor
Department of Physical Medicine
  and Rehabilitation
The Johns Hopkins University
  School of Medicine
Baltimore, Maryland

Melanie Brown, MD
Medical Director for Brain Injury
  Rehabilitation
Department of Physical Medicine
  and Rehabilitation
Sinai Hospital of Baltimore
Baltimore, Maryland

Maggi A. Budd, PhD, MPh
Clinical Rehabilitation
  Neuropsychologist
Department of Spinal Cord Injury
VA Boston Health Care System
Boston, Massachusetts
Clinical Rehabilitation
  Neuropsychologist
Department of Psychiatry
Harvard Medical School
Cambridge, Massachusetts

Michael Lang Bushby
Lifebridge Health
Courtland Gardens Nursing &
  Rehabilitation Center
Baltimore, Maryland

SriKrishna Chandran, MD
Chief Resident
Department of Physical Medicine
  and Rehabilitation
The Johns Hopkins University
  School of Medicine
Baltimore, Maryland

Maria Eppig, DO
Resident Physician
Department of Physical Medicine
  and Rehabilitation
Sinai Hospital of Baltimore
Baltimore, Maryland

**Dorianne Rachelle
Feldman, MD**
Assistant Professor
Department of Physical Medicine
and Rehabilitation
The Johns Hopkins University
School of Medicine
Baltimore, Maryland

Heidi A. Frere, DPT
Senior Physical Therapist
Rehabilitation
Children's Memorial Hospital
Chicago, Illinois

Jarrod David Friedman, MD
Pain Management Physician
Boca Raton, Florida

Melissa Gong, DO
Chief Resident
Department of Physical Medicine
and Rehabilitation
Sinai Hospital of Baltimore
Baltimore, Maryland

**Marlís González-
Fernández, MD, PhD**
Department of Physical Medicine
and Rehabilitation
The Johns Hopkins University
School of Medicine
Baltimore, Maryland

**Mark S. Hopkins, PT, CPO,
MBA, BS**
Clinical Director
Dankmeyer, Inc.
Adjunct Faculty
Department of Physical Medicine
and Rehabilitation
The Johns Hopkins University
Medical School
Baltimore, Maryland

Maribeth Gorman Jankowski, BS
Senior Occupational Therapist
Department of Occupational
Therapy
Children's Memorial Hospital
Chicago, Illinois

John M. Jones, DO, MEd
Chair, Osteopathic Principles and
Practice
William Carey University College
of Osteopathic Medicine
Hattiesburg, Mississippi

Phong Kieu, MD
Senior Resident
Department of Physical Medicine
and Rehabilitation
The Johns Hopkins University
School of Medicine
Baltimore, Maryland

Barbara J. de Lateur
Distinguished Service Professor
Department of Physical Medicine
and Rehabilitation
The Johns Hopkins University
School of Medicine
Baltimore, Maryland

Scott J. Lepre, MD
Clinical Associate
Department of Physical Medicine
and Rehabilitation
The Johns Hopkins University
School of Medicine
Baltimore, Maryland

Zachary Martin, MD
Plastic and Reconstructive
Surgery
Good Samaritan Hospital
Baltimore, Maryland

Rosemary Martino, MH, MSc, PhD
Associate Professor
Department of Speech Language
    Pathology
University of Toronto
Affiliated Scientist
Health Care and Outcomes
    Research
Toronto Western Research
    Institution
Toronto, Ontario, Canada

Robert Samuel Mayer, MD
Vice Chair, Education
Department of Physical Medicine
    and Rehabilitation
The Johns Hopkins University
    School of Medicine
Baltimore, Maryland

Nathan J. Neufeld, DO
Resident Physician
Department of Physical Medicine
    and Rehabilitation
The Johns Hopkins University
    School of Medicine
Baltimore, Maryland

Bryan O'Young, MD
Clinical Associate Professor
Department of Rehabilitation
    Medicine
New York University School of
    Medicine
Attending Physician
Rusk Institute of Rehabilitation
    Medicine
New York University Langone
    Medical Center
New York, New York

Andrew Sears, PhD
Professor and Chair
Department of Information
    Systems
University of Maryland
Baltimore, Maryland

Lauren T. Shapiro, MD
Instructor
Department of Physical Medicine
    and Rehabilitation
The Johns Hopkins University
    School of Medicine
Baltimore, Maryland

Kenneth H. Silver, MD
Vice Chair, Clinical Affairs
Department of Physical Medicine
    and Rehabilitation
The Johns Hopkins University
    School of Medicine
Baltimore, Maryland

Kerry J. Stewart, EdD
Professor of Medicine
Division of Cardiology
Director
Clinical and Research Exercise
    Physiology
Director
Hopkins Institute for Clinical and
    Translational Research Exercise
    and Body Composition Core
The Johns Hopkins University
    School of Medicine
Baltimore, Maryland

Katherine Dawn Travnicek, MD
Resident
Department of Physical Medicine
    and Rehabilitation
Johns Hopkins School of
    Medicine
Baltimore, Maryland

Sue Carol Verrillo, BSN, MSN, RN

Nurse Manager
Department of Physical Medicine
    and Rehabilitation
The Johns Hopkins Hospital
Baltimore, Maryland

Christine L. Yantz, PhD

Psychologist
Department of Psychology
Gaylord Specialty Healthcare
Wallingford, Connecticut

Mark A. Young, MD

Department of Physical Medicine
    and Rehabilitation
The Johns Hopkins University
    School of Medicine
Chair, Physical Medicine and
    Rehabilitation
The Workforce and Technology
    Center
Maryland Division of
    Rehabilitation Service
State of Maryland Department
    of Education
Baltimore, Maryland

Michael J. Young

University of Maryland
Baltimore, Maryland

Richard D. Zorowitz, MD

Associate Professor
Department of Physical Medicine
    and Rehabilitation
The Johns Hopkins University
    School of Medicine
Chairman
Physical Medicine and
    Rehabilitation
Johns Hopkins Bayview Medical
    Center
Baltimore, Maryland

Physical Medicine and Rehabilitation Pocket Companion

1

Rehabilitative Strategies

Barbara J. de Lateur

The goal of rehabilitation, the guiding principle, and the rehabilitative strategies to accomplish the goal collectively provide a theoretical construct that will allow the practitioner to systematize the approach to the rehabilitation of individual patients, regardless of diagnosis. With this construct in mind, rehabilitative tactics can be applied.

■ GOAL

The goal of rehabilitation is to optimize the health, function, and ability to participate in desired activities in the family, work, recreation, and community.

■ GUIDING PRINCIPLE

Woven throughout rehabilitation is the guiding principle of anticipatory management. Although no 2 patients with any given disease or injury are exactly alike, there are enough similarities that certain patterns can be discerned in the natural history of the condition. Patients and providers can thus be spared the distress of enduring typical complications, which may cause a deterioration of health and prevent or delay return to function and participation.

■ STRATEGIES

I would suggest that the first and the best rehabilitative strategy, whenever possible to apply, is primary prevention. This is not ordinarily considered a part of rehabilitation and is certainly not the province solely of rehabilitative medicine, but surely prevention is preferable to "picking up the pieces" after a stroke, spinal injury, traumatic brain injury, heart attack, malaria, burn, or other condition has occurred.

The second strategy is reduction of the pathologic process to a minimum. Here, early care is of great importance to the ultimate functional outcome.

The third strategy, and the first one commonly considered a rehabilitative strategy, is prevention of secondary complications (sometimes expressed as secondary disability). This strategy often challenges time-worn concepts of bed rest as a treatment and, instead, promotes early mobilization to prevent pressure sores, deconditioning, contractures, loss of bone mass, and depression, to name a few.

The fourth strategy is enhancement of the function of the affected systems—basically attempting to repair the damage done. Attempting to strengthen weakened limbs in a patient with stroke would be an example of this strategy.

The fifth strategy is enhancement of the function of the unaffected systems. This overlaps with the sixth strategy, which is compensation or compensatory techniques. Examples of these strategies include strengthening the upper body of a person with paraplegia (fifth) and strengthening the less affected side of a person with stroke (sixth).

The seventh is cognitive and behavioral intervention. A person with spatial-perceptual impairment may learn to "talk himself through" a transfer or dressing or other task.

The eighth strategy is environmental adaptation. This may be temporary, employed before the first 7 strategies have had their full effect. More often, they change as rehabilitation progresses.

■ TACTICS

The tactics or techniques employed in rehabilitation are numerous. They are what are usually considered rehabilitation. The tactics and techniques are the means by which the goal is achieved and the strategies accomplished. In earlier times of multidisciplinary rehabilitation, certain tactics were considered the territory of certain disciplines. I would submit that in true interdisciplinary rehabilitation, practitioners of one discipline may have primary responsibility for one strategy and the associated tactics, but other team members will be actively involved. For example, the psychologist may have primary responsibility for helping the patient incorporate certain behaviors in his/her repertoire (such as frequent pressure-relief maneuvers in the patient with spinal cord injury), but other team members, including family and friends, will need to reinforce the behaviors by a smile or the word "Good" when a wheelchair pushup is observed. Wheelchair transfers may be taught in the physical or occupational therapy gym, but nursing will need to ensure that the patient does these transfers in her room. This interdisciplinary approach helps the patient transition from "can do" to "does."

■ ACKNOWLEDGMENTS

I was introduced to the concept of rehabilitation strategies some 40 years ago by Walter C. Stolov. He began them with "Prevention of secondary disability." Dr. Justus F. Lehmann added the strategy "Reduction of the pathology to a minimum." I bear the responsibility of adding "Primary Prevention." Many physicians employ the concept of "Secondary Prevention," by which they mean prevention of another stroke or prevention of a relapse in multiple sclerosis. In certain contact sports, such as American football, it may mean prevention of a second, third, or fourth (or more) concussion. I have applied strategies 3 through 8 to trauma in "Orthopaedic Trauma Protocols" S.T. Hansen, Jr. and Marc F. Swiontkowski, eds, New York: Raven Press; 1993, pages 43–49.

Rehabilitation Documentation

Kenneth H. Silver

■ INTRODUCTION

Well-written, accurate, and comprehensive documentation is key to optimal patient assessment and management as well as serving as justification for a patient's admission to, and continued stay, on a comprehensive inpatient rehabilitation service. Recent changes in Medicare oversight of inpatient rehabilitation facilities (IRF) have heightened the necessity for physicians and other rehabilitation care providers to improve documentation in order to avoid denial of payment by auditors (1,2). Documentation at the preadmission, admission H&P, daily progress note, team conference, and discharge summary levels should support that services are reasonable, appropriate (in terms of efficacy, duration, frequency, and amount) for treatment of the patient's condition, as well as necessary to furnish the care on an inpatient hospital basis, rather than in a less intensive facility such as a skilled nursing facility (SNF) or on an outpatient or home-based basis. Templates, both electronic and written, are useful to facilitate the completion of such documentation requirements.

■ HISTORY AND PHYSICAL ADMISSION NOTE

The history and physical admission note (H&P) should clearly communicate the assessment and treatment plan of the admitting physician. The reviewer must be able to ascertain the reason for admission, the prior level of function, the therapies required, the anticipated course of treatment, and the expected goals (3,4).

More specifically, the H&P serves as the detailed review of a rehabilitation patient's

■ Actively treated conditions

■ Newly recognized conditions

■ Resolving/resolved conditions

■ Rehabilitation diagnosis (primary functional limitation, primary impairment, and cause)

■ Complications and coexisting conditions

- Symptoms that will require treatment

- Chronic medical conditions

- Potential conditions that require preventive measures, restrictions, and/ or precautions

- Other functional deficits

In addition, the H&P should support the medical and rehabilitation necessity of the IRF admission by

- Describing the reason for admission to an IRF

- Providing evidence of the complexity of the planned interdisciplinary program

- Listing the interventions to be provided by each discipline (ie, Physical, Occupational, Speech Therapies, Nursing, Rehabilitation Nursing, and Case Management)

- Providing evidence that the patient will be able to tolerate, benefit from, and participate in the intensity of approximately 3 hours of therapy per day

- Detailing the need and plan for cross-disciplinary reinforcement of the medical, nursing, and therapy programs

- Demonstrating the complexity of medical and rehabilitation conditions that require both nursing assessment 24 hours a day and frequent physician visits and oversight

- Identifying the anticipated impact of coexisting medical conditions on the rehabilitation plan and how those medical issues alter the approach to treatment

The following characteristics apply to all documentation in the inpatient rehabilitation service, including the H&P: legibility, completeness, timeliness (payor and institutions may require certain documents to be in the patient's record within 24 or 48 hours), and authentication (physicians' and other clinicians' signatures are required on all their own documentation). As well, attending physicians need to co-sign and often document more detailed information along with documentation for other clinicians whose work they are responsible for (ie, residents and physician extenders). Additionally, the appropriate method to make corrections and alterations of the document should be corrected in the following manner: put a line through the documentation made in error; write the word error above the line; initial and date just after the word error; and finally, erasures, whiteout, or other cover-up techniques should never be used in patient medical records—they call into question the credibility of the entire record.

The physiatric history and physical admission note utilize the standard medical H&P as a platform from which to additionally document an assessment of the patient's impairments, disabilities, and handicaps, as well to formulate a management plan of coordinated, multidisciplinary rehabilitation care. Key to a comprehensive Rehabilitation H&P is a detailed account of the patient's medical history that focuses on past and present medical conditions as well as past and present functional limitations and the resources available to maximize independence and functionality postdischarge. (see Table 2.1).

The physical examination component of the admission note should be the documentation of a thorough examination that emphasizes the patient's neurological, musculoskeletal, and psychological status, while also examining more specifically aspects of gait, balance, and upper and lower extremity function. The physical examination needs to be tailored to the condition for which the patient is being admitted. For instance, an orthopedic patient with a total joint replacement does not necessarily require a comprehensive neurological examination.

The summary portion of the H&P admission note should include an active medical and functional problem list, along with a management plan that details the coordinated, multidisciplinary approach required for patients admitted to an IRF. The management plan should speak to

TABLE 2.1 ■ The Admission Inpatient Rehabilitation document should contain the following categories of the patient's history.

Date of Admission
Referring Physician/Institution/Service Information
Consulting Physicians from Referral Institution
PCP
Reason for Admission
Primary Medical Diagnosis
Rehabilitation/Functional Diagnoses
History of Present Illness
Past Medical History
Past and Recent Medications Including Allergies
Social History Including
   Occupation
   Where patient lives or plans to live
   Type of residence including stairs, floor levels, outside access
   Family resources
   Tobacco, alcohol, illicit drug use history
Family Medical History
Functional history (prior to and current) including levels of proficiencies in upper and lower extremity ADLs, mobility, toileting, cognition, comprehension, and expression
Bladder and Bowel Function (prior to admission and current)
Diet and swallowing history (prior to admission and current)
Comprehensive review of systems
Laboratory and imaging data

justifying the admission as it relates to medical necessity standards. The H&P summary should also highlight the patient's anticipated activity and participation limitations, focusing on:

- Estimated length of stay
- Anticipated discharge setting
- Discharge functional goals
- Precautions (falls, cardiac, seizure, sternal, orthopedic).

If a resident physician or a physician extender (PA or NP) is involved, there should be a separate section for the PM&R attending physician's history, physical examination, and assessment information.

DAILY PROGRESS NOTES

Progress notes must demonstrate frequent, direct, and medically necessary physician involvement for the entire IRF stay. This documentation should include any revisions to the expectations of the anticipated course and predicted functional gains. In addition to serving as an accurate current assessment of the status of the patient's medical problems and functional/rehabilitation progress, the progress note identifies the continuing necessity for a coordinated and comprehensive inpatient rehabilitation approach. This is accomplished by documenting a daily management plan that links specific medical or rehabilitation issues to prescribed treatments and involvement of the multidisciplinary team. For instance, the development of orthostatic hypotension in a stroke patient would require in addition to a medical plan for further medical assessment and treatment, documentation of how the therapist should modify the therapeutic plan for gait therapy and monitor vital signs, and nursing should institute and monitor response to compression stocking/wrapping. In addition, the daily note should include information regarding the patient's progress toward the stated rehabilitation goals, and if he/she was unable to attend or participate in rehabilitation therapies, the reason should be indicated. As inpatient rehabilitation reimbursement becomes subject to strict reviews of medical necessity documentation, it is imperative that the daily progress note document the continuing justification for the patient to remain on the rehabilitation service. This includes evidence in the note that progress is being made toward goal attainment, the patient is able to tolerate the intensity of services prescribed, and that coordinated multidisciplinary care requiring 24-hour rehabilitation nursing and frequent physician presence is being given.

A Physiatric Daily Progress note may be written in a SOAP format (symptoms, objective, assessment, plan) with inclusion of the patient's functional/rehabilitation status and progress in addition to addressing the active medical problems and plan of care. Typically this includes

1. Chief complaints and status of present illness

2. Relevant review of systems

3. Physical examination findings including vital signs

4. Results of recent and pertinent laboratory tests and imaging

5. An impression that focuses on the status of active medical problems and rehabilitation issues including the degree of progress accomplished

6. A plan of management for those active medical and rehabilitation problems with sufficient specificity as to both the individualized and coordinated nature of plan. For example, daily documentation for a patient whose leg spasticity is worsening may include not only the medical assessment of the type and degree of spasticity and the medication to be prescribed but also that management of the spasticity will additionally focus on nursing carrying through a stretching program in bed with appropriate splint application, and physical therapy will use ice and electrical stimulation to reduce tone and increase ankle range of motion.

DOCUMENTATION OF DISCHARGE FROM THE REHABILITATION INPATIENT SERVICE

Hospital discharge or transfer of service summaries serve as the primary documents communicating a patient's care plan to the receiving medical or surgical service, subacute rehabilitation unit or facility, or an outpatient primary care or specialist provider. At times, these documents are the only form of clinical information that accompanies the patient to the next setting of care. Therefore, these summaries need to be of high quality including sufficient enough detail to permit safe and effective care to resume after the handoff from one practitioner to the other. The Joint Commission has published standard that specify expected components of hospital discharge summaries that include (5):

1. Reason for hospitalization (chief complaint and history of present illness)

2. Significant findings during the stay (primary diagnoses)

3. Procedures and treatments provided (hospital course, procedures and consultations)

4. Patient's discharge condition (the patient's health status at discharge)

5. Patient and family instructions if appropriate (discharge medications, activity orders, therapy orders, dietary instructions, plans for medical/surgical follow-up)

6. Attending physician signature of the discharge summary

Although the above applies to all types of medical and surgical discharges or transfer notes, the physiatric version needs to additionally focus on conveying critical information pertaining to the rehabilitation needs of the patient. The discharge summary reviews both the medical and the rehabilitation aspects of the hospital stay including functional deficits, barriers to further progress, progress/attainment of rehabilitation goals, and the type of discharge setting.

For program summaries of patient's being discharged to the home setting, it is critical to specify equipment already provided or being delivered including assistive devices, dwelling modifications suggested, the degree of physical assistance needed, and specifications for the frequency and duration of nursing and therapy services prescribed, either in the home or in an outpatient facility, and documenting appropriate training and education of the patient and family.

For those patients being discharged to a skilled nursing facility/subacute rehabilitation program, rehabilitation instructions should focus on a detailed plan of medical and rehabilitation care that the receiving team of nurses and therapists can easily understand and institute. Recommendations for equipment and rehabilitation services have to be consistent with resources likely to be available in noncomprehensive rehabilitation settings.

Patients being transferred off a comprehensive rehabilitation service due to a need for urgent or more complex medical and surgical management should be accompanied by a Transfer Summary, which follows the principles of the rehabilitation discharge summary mentioned above. However, transfer summaries need to include detailed documentation as to why the patient requires changing services with up-to-date summary of the recent hospital course, up-to-date lists of medications, procedures, and laboratory and imaging findings. This transfer information needs to be sufficiently clear and comprehensive that the physician and nursing team assuming care can do so expeditiously and safely. Moreover, the summary must also detail recommendations for continued rehabilitation management as best can be accomplished on an acute medical–surgical service. Particular emphasis needs to be placed on bladder and bowel management, and skin care, as well as the importance of early mobilization and preserving joint range of motion. Suggestions should be made to restart rehabilitation therapies as soon as is medically feasible.

■ ELECTRODIAGNOSTIC REPORTS

Electromyography (EMG) and nerve conduction studies (NCS) performed by appropriately trained and experienced individuals are used to evaluate patients with neuromuscular disease and to diagnose the presence, distribution, and severity of neurological system pathology. The report that the electrodiagnostician produces after completion of the test serves as a communication instrument to the referring physician documenting the results and conclusions of the electrodiagnostic evaluation. EMG and

NCS need to be performed and reported with consideration of the clinical context, not merely as isolated tests—in essence, an electrodiagnostic consultation. Electrodiagnostic studies should always be considered as an extension of the physical exam. The final diagnoses and subsequent clinical decisions made should reflect that. Thus, the EMG report should strive not to portray generalizations (ie, "suggest clinical correlation"), but rather to make a determination as to whether or not the results explain the patient's signs and symptoms. This is only possible if the electromyographer has discussed the history with the patient and done at least a focused physical examination.

The question arises what information should be included in the report and what is the best way to present that information. It is paramount that the electromyographer's final report be a concise and clearly written summary of relevant findings and interpretation. It is desirable that the report not be a lengthy list of every subtest result, irrespective of the clinical significance of those findings. This type of report is often due to the electromyographer's lack of certainty as to the clinical relevance of a given result. The EMG report should be concise, to the point, and understandable to the less sophisticated reader.

A good-quality EMG report should always include the actual waveforms of sensory, motor, and F-wave tests. This is in addition to the numerical data that are usually included in tabular format. Another important indicator of a good-quality study and report is the inclusion of temperature data. Whether or not the ideal temperature can be obtained, an EMG report without a temperature recorded offers incomplete and possibly inaccurate information.

The model report should include a description of the clinical problem for which the patient was referred, the electrodiagnostic tests performed and their results, and the diagnostic interpretation of the data. If the report only contains a conclusion but without supportive data, it is difficult for the referring clinician to determine whether the test results support the conclusions made and whether the diagnosed condition is worsening, improving, or stable. Normal reference values included adjacent to the specific results are desirable to allow the reader to verify why certain findings were reported as abnormal.

List of recommended components of a complete electrodiagnostic report (6–8):

1. Patient's demographic data (name, age/birth date, gender)

   Also consider: height, weight, handedness

2. Clinic-based information: Hospital/patient number, electromyographer's name, referring physician, name of assisting technician or resident physician, testing location, date

3. Limb temperatures

4. Medical history including presenting problem, relevant past medical history, relevant medications (especially anticoagulants)

5. Brief physical examination findings

6. Other: obstacles to performing the complete test (ie, contraindications to performing parts of the test such as nerve conduction in face of a cardiac pacemaker, or needle EMG of certain muscles because of anticoagulation, or inability to test certain muscles/nerves due to difficulty in positioning)

7. Use nonnarrative, tabular formats to present NCS and Needle-EMG data

8. Nerve conduction study results. List the nerves and the side (right or left) studied, and include results for the following test parameters:

- name of nerve studied

- sites of stimulation

- distance between the distal stimulation site and the recording site, and distances between the various stimulation sites

- sensory peak distal latencies and peak-to-peak (or baseline-to-peak) amplitudes

- depending on preference, calculated sensory conduction velocity (determined from onset latencies)

- motor onset latencies and baseline-to-negative peak compound muscle action potential (CMAP) amplitudes

- calculated motor conduction velocities for specified nerve segment (ie, ulnar across elbow segment)

Example of Motor Nerve Conduction Table of Results

Nerve	Side	Site (stim–record)	Distance (cm)	Latency (ms)	Amplitude (mV)	Segment	Conduction Velocity (m/s)
Ulnar	Right	Wrist (W)-ADM	8	3.8	8	—	—
		Below elbow (BE)	28		7	BE–W	56
		Above elbow (AE)	12		6.5	AE–BE	62

9. Other Nerve Conduction

- F-wave studies
  - Name of nerve studied (ie, ulnar)
  - Side of test
  - Stimulation and recording sites
  - Report minimum F-wave latency
- H-reflex studies
  - Name of the nerve studied (ie, tibial)
  - Side of test
  - Stimulation and recording sites
  - Report minimum H-reflex latency
  - (recorded H-wave amplitude is optional)
- Repetitive nerve stimulation
  - Sites of nerve stimulation and muscle recorded from
  - Indicate if stimulation was performed at rest or after exercise, and if after exercise, the duration of the exercise and the time since the exercise
  - Indicate the rate of stimulation (ie, 3/s) and the number of stimuli in the pulse train
  - Report the initial CMAP (M) amplitude, and the increment or decrement is calculated (% change of amplitude or area of the fourth or fifth M-wave to the first).

10. Needle electromyography

- Describe insertional, spontaneous, and voluntary activity for each muscle studied
- It is helpful, but optional, to associate each muscle tested with a corresponding peripheral nerve or root level of innervation
- State whether the test utilized a monopolar or concentric needle
- Divide the needle EMG findings per muscle according to spontaneous activity and voluntary activity
  - Spontaneous activity should include insertional activity (increased, decreased, or normal); fibrillations (0-4+); positive sharp waves (0-4+); fasciculations, complex repetitive discharges, other abnormal spontaneous activity noted (ie, myokymia, myotonia, cramps)
  - Voluntary activity should be divided into motor unit action potential (MUAP) amplitude and duration (increased, normal, or

decreased), polyphasicity (normal or increased), and recruitment or firing pattern (normal, early, decreased). Indication of the fullness of the interference pattern with maximal effort should be described (full, incomplete, discrete, or single unit pattern)

iii. Indication of factors limiting the needle examination of that muscle (ie, unable to relax; did not tolerate secondary to pain)

Example of Needle EMG Table of Results

☐ At rest   ☐ With activation

Muscle	Innervation	Insertional	Fib	PSP	Fasic	CRD	Other
APB	Med/C8	increased	2+	2+	none	Occ	none

(Continues below)

Ampl	Duration	Polys	Recruitment	Interference	Comments
increased	Increased	increased	decreased	incomplete	Pain limited

11. The summary of results section of the report should not be a regurgitation of detailed individual data elements (already included in the table format presentation) but instead be a summarization of the findings with an attempt at recognized patterns of the results (9)

• For instance, "NCS show generalized borderline motor nerve conduction velocities with low amplitude sensory and motor responses. There is disproportionate focal slowing of conduction across the left elbow without amplitude loss comparing above and below elbow stimulation sites. Concentric needle examination demonstrated low-grade spontaneous activity in distal leg and arm muscles, with mildly increased MUAP amplitudes in several distal foot muscles."

12. The interpretation section of the report should tie the summary of results into a probable electrophysiological diagnosis, noting whether the findings are normal or abnormal. (ie, This is an abnormal electrodiagnostic examination. The EMG findings suggest mild to moderate predominantly axonal, sensorimotor peripheral neuropathy with superimposed focal compression ulnar neuropathy at the right cubital tunnel).

■ **REFERENCES**

1. US Department of Health and Human Services, Centers for Medicare & Medicaid Services. Proposed Rule: Medicare: inpatient rehabilitation facility prospective payment system (2008 FY); update, [07-2241]. *Fed Regist.* 26230–26279.

2. The Medicare Recovery Audit Contractor (RAC) Program: an evaluation of the 3-year demonstration. June 2008, CMS. http://www.cms.hhs.gov/RAC/Downloads/RAC%20Evaluation%20Report.pdf

3. Ganer B, Erickson R, et al. Clinical evaluation. In: Joel AD, Gans BM, Walsh NE, Bockenek WL, eds. *Physical Medicine and Rehabilitation: Principles and Practice*. 4th ed. Lippincott Williams & Wilkins; 2004.

4. Odell M, Lin C, Panagos A, Fung N. The physiatric history and physical examination. In: Braddom, ed. *Physical Medicine and Rehabilitation*, 3rd ed. Elsevier.

5. Kind JHA, Smith MA. Documentation of mandated discharge summary components in transitions from acute to subacute Care. http://www.ahrq.gov/downloads/pub/advances2/vol2/Advances-Kind_31.pdf

6. Jablecki C, et al. Reporting the results of needle EMG and nerve conduction studies: an educational report. *Muscle Nerve*. 2005.

7. American Association of Neuromuscular and Electrodiagnostic medicine. Recommended policy for electrodiagnostic medicine. *Muscle Nerve*. 1999; 22:S101–S104.

8. Dumitru D, Zwarts MJ. The electrodiagnostic medicine consultation: approach and report generation. In: Dumitru D, Amato AA, Zwarts MJ, eds. *Electrodiagnostic Medicine*. 2nd ed. Philadelphia, PA: Hanley & Belfus; 2002:515–540.

9. Smith B. What good is EMG to the patient and practitioner? *Semin Neurol.* 2003;23(3):335–342.

3

Outpatient Rehabilitation: Clinics and Practice

Jarrod David Friedman

■ INTRODUCTION

Outpatient medicine is a key component of a physiatric practice. Clinics can be both a primary and secondary site in the care of our patients. An outpatient physician does not have to practice within a hospital setting or a university setting. Unlike an inpatient practice, the majority of outpatient clinics are not part of a university or hospital setting. This short chapter will give you some basic important information regarding outpatient clinics and outpatient medicine.

■ STATISTICS

Outpatient visits outnumber inpatient visit at a ratio of 3:1. According to the CDC US Health Report in 2009, US hospitals saw 102.2 million outpatients compared with 34.9 million discharges from US hospital inpatient care facilities in 2006 (1). The same report notes that in 2007, Medicare-reported physicians saw 994 million patient visits to their outpatient physician offices, whereas US hospital outpatient facilities saw only 89 million visits (1). In general, physicians who plan to practice in an outpatient setting see and handle larger volumes of patients than inpatient attending physicians and must be capable of handling a higher patient load and be efficient doing so while ensuring that the health care they deliver is of the highest quality.

Despite the significantly higher volume of patients seen in the outpatient setting, the cost of care is lower. According to the CDC, 2007 National healthcare expenditures in the US totaled $2.2 trillion. Hospital costs accounted for 31% of these expenditures, while outpatient clinic costs accounted for 21% (2). This does not speak for the complexity of outpatient care, very much to the contrary. Outpatient care can be very complex, and the skills needed to handle an outpatient practice effectively require not only broad medical and physiatric knowledge base but also an understanding of good business practices.

■ **OUTPATIENT PRACTICES**
Physiatrists have a wide array of subspecialties to choose from. From neurologic disorders to musculoskeletal disease or even cardiopulmonary disease and the choice between pediatric and adult populations, physiatry can accommodate a wide variety of interests (Table 3.1). Specialization within physiatry is not necessary if a physician is interested in seeing a wide variety of patients with a host impairments and disability.

Only through experience can an individual choose which focus or subspecialty best suites his or her personality and intellectual interest. Anyone thinking of pursuing a career in outpatient physiatry is encouraged to obtain exposure to as many different fields as possible.

■ **THE OUTPATIENT TEAM**
A hallmark of acute inpatient rehabilitation is the provision of multidisciplinary care with a team approach. The outpatient setting is no different. Understanding and learning the different components is very important to best serve patients in an outpatient setting. The role of the physiatrist as coordinator of care becomes crucial in the outpatient setting when the care provided by different disciplines is in multiple locations.

In order to understand outpatient practice, it is useful to understand how a patient moves in and out of a given clinic. This is referred to as clinic flow dynamics. Although each clinic is different, the basic design is usually similar (Figure 3.1).

Clinic flow and the other logistical issues that will be mentioned might be considered obvious to some, while others find it difficult or think it is irrelevant. However, because many of these issues affect outpatient practice and are seldom taught during residency or medical school, we will provide a brief introduction.

■ **CLINIC FLOW AND CLINICAL PRACTICE**
Clinic flow and efficiency can have a significant impact on clinical practice for multiple reasons:

1. Clinic flow affects patient satisfaction and referrals

Understanding clinic flow can help to minimize or even prevent patient and physician frustration and dissatisfaction. For example, if a colleague needs a patient scheduled quickly into your clinic and you are not fully aware of the clinic's registration process or availability of appointments, you may tell him to just call the clinic without realizing that the process can take 15 minutes to 1 hour on the phone talking to 3 different people. Potentially, the next open appointment is 4 weeks away or worse than that, the clinic doesn't accept the patient's insurance. These issues lead to frustration on the referring physicians' part and can inevitably lead to less referrals. By understanding who schedules your patients and the registration process, you can better

TABLE 3.1 ■ Types of clinics.

Common Clinics	Subtypes
Amputee	
Balance disorders	
Brain Injury	
Cancer	
Cardiopulmonary	• Cardiac • Pulmonary
EMG/NCV	
Independent medical evaluation/ disability evaluations	
Gait	
General outpatient physiatry	
Musculoskeletal	• Arthritis and joint osteoporosis, etc.
Occupational/work	
Orthotics and prosthetics	
Pain management	• Interventional • Noninterventional
Palliative care	
Pediatrics	• Numerous subclinics exist: Cerebral palsy, gait, JRA, neuromuscular clinic, etc.
Scoliosis	
Spasticity	• May be part of a spine, stroke, or brain injury clinic or independent
Spine	• Spinal cord injury • Scoliosis • Conservative pain focus: Radiculopathy, degenerative or herniated disc disease
Sports medicine	
Stroke	
Wheel chair clinic	

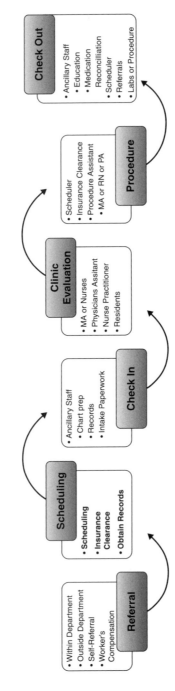

FIGURE 3.1 ■ Basic outpatient clinic flow.

direct a colleague or a patient to the right person to facilitate flow. Knowing clinic flow is necessary to correct issues related to your patients' needs and treatment as they arise, thus minimizing or preventing patient and referring physician frustration and dissatisfaction.

2. Clinic flow affects availability of clinical services

If no clear procedures are in place for "walk-in's," urgent appointments, late-cancellations, and so on. clinical productivity is affected. Processes should be in place to fill all available appointment times and to reduce the time between the initial call and the scheduled appointment.

3. Clinic flow affects overall work satisfaction

Delays can be very frustrating to clinic staff and physicians alike. For example, a patient is scheduled for a follow-up appointment specifically to discuss laboratory or radiological results. On the day the patient comes for the appointment, the results are not available. The staff has to make last-minute phone calls or computer entries, which takes time and prevents them from performing other duties, slowing down the clinic flow, prolonging the clinic day, and delaying care of other patients. Clinic-flow analysis studies show that delays in an outpatient clinic are a key issue in patient and physician dissatisfaction (2). Constant delays unnecessarily reduce patient volumes, affecting overall productivity and staff satisfaction. By understanding clinic processes, problems can be minimized and processes optimized.

It is important to learn from experience and develop a practice style based on the specific practice's needs. The goal should always be efficiency while maintaining the highest quality of service and patient care.

There are also some basic questions that should be asked when working in a new outpatient clinic (Table 3.2). These questions can guide the evaluation process. Investing the time to understand these issues as related to clinic flow dynamics is key in the delivery of patient care.

■ REFERRAL SOURCES

No physician can practice without patients. Physiatrist patient volumes are highly dependent on referrals. Understanding and maintaining referral sources is very important within the practice of physiatry. Referral sources can be both direct and indirect (Table 3.3).

Direct referrals are when a patient schedules a visit without another health care providers' intervention (self-referred). They might have been given your name by a friend, seen an advertisement, or read an informational brochure or an article. Indirect referrals are when another physician or health care provider refers a patient for evaluation.

Reasons for referrals from other physicians or health care practitioners vary. Most commonly, a specialized evaluation or procedure is requested. Factors that may affect referrals include rapport with referral

TABLE 3.2 ■ Common questions that can help you become familiar with clinic-flow dynamics.

Questions to Ask

1. How does the flow of your clinic work?
2. What is each person's responsibility? That is, who checks in, who brings patients to clinic rooms, who takes vital signs?
3. How long does your check-in process take? What is involved?
4. What is the average wait time until a patient is actually ready for you to see them?
5. What is the average wait time for new and return patients? Is the process the same or different? Can you add patients easily on to your schedule? That is, urgent visits or important referrals.
6. What procedures require insurance clearance? What do not?
7. What labs or x-rays can be done within your clinic? If any, what is the wait time?
8. How many clinic rooms do you have to use? Do patients wait in the rooms or another area for procedures, labs etc?
9. Given the requirements in some areas for medication reconciliation forms to be given to patient prior to leaving the clinic, how is this handled and how are medication prescriptions tracked and followed?
10. Who is in charge of the ancillary staff? If you have a problem, who is in charge of resolving it?

sources and availability of services (wait times). To establish relationships for continued referrals, it is important to understand the needs of the health care providers in the local community. Educating referral sources on how a particular practice can meet their needs will lead in turn to more referrals.

Once a patient has been seen, several steps will ensure continued referrals (Table 3.4):

1. All the questions in the referral and any specific requests should be answered.

2. Notes should be legible, easy to read, and organized.

3. Plan of care should be clear and simple. Respect the referring physician's time.

4. Make sure clinical reasoning is clearly stated for each recommendation. Notes are frequently reviewed by payers to determine if procedures or medications are medically necessary.

5. Communicate to the referring physician or support staff the results of your evaluation or testing/procedure promptly and without delay. This is extremely helpful and allows building a better relationship with referral sources.

TABLE 3.3 ■ Common referral sources.

Main Type of Referral	Sources Subtype
DIRECT	
1. *Self-referral*	
	• Another patient
	• Internet search
	• Yellow pages
	• Newspaper, radio or TV information, or article
	• TV or radio ad
INDIRECT	
2. *Consults from another physician or practitioner*	
	• Cardiology
	• Geriatrics
	• Neurology
	• Neurosurgery
	• Oncology
	• Orthopedics
	• Primary care
	• Pulmonary
	• Rheumatology
3. *Follow-up from an inpatient admission*	
	• Your own patient
	• From MD within your group.
	• From MD outside your group.
4. *Referral for specific test or procedures*	Such as
	• Driving evaluation
	• Gait analysis
	• Intramuscular injection
	• NCV/EMG
	• Neurocognitive testing
	• Peripheral joint injection
	• Swallowing evaluation
	• Spinal injection
	• Urodynamics
5. *Workers' compensation*	
	• Direct from a company
	• Insurance career
	• Law firm
	• Self-referred

TABLE 3.4 ■ Referrals appreciate prompt accurate communication of your evaluation and/or test results.

Notes
1. Answer referral questions clearly
2. Legible notes
3. Organized concise notes & plan
4. Recommendations clearly stated
5. Goals clearly stated

COMMUNICATION
1. Send notes promptly
2. Ensure accuracy of notes
3. Make phone calls when necessary

■ GOALS OF AN OUTPATIENT PROGRAM

Understanding the clinic's philosophy and goals and the specific practitioner's goals is very important. Table 3.5 describes some common goals of an outpatient program. Understanding and clearly defining the goals of a clinic and practice are paramount to servicing patients and ensuring the highest quality of care and quality of life for the patient.

BASIC STEPS IN AN OUTPATIENT CLINIC

We discussed briefly clinic flow dynamics, but patient and physician flow dynamics are different (Figure 3.2).

The goal of this diagram is to help understand the steps involved in outpatient care because, regardless of the type of practice, an outpatient practice thrives on the delivery of high-quality care efficiently. This is very important in today's health care system, where we are to provide excellent care while being cognizant of reducing cost.

These steps are also important and a necessity for patient satisfaction. A smooth and efficient outpatient program is less frustrating for patients and health care practitioners.

Special considerations:

1. Patient referral sheet obtained and reviewed. (Ideally prior to appointment)

A patient referral sheet is the most common source of information when we see a patient. It is the basic form of communication from one department to another. In some settings, this is computerized; for others and many in nonhospital affiliated systems, the process still involves a piece of paper. It is usually faxed or emailed before the appointment, but on occasion it is brought in by the patients on the day of service. This referral sheet serves as confirmation to third-party payers of the referring practitioner's

TABLE 3.5 ■ General principles of outpatient practice.

1. Always note and determine the patients goals.
   - Document goals
   - Determine if these goals are reasonable
   - If the goals are not reasonable, educate and establish reasonable goals with your patient.
   - Review and update goals during each visit.
   - Document when goals have been accomplished or reached.

2. Determine current pathologies.

3. Determine biomechanical dysfunction and neurologic impairments both direct and indirect.
   - Current
   - Future (when possible)
     - Example
       - Spinal Fusion: Commonly have pain in the future above and below the levels of fusion. This is likely secondary to biomechanical strain at these areas. Goal is to minimize through preventative education and biomechanical retraining to not overrotate or strain the areas above and below the fusion during activity and utilization of adaptive equipment to accomplish everyday tasks.

4. Determine methods and needs to optimize function.
   - Diagnostic testing
     - Balance testing
     - Functional evaluation
     - Neurocognitive evaluation
     - Functional radiological testing
     - Urodynamics testing
       EMG/nerve conduction
       Swallowing study
   - Equipment needs
     - Adaptive equipment
     - Bracing
     - Car adaptations
     - Ergonomics at home and work
     - Home equipment
     - Orthotics
     - Prosthetics
     - Work adaptation
   - Exercise
   - Interventional procedures: Injections, surgeries
   - Life style adaptation
   - Nutrition
   - Weight loss plan: Should include percentage of body fat
   - Smoking and drug cessation plan when relevant

(Continued)

TABLE 3.5 ■ *(Continued)*

5. Educate patient and family

6. Improve or at a minimum attempt to maintain current function and quality of life

7. Optimize and record medical history and current and past medications
   • Determine how they may contribute to
     • Functional impairment or improvement
     • Quality of life impairment improvement

intent and may be the only means to legally show that you were asked to see the patient and may be reviewed by insurance companies or third parties for determination of payment for the services provided. It is important to review this sheet (personally or by an experienced staff member) to ensure that the questions to be answered are within the scope of the practice. Health care and patient advocates have noted inappropriate evaluations and referrals as a source of medical waste. Thus, this step will avoid unnecessary evaluations and improve utilization of health care resources.

2. Clinic registration and insurance clearance

This step is straightforward, but it can take a significant amount of time because of the paperwork and data entry required. This time is useful to ensure that patients brought and have filled out clinical information forms and have other supporting documents available. This step provides another checkpoint in clinic flow to help ensure that the face-to-face time spent in patient care is optimal.

3. Patient intake

Patient intake is the step that involves the initial data gathering performed before seeing the primary provider. In most outpatient clinics, this step is performed by physician extender (Table 3.6, physician extenders). Physician extenders improve clinic efficiency and can obtain basic information as

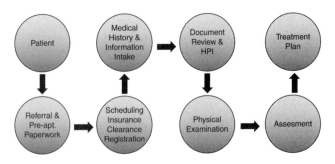

FIGURE 3.2 ■ Basic patient flow.

TABLE 3.6 ■ Physician extenders.

Physician Extenders
• Medical assistant
• Registered nurse
• Nurse practitioner
• Physician assistant
• Medical students
• Resident
• Fellow

described in Table 3.7. This information is then confirmed by the primary physician to ensure accuracy as well as interpret its relationship for inclusion in the evaluation. The physician should also obtain further details if needed.

4. Main evaluation

The role of the physician in the outpatient setting is very similar to the role as an inpatient practitioner. A significant difference is that in the inpatient setting the primary diagnosis is usually known and we concentrate on treating the physiologic and biomechanical dysfunction associated with the patient's individual pathologies and known or unknown diagnoses. A significant portion of an outpatient practice setting is the evaluation of patients for the purpose of providing a diagnosis or to determine if a procedure is indicated.

A patient referred from an inpatient program usually has a clear diagnosis, and the effort is to focus on continued rehabilitative efforts building upon what was already started on an inpatient basis or to take rehabilitation to the next step. The primary focus is on function and quality of life while continuing to manage the patient's pathologies and disease processes and working to prevent or minimize progression.

Outpatient intake information (ie, HPI, medical history, and functional history) is similar to other care settings. The main difference is likely to be that the diagnosis, biomechanical dysfunction, and impairments are not known. Subsequently, the assessment and plan will differ. The assessment will need to restate the complaint and biomechanical or neurologic dysfunction along with the patient's stated goals (ie, I want to be pain-free, I want to eat regular food, or talk normal etc.) (Table 3.8). The assessment should be logical and orderly. If the pathologic diagnosis is not known, your assessment will need to justify your suspected diagnosis, the rationale for the differential diagnosis, subsequent evaluation, and treatment.

The differential diagnosis should be ordered starting with the most likely diagnosis. In patients who have multiple issues causing or related to the patient compliant, list the potential pathologies associated to each complaint. It is prudent to include in this section active comorbidities

TABLE 3.7 ■ Basic patient information.

	Extender	**Physician Inquiry**
Basic Vitals		
	• Age • Height • Weight • Temp • HR • BP • RR • Pulse Ox • Pain (VAS 0-10)	
Current Medication	• Prescription meds • Supplements • Allergies	Inquiry about allergy details. Previous meds: Opioids, anesthetics, neurologics
ROS	• Standard systems	Physician should review this and ask more focused questions related to patient problem

History	• Family
	• Medical
	• Surgical
	• Obstetrical
	• Home equipment
	• Orthotics/prosthetics
	• Mental health
	  • Hospitalization
	  • Drug use/Hx
	  • ETOH
	  • Nicotine
	  • Illicit drug use
		Mood, impulsivity, sleep, buying habits, concentration, suicidal thoughts, etc., especially in pts with risk factors or central neurologic

	• Social history	Housing, education, religion, work hx, work environment, driving/transport, children/support
	• Legal history	• Active or settled case • Situation: MVA, work, or personal injury • Record all details and time frame

TABLE 3.8 ■ Physician's evaluation.

HPI	Summary of symptoms and historical data
	• Seek information from as many sources as possible • Patient • Family members • Medical records
Documentation	(Review all supportive documentation) May or may not be part of HPI.
	• Hospital history and physical • Hospital discharge summary • Referring notes • Diagnostic studies
Physical Examination	(Clinical findings)
	• *Initial:* Complete but pertinent examination • *Follow-up:* May be more focused
Assessment	(Thought process)

	1. State the reason for the visit
	  a. No need to restate the entire history
	  b. Review key issues and facts concisely
	2. Ensure you state the patient-stated goals. Report your opinion and why goals are
	  a. Reasonable
	  b. Unreasonable
	3. List outpatient current impairments
	  a. Biomechanical
	  b. Neurologic
	  c. Musculoskeletal

Diagnoses	
	• List in order of significance.
Treatment Plan	

	• Diagnostic testing
	• Medications
	• Equipment
	• Therapies
	  • Physical
	  • Occupational
	  • Psychology
	  • Speech
	  • Complementary
	• Interventions
	• Other consults/referrals
	• Prognosis: Short/long term
	• Work status
	• Follow-up recommendations

and relevant important lifestyles or behaviors (ie, obesity, smoking, sedentary lifestyle, illicit drug use, among others).

In order to confirm the diagnostic impression, additional diagnostic testing is usually necessary. In cases where the diagnosis is already known, diagnostic testing may or may not be necessary. A justification statement for diagnostic tests is highly recommended (both for patient care and payment justification or even approval). Other plans should be listed out in an organized fashion with justification.

Proper communication and patient education is the final step and the most important. After reviewing with the patient the diagnosis and plan, the checkout process occurs.

The process and flow in outpatient physiatry is simple and yet covers a wide array of pathologies and disabilities. Currently, there is high demand for qualified board-certified physiatrists. As diagnostic and therapeutic technology continues to improve, the need for outpatient physiatrists will only continue to increase. Our field has the unique ability to combine the best of both diagnostic and therapeutic interventions on both inpatient and outpatient environments. The strengths of physiatric practice lies in our ability to integrate information, manage patients, and optimize biomechanical and physiological function while improving and/or maintaining quality of life.

■ **REFERENCES**
1. National Center for Health Statistics. *Health, United States, 2009: With Special Feature on Medical Technology.* Hyattsville, MD; 2010.
2. Johns Hopkins Bayview Hospital Patient Satisfaction Survey, 2009.

Nursing Home Care and Subacute Rehabilitation

Kenneth H. Silver

Frequently, patients unable to return home following acute hospitalization are discharged for subacute rehabilitation in skilled nursing facilities (SNFs) rather than being admitted for more intensive and coordinated treatment in an inpatient rehabilitation facility or unit (IRF/U). Subacute rehabilitation is well suited for individuals ready for discharge from an acute hospital service who may not yet be physically able to participate in full-day intensive therapy, such as elderly patients following hip fracture who are restricted from weight-bearing for 6 weeks, or stroke patients lacking the physical stamina or cognitive capabilities to benefit from 3 hours of rehabilitation therapy services daily. SNF-based rehabilitation programs may also be recommended for those who have made some progress in an IRF/U but require a longer period of lower intensity. rehabilitation to master additional tasks consistent with a safe return to the home setting. Subacute rehabilitation may also be appropriate for those recovering from unilateral hip or knee surgery, fractures, and other orthopedic conditions that do not require multidisciplinary, coordinated care and frequent treatment by a physician. Generally, individuals not ready for home-discharge, not requiring frequent physician management, not in need of, or unable to benefit from or tolerate more intensive, inter-disciplinary therapies, who are medically stable, motivated to participate and who show reasonable potential to achieve their rehabilitation goals within a relatively short time are candidates for subacute programs. Patients are typically admitted directly from an acute-care hospital once their condition has stabilized. Presently in subacute facilities, patients are grouped according to the amount of rehabilitation they required. These resource utilization groups (RUGs) are based on data from resident assessments and fall into 5 categories ranging from "Ultra High" with a minimum of 720 minutes of two therapy disciplines weekly to "Low" with a minimum of 45 minutes weekly of one therapy discipline provided over at least 3 days.

It has been reported that one third of all Medicare patients discharged from acute-care hospitals require postacute care. Thirteen percent of these patients are sent to SNFs, 11% to home care services, and 5% to IRF or LTAC. Despite the availability of different settings along an apparent continuum of service intensity, only 4% of the beneficiaries discharged used more than one postacute setting (1). The need to clearly differentiate among the various levels and sites of rehabilitation care is an ongoing challenge in ongoing challenge in field of Physical Medicine and Rehabilitation, made more difficult by evolving regulatory oversight from the Centers of Medicare and Medicaid Services (CMS) (2). The rapidly changing health care system has resulted in the modification of the traditional pathways through the continuum of rehabilitation medicine. As of this writing, most states in the country use a compliance rate of 60% for determining a hospital's eligibility for payment as a rehabilitation hospital or unit as a result of CMS's "75% rule"—enacted in 2004 as a gradual phase-in requiring that 75% of patients on a comprehensive IRU carry 1 of 13 core diagnoses as the reason prompting admission (3). In addition, comprehensive rehabilitation programs are now being asked to return payments for hospital stays retroactively audited by CMS and found not to meet new "medical necessity" guidelines (4). Both the "60% rule" and "medical necessity" denials have forced IRF/Us to reduce or curtail admissions for patients with unilateral knee or hip replacements among other diagnoses, raising concern that such policies effectively limit access to appropriate rehabilitative care for some patients. Given the push by payers to discharge acutely hospitalized patients with rehabilitation needs to less-intensive settings (usually an SNF), it is critical that professionals in the rehabilitation field differentiate among the sites of care to ensure medically sensible placement of patients and appropriate reimbursement. Triage should result in selecting the right patient for the right treatment setting at the right time. A primary goal at completion of rehabilitation is the patient's return to living in the community, which could mean living at home independently, living with family, receiving home health care, or living in an assisted-living residence (Table 4.1). It is also important to consider that when patients are discharged to a subacute or long-term nursing facility, the option exists for transfer back to an inpatient comprehensive rehabilitation facility or unit. This would be relevant only if improvement in their physical/cognitive status is consistent with participation in more intensive and complex rehabilitation training. For example, a transfer back to an IRF from a SNF program may be indicated for a stroke patient who initially could not tolerate intensive rehabilitation because of severe concurrent debility and lethargy, but has now after 3 weeks of subacute care has gained sufficient strength, endurance, and alertness to undertake 3 hours of an interdisciplinary therapy program.

As a general overview, the most intensive rehabilitation services today are provided at comprehensive IRUs within acute-care hospitals or at freestanding rehabilitation hospitals. Less-intense rehabilitative services are also administered in SNFs, at outpatient rehabilitation facili-

TABLE 4.1 ■ Across-discipline comparison of IRF and skilled care.

Medical Discipline	Inpatient Rehabilitation	Subacute Rehabilitation
Physician	• Some active medical conditions not fully resolved • Needs physician to oversee medical/rehab needs 5–7 d/wk	• Sufficiently resolved medical issues to be able to be managed by physician infrequently or off-site
Nursing	• Rehab nursing that deals with medical issues and promotes goals attainment • Higher compliment of RN/LPN staff • Documented patient/family education • Minimum 6 h/d	• Predominantly medical focus for staff • Little or no family/patient education • Predominantly staffed with LPN overseeing aides • 4 h/d
Therapy	• Two or more therapists (at least PT and OT) • At least 3 h/d, 5 d/wk = 15 h/wk • Groups <20% of therapy sessions	• May or may not receive therapies • Only one therapy type permitted • No minimum amount, maximum 6 h/wk

Abbreviation: IRF, inpatient rehabilitation facility; LPN, licensed practical nurse; OT, occupational therapist; PT, physical therapist; RN, registered nurse.

ties, or at home through home health care. In addition, some patients who cannot tolerate 3 hours of daily rehabilitation therapy but still have long-term (>25 d length of stay) complicated medical and rehabilitative needs are discharged to chronic care in a long-term acute-care hospital (LTACH), for example, respiratory disease with ventilator-dependency, complicated wound care, and multisystem organ failure (5,6). Also, patients who have lower-level rehabilitation needs, require only maintenance range of motion exercises and mobilization out of bed, and who have projected long-term institutional care needs may be discharged from the acute hospital directly to long term care in the nursing home setting.

The choice of the appropriate pathway for obtaining postacute rehabilitation care is typically made by the acute hospital's case manager or social worker, as a result of consultation with the treating physical or occupational therapist (PT/OT), the attending physician, the patient, and the patient's family. In some hospitals, rehabilitation medicine consultants, typically physiatrists, are available to make these recommendations (Figure 4.1).

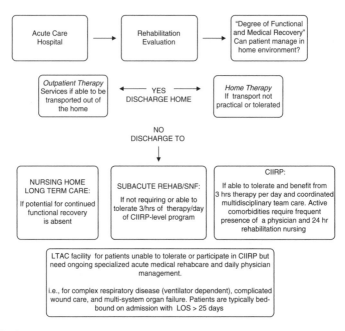

FIGURE 4.1 ■ Determination of rehabilitation destinations.

Complicating this basic decision tree for rehabilitation program placement are the newer realities of admission justification along the "75% rule" and "medical necessity" guidelines. This requires the receiving IRF provide preadmission scrutiny of the referred patient ensuring IRF/U appropriateness. Consequently, admission staffs at IRFs have recently had to develop more sophisticated and detailed screening tools and documentation forms to help clarify the medical and rehabilitation justification for comprehensive integrated inpatient rehabilitation program (CIIRP) admission (see chapter on Hospital Forms).

A number of criteria typically guide which patients are admitted to SNF subacute rehabilitation versus CIIRP. The following factors help distinguish the 2 postacute-care settings:

IRF/U entry criteria

1. Require at least 3 hours of any combination of physical, occupational, and speech therapy per day (the 3 h rule).

2. Require frequent care by a physician with rehabilitation training or experience related to the need to manage active medical comorbidities.

3. Require 24-hour care by a registered nurse with rehabilitation training or experience.

4. Require a coordinated care plan provided by a multidisciplinary team.

5. Be expected to achieve significant improvement over a reasonable period of time.

6. Have realistic rehabilitation goals that focus on achieving the maximum level of independent function.

7. Have a reasonable length of stay.

8. Generally (per 60% rule), patients' admitting diagnosis should predominantly be one of the following 13 categories:

- Stroke
- Hip fracture
- Amputation
- Major multiple trauma
- Brain injury
- Spinal cord injury
- Congenital deformity
- Neurological disorders
- Burns
- Polyarticular rheumatoid arthritis
- Systemic vaculitides with joint inflammation
- Severe osteoarthritis of > -3 weight-bearing major joints,
- Complex total joint replacement (bilateral hip or knee, morbid obesity, or > -85 years old)

SNF Rehabilitation (subacute rehabilitation) entry criteria (7):

1. No regulations for rehabilitation intensity or diagnoses.

2. Daily skilled nursing and/or rehab nursing.

3. 24-hour nursing service.

4. Prior minimum 3-day inpatient hospital stay for related illness or injury.

5. Practically, the required services can only be provided on an inpatient basis.

6. MD supervises care, with a required visit, other than for admission, only every 30 days or as required if a patient is experiencing a change in medical status. It is important to note that some subacute units in SNFs retain physiatrists who either provide PM&R consultation services or serve as the attending physician or even medical directors of these programs, often seeing the patient more frequently, between 1 and 3 times weekly.

More specific differences between IRF and SAR/SNF levels of care include the following:

1. An SNF is less likely than an IRF to have doctors and registered nurses on site at all times.

2. An SNF is more likely to have therapy aides or assistants provide rehabilitation treatments instead of licensed therapists.

3. Patients in an SNF are less likely to be discharged home and more likely to transition during their stay to long-term residents in that facility.

4. An IRF is more likely to have hospital-level resources on site such as laboratories, a pharmacy, or radiology rather than pharmacy and laboratory contracts, and portable x-ray machinery typical of most SNFs.

5. SNFs typically have a limited amount of space and equipment dedicated to rehabilitation therapies in contrast to more spacious and well-equipped gyms seen in IRF.

6. SNFs are not as able to respond quickly to changes in a patient's medical status as are IRFs where highly skilled licensed professionals are always available.

7. IRFs have greater degrees of standardization of their rehabilitation programs and activities than SNFs due to licensing requirements.

TABLE 4.2 ■ Intensity/complexity of rehabilitation care comparisons.

	Acute Rehab	Subacute NH	Long-term Care NH
Therapy available	5–7 d/wk	3–5 d/wk	1–3 d/wk
Therapy intensity	2–4 h/d	1–3 d/wk	30 min–1 h/d
Care plan conferences	Every 7–14 d	Every 30 d	Every 90 d
Av LOS	8–20 d	20–35 d	1–2 yr
MD visits	1/d	2–3/wk	1/mo
Nursing h/d	4.5–8.0	3.5–6.0	2.0 minimum; 3.2 av.
Nurse training req.	Rehab certified	Not specified	Not specified
Interdisciplinary care	Yes (required)	Occasionally (Not required)	No

8. Outcome measurements differ between the 2 care settings, with IRFs using IRF—PAI (Patient assessment instrument) along with access to aggregated local, regional, and national data to manage their programs. SAR in SNF collect similar data but usually lack the sophisticated program evaluation tools.

Cost-effectiveness of care in subacute rehabilitation programs is still controversial. Comparative analyses between the 2 settings are difficult and must take into account both the direct costs as well as indirect

A. *Positive answers would support a comprehensive integrated inpatient rehabilitation program:*

  1. Is the functional loss significant?

  2. Does the patient have the ability or willingness to participate in multiple therapies per day?

  3. Would the amount of achievable improvement likely alter postdischarge independence, improve safety, or decrease secondary complications?

  4. Do support services exist to facilitate eventual community discharge or would functional improvement materially benefit the patient in a subsequent institutional setting (ie, SNF or NH)?

  5. Are acute medical problems sufficiently controlled to allow primary focus on and involvement in the rehabilitation program?

B. *Negative answers would support a subacute rehabilitation program (SNF):*

  1. Does the patient require rehabilitation nursing and/or more frequent or more accessible medical oversight than nonhospital level of rehab can provide?

  2. Does the patient require multiple therapies coordinated within a common treatment plan, frequently reviewed and revised based on multidisciplinary input?

  3. Is there need for cross-disciplinary reinforcement of therapies?

  4. Does the rate of change of the patient's condition require frequent reevaluation/adjustment of the medical and rehabilitation care plan?

  5. Would the time course for the achievement of goals be significantly affected by level of care chosen?

  6. Is there a requirement for specialized equipment or assistive devices in the training or education program?

  7. Will greater than 3 hours of therapy per day achieve goals more effectively than less than 3 hours daily?

  8. Do behavioral health or psychological needs require regular assessment and treatment?

subsequent costs such as hospital readmissions due to suboptimal medical stability. Some feel that much of the care provided in IRFs can be equally provided in SNFs; however, no accurate data exist to support such a policy. In fact, a number of studies have suggested that for certain diagnoses, subacute care increases relative costs, lessens likelihood of discharge home, and increases risk of poor outcome and rehospitalization. Even though costs are considerably low on a daily basis in SNFs, the evidence comparing health outcomes is mixed (1,8–11). Comprehensive stroke rehabilitation in IRFs has been shown to improve functional outcomes with a higher rate of return to community patients compared with patients treated at an SNF. Similarly, stroke patients discharged to SNFs had a higher mortality rate than that of patients referred to home health or IRF (12). Outcomes for patients following orthopedic procedures are less clear, with no difference found in recovery of activities of daily living or return to community for patients with hip fracture treated in subacute SNFs compared with IRFs. However, others found that hip fracture patients experienced the most functional improvement when discharged to an IRF compared with SNF or home care and had significantly shorter lengths of stay (13). The broad field of physical medicine and rehabilitation could benefit by more health services and outcomes research initiatives in this area.

It is important to consider that when patients are discharged either from acute medical or surgical services or from IRF/U to subacute or longer term nursing facilities, admission or readmission to hospital level rehabilitation may be indicated when or if clinical circumstances improve. For example, a transfer back to an IRF from an SNF program may be relevant for patients who need to gain strength and endurance before undertaking more complex and intensive rehabilitation (3 h/d).

■ REFERENCES

1. Walsh MB, Herbold J. Outcome after rehabilitation for total joint replacement at IRF and SNF: a case-controlled comparison. *Am J of Phys Med Rehab*. 2006;85(1):1–5.
2. Gans B. There is a difference: distinguishing between IRH/U and SNF rehabilitation. *Focus on Rehabilitation*, Summer 2008;7(2):6.
3. Centers for Medicare & Medicaid Services. Proposed Rule: Medicare: Inpatient rehabilitation facility prospective payment system (2008 FY); update [07–2241]. *Fed Regist*. 26230–26279.
4. The Medicare Recovery Audit Contractor (RAC) Program: an Evaluation of the 3-Year Demonstration. June 2008, CMS. http://www.cms.hhs.gov/RAC/Downloads/RAC%20Evaluation%20Report.pdf
5. Zollar C. CMS publishes long-term care prospective payment system. *AMRPA Magazine*. 2002;5(7):37–42.
6. Seneff MG, Wagner D, Thompson D, et al. The impact of long-term acute-care facilities on the outcome and cost of care for patients undergoing prolonged mechanical ventilation. *Crit Care Med*. February 2000;28(2):342–350.

7. Harris J. Guest Column: Rehabilitation Continuum of Care. 1997;38–39. www. wheelchairnet.org/WCN_Prodserv/Docs/TeamRehab/RR_97/9709art3.PDF

8. Prvu Bettger JA, Stineman MG. Effectiveness of multidisciplinary rehabilitation services in postacute care: State-of-the-science. A review. *Arch Phys Med Rehabil.* 2007;88:1526–1534.

9. Deutsch A, et al. Outcomes and reimbursement of inpatient rehabilitation facilities and subacute rehabilitation programs for Medicare beneficiaries with hip fracture. *Med Care.* 2005;43:892–901.

10. Deutsch A, et al. Poststroke rehabilitation: Outcomes and reimbursement of inpatient rehabilitation facilities and subacute rehabilitation programs. *Stroke.* 2006;37:1477–1482.

11. Kane RL. Assessing the effectiveness of postacute care rehabilitation. *Arch Phys Med Rehabil.* 2007;88:1500–1504.

12. Kane R, Chen Q, Finch M, et al. Functional outcomes of posthospital care for stroke and hip fracture patients under Medicare. *J Am Geriatr Soc.* December 1998;46:1525–1533.

13. Munin M, Seligman K, Dew M, et al. Effect of rehabilitation site on functional recovery after hip fracture. *Arch Phys Med Rehabil.* 2005;86:367–372.

Physical Therapy

Heidi A. Frere

■ WHAT IS A PHYSICAL THERAPIST?

A physical therapist (PT) specializes in the evaluation and treatment of patients with functional limitations, impairments, and disabilities. Since 2002, all PT programs have been accredited at a master's degree level; however, the Commission on Accreditation in Physical Therapy Education (CAPTE) will mandate all PT programs to offer the Doctor of Physical Therapy (DPT) degree effective December 31, 2015 (1). The American Physical Therapy Association (APTA) reports that 96% of the professional PT programs already offer the DPT degree, as of February, 2010 (2). The DPT is a clinical doctorate which augments the Master of Physical Therapy (MPT) degree with continued training in differential diagnosis, pharmacology, radiology/imaging, and evidence based practice (3). The DPT appeared to emerge concomitantly with the need for direct access to physical therapy without a physician referral. The rationale for direct access is for patients to receive more timely treatment while decreasing health care costs. The APTA reports that 45 states and the District of Columbia have recognized direct access to physical therapy without a physician referral (4).The expectation is for the PT to refer to a physician when the patient's condition is outside the scope of PT practice. Many states have provisions related to direct access to PT. Please refer to individual state laws for details.

A physical therapist assistant (PTA) works under the direction and supervision of a licensed PT. The PTA provides select treatment interventions for the patient, collects data relevant to the treatment, and modifies select interventions to ensure patient safety or to progress the patient as directed by the PT (5). PTAs must earn an associate's degree from an accredited program. A passing score on a national examination is required for licensure for both Physical therapists and PTAs in most states (6).

■ WHERE DO PHYSICAL THERAPISTS PRACTICE?

Physical therapists practice in a variety of settings, working with patients that span age ranges from the neonate to the elderly. They may work in acute care hospitals; acute, sub-acute, or day rehabilitation centers; skilled nursing facilities; or outpatient facilities to name a few. The American Board of Physical Therapy Specialties (ABPTS) recognizes board-certified specialists in the following areas: cardiovascular and pulmonary, clinical electrophysiology, geriatrics, neurology, orthopedics, pediatrics, sports, and women's health physical therapy.

■ **WHAT TYPES OF DISORDERS ARE APPROPRIATE FOR REFERRALS?**

Physical therapists work with a wide variety of diagnoses which vary based upon the setting and area of specialty. Broadly speaking, Physical therapists work with impairments involving the neuromuscular, musculoskeletal, integumentary, and cardiovascular/pulmonary systems (7). Examples of PT problems appropriate for referral are grouped by system and listed below. This list is adapted from the APTA's *Guide to Physical Therapist Practice* (8).

Neuromuscular

Impaired motor control

Impaired neuromotor development

Impaired balance and coordination

Compensatory movement strategies

Gait deviations

Musculoskeletal

Postural alignment deviations

Impaired functional mobility (ie, bed mobility, transfers, ambulation, stair climbing, etc.)

Decreased joint mobility/ROM

Decreased strength

Decreased agility (ie, pivoting, running, jumping, climbing, etc.)

Integumentary

Impaired integumentary integrity associated with superficial, partial-thickness, and/or full-thickness skin involvement

Cardiovascular/Pulmonary

Decreased endurance

Deconditioning

Impaired ventilation

Decreased ribcage or thoracic spine mobility

■ PHYSICAL THERAPY ASSESSMENT AND TREATMENT

The *Guide to Physical Therapist Practice* describes the approach to patient management as follows: examination, evaluation, diagnosis, prognosis, and intervention.[9] PT examination begins by obtaining a detailed history from the patient followed by a systems review. It is important to assess the impact of the patient's medical history on his or her function.[10] The systems review may indicate a need for a referral to a physician or other health care provider.[11] If the patient's medical condition is well managed and it is safe to continue the PT assessment, the PT will evaluate the patient, performing objective tests and measures to identify areas of functional limitations, and make clinical judgments based on the data gathered during the exam.[12] The PT diagnoses the PT problems and prioritizes them based on the systems involved and the severity of limitation. A prognosis is made by determining the maximal level of function the patient may expect to attain and the time frame involved to complete this task.[13] PT intervention is then implemented accordingly.

GOALS

PT treatment goals differ based upon the patient setting. It is important to discuss the patient's and/or family's goals for the patient's functional mobility so that they are incorporated into the PT goals appropriately.

INPATIENT

Inpatient PT goals focus on patient and family education as well as safe mobility to promote a safe discharge home. It is not necessarily a return to prior level of function. The patient may require follow-up with inpatient rehabilitation or outpatient physical therapy to accomplish the goal of return to maximal level of function. Safe mobility may include bed mobility, transfers, ambulation, and stair climbing and involves education of the patient's caretakers if the patient requires assistance to complete a task. If the patient has stairs at home, it is important that the patient is able to perform stair climbing prior to his/her discharge home to promote safety in the home environment.

OUTPATIENT

The focus of outpatient PT is to habilitate the patient to achieve developmental skills previously unattained, or to rehabilitate the patient to return to his/her maximal level of function. This may include return to sports in the athlete's case.

Things to consider when writing an order for PT:

■ Prescriptions need to include diagnosis/reason for referral

■ Please note that a physician prescription is typically required for modalities including ultrasound, iontophoresis, and electrical stimulation. Please see state laws for guidelines in your area.

■ If indicated, identify ROM or weight bearing restrictions—be as specific as possible.

■ If weight bearing or ROM restrictions are to be placed, specifically state length of time restrictions are to be maintained or criteria for lifting or progressing the restrictions.

■ If indicated, specify cardiac precautions or vital sign parameters

■ If indicated, note any positioning restrictions, including possible bracing needs.

Prescriptions are individualized. Please add or delete information as appropriate to meet the needs of each patient.

SAMPLE OUTPATIENT PRESCRIPTION

CHARLIE P. LENERT, M.D.

Date of Prescription: 7/15/2010

Physical Therapy: Evaluate and treat

Frequency: 2×/week × 6 weeks

Diagnosis: h/o left femur fracture s/p ORIF 6/1/2010

Precautions: weight bearing as tolerated LLE

Activities: Strengthening, Active ROM and gentle PROM okay. Progress to full weight bearing.

Modalities: Ice as needed

Charlie P. Lenert, M.D.

Charlie P. Lenert, M.D.

■ SUGGESTED READINGS

■ American Physical Therapy Association. Guide to physical therapist practice. second edition. *Phys Ther.* 2001;81(1):9–746.

■ *www.apta.org*

■ REFERENCES

1. Retrieved August, 2010, from *http://www.apta.org/AM/Template.cfm?Section= Professional_PT&TEMPLATE=/CM/ContentDisplay.cfm&CONTENTID=16984*

2. Retrieved August, 2010, from *http://www.apta.org/AM/Template.cfm?Section= Professional_PT&TEMPLATE=/CM/ContentDisplay.cfm&CONTENTID=16984*

3. Retrieved August, 2010, from *http://www.apta.org/AM/Template.cfm?Section= Professional_PT&TEMPLATE=/CM/ContentDisplay.cfm&CONTENTID=16984*

4. Retrieved August, 2010, from *http://www.apta.org/AM/Template.cfm?Section= Top_Issues2&CONTENTID=69716&TEMPLATE=/CM/ContentDisplay.cfm*

5. Retrieved August, 2010, from *http://www.apta.org/AM/Template.cfm?Section= Prospective_Students&TEMPLATE=/CM/HTMLDisplay.cfm&ContentID= 74688*

6. Retrieved August, 2010, from *http://www.apta.org/AM/Template.cfm?Section= Prospective_Students&TEMPLATE=/CM/HTMLDisplay.cfm&ContentID= 74690*

7. Retrieved August, 2010, from *http://guidetoptpractice.apta.org/content/current*

8. Retrieved August, 2010, from *http://guidetoptpractice.apta.org/content/current*

9. Retrieved August, 2010, from *http://guidetoptpractice.apta.org/content/1/SEC4. extract*. Retrieved August, 2010.

10. Massery, Mary. Advanced Pulmonary Course, 2010. Unpublished.

11. Retrieved August, 2010, from *http://guidetoptpractice.apta.org/content/1/ SEC4.extract*

12. Retrieved August, 2010, from *http://guidetoptpractice.apta.org/content/1/ SEC5.extract*

13. Guide to physical therapist practice. *Phys Ther* 1995;75(8): 713–716.3

6

Occupational Therapy

Maribeth Gorman Jankowski

■ WHAT IS AN OCCUPATIONAL THERAPIST?

Occupational therapists (OTs) are professionals who assess, treat, and educate individuals who have difficulties with the skills of everyday living including, but not limited to, self-care skills, fine motor skills, visual motor skills, social interactions, and sensory processing. An OT must graduate from a program that is accredited by the Accreditation Council for Occupational Therapy Education (ACOTE), complete a minimum of 24 weeks of clinical training, and sit for the national certification examination administered by the National Board for Certification in Occupational Therapy (NBCOT) to use the OTR title. Most states also require state licensure, which may or may not include passing a test, and most states require ongoing professional continuing education.

Occupational Therapy programs are Master's or Doctorate degree level programs; both may be entry-level or postprofessional.

An occupational therapy assistant (OTA) is a professional who works under the supervision of an OT to assist in the treatment of a patient. The OTA must graduate from a program that is accredited by the Accreditation Council for Occupational Therapy Education (ACOTE), complete a minimum of 16 weeks of clinical training, and sit for the national certification examination administered by the National Board for Certification in Occupational Therapy (NBCOT). Passing the certification exam allows the professional to use the COTA title. OTA programs consist of a 2-year associate's degree or a 1-year certificate from an accredited college or technical school. Most states also require state licensure which may or may not include passing a test, and most states require ongoing professional continuing education (1).

■ WHERE DO OCCUPATIONAL THERAPISTS PRACTICE?

By the end of 2009, there were 107 000 OT jobs in the United States (2). The skills of an OT can be applied in a variety of areas including, but not limited to, acute care, inpatient rehabilitation, subacute rehabilitation, skilled nursing facility, day rehabilitation, mental health units and hospitals, schools, and a variety of outpatient settings. Each setting provides a distinct level of care, thus requiring a different intensity and purpose of therapy. As mentioned above, various settings may require a specialty level of training for the therapist. It is not common practice to have an OT who treats the adult and geriatric population, also have the skill set to treat the pediatric population. Just as a pediatric therapist may not have the skill set to work with the adult and geriatric population to best serve their specific needs. OTs may also conduct research in any of the above named settings.

The following are examples of the role an OT plays in various settings:

Neonatal Intensive Care Unit (NICU): work with parents, caregivers, and hospital staff to position the infant to promote typical movement patterns while limiting atypical patterns from developing, encouraging developmentally appropriate stimulus to foster typical development while promoting a sensory sensitive environment, and in some NICUs working on feeding skills. Please be aware that the roles between OT, physical therapy (PT), and speech-language pathology (SLP) in this environment may vary slightly. Specific skills such as feeding may be addressed by different disciplines in a particular unit. Inquiring about the discipline performing specific training in a particular unit might be necessary.

Acute Care Hospital: (Adults) work with patients and caregivers to promote return to independence in everyday skills such as dressing, bathing, grooming, and eating. This includes working on strength and endurance tasks, muscle reeducation, and also task modifications including use of adaptive equipment as appropriate. The focus is to prepare the patient for return to home with possible referral to outpatient therapy or to prepare for a transfer to a rehabilitation unit or hospital for maximal recovery.

Pediatrics: work with the children and their caregivers to promote age-appropriate skills in the areas of self-care (dressing, bathing, grooming, eating, etc), play, and visual motor skills. As in the adult population, OT in acute care is to prepare for the next level of care whether it is return to home or to a more intensive therapy program.

It is not a standard practice to refer for rehabilitation services in an acute care setting to "continue" OT if the adult or child has been receiving outpatient services and is admitted for an acute medical issue (ie, child with C.P. admitted for respiratory infection who receives outpatient OT does not need OT in the acute setting because she/he is missing their outpatient appointment or parent is requesting OT to continue). It would be appropriate if the acute care admission resulted in a change of functional status and the patient needed OT to teach/train the caregivers and/or patient strengthening exercises or adaptive techniques to return to prior level of function.

Rehabilitation Settings (unit in Acute Care Hospital or Rehab hospital): This is an intensive, therapy-focused environment. Depending on state and federal regulations, there is a daily minimum of therapy hours a patient must participate in to be in this setting. The hours are typically divided amongst OT, PT, SLP, and possibly psychology services. The OT's role in this environment is functional independence. This means the goal is for the patient to return to an age-appropriate level of functioning. For adults, they will be able to complete their self-care skills (dressing, bathing, grooming, toileting, eating, and transfers), as well as participate in job-related activities and leisure activities safely and as independently (with possible modifications and/or equipment use) as possible. With the ever-changing regulations, more rehabilitation programs are restricted on admission days based on diagnosis and on progress with therapy. Patients who are unable to meet their goals of independence can transition to either subacute or to outpatient settings.

Subacute Care: OTs work with patients whose progress is at a slower pace than allowable on a rehabilitation unit. In this environment, the OT's focus is consistent with that on a rehabilitation unit, but the goals are typically lower level of functional outcome.

Outpatient Settings: There are a variety of outpatient settings including outpatient rehab clinics, schools, home health, hand clinics, and day rehab centers. The general role of the OT in these settings is to foster age-appropriate functional skills.

For adults, it is typically an exercise program to work on strength and endurance, muscle reeducation with possible use of modalities to assist return of muscle strength, return to work programs (ergonomics, work simplification, joint protection), and higher level self-care skills (ie, cooking, laundry, balancing a checkbook, community reentry, and in some cases, driving). In some but not all clinics, it is the OT's role to do splinting as well.

For pediatrics, it can be an exercise program to work on strength and endurance, upper extremity muscle reeducation or muscle activation, promotion of typical patterns of movement, promotion of typical development and typical patterns of development, fine motor skill development (eg, handwriting skills, shoe tying and other fasteners, manipulation skills), eye–hand coordination skills, visual motor skills, and self-care skills. In some clinics, the OT will work on feeding, while in other clinics the speech therapist will work on feeding, and there are even some clinics where it is a combined OT and speech domain to work on feeding skills. There are also therapists trained in the area of sensory processing dysfunction (also known as sensory integration or SI). There are some clinics devoted solely to this population.

■ WHEN IS IT APPROPRIATE TO REFER TO OCCUPATIONAL

It is appropriate to refer to occupational therapy when the patient demonstrates a decline in baseline function that impacts his or her level of independence with everyday skills. This decline in function or loss of skill may be a result of an injury (neurological or orthopedic), a progressive disease (eg, arthritis, multiple sclerosis, Alzheimer's disease), or an acute medical process such as cancer. It is also appropriate to refer to occupational therapy to focus on acquisition of skills that were either not present or dysfunctional from birth. This is most common in the pediatric population for conditions such as developmental delays, cerebral palsy, spina bifida (MM), sensory processing dysfunction, visual impairments, and birth injuries (eg, brachial plexus injuries, HIE).

It is important to note that each state has its own requirements for a proper referral to occupational therapy. There are some states that have no specific requirements while others mandate a prescription from an authorized referral source such as a medical doctor, psychologist or psychiatrist, a dentist, an optometrist, or a podiatrist.

Things to Consider When Writing an Order for OT

■ Occupational therapy and Physical therapy are 2 separate disciplines who often work in tandem, however require separate orders

■ Use terminology and abbreviations per hospital standards

■ Include diagnosis/reason for referral

■ If indicated, identify ROM or weight-bearing restrictions

■ If indicated, specify cardiac precautions or vital sign parameters

■ If indicated, note any positioning restrictions, including possible bracing needs (Please see the sample prescription on page 42 of the Physical Therapy chapter).

■ WHEN IS A PATIENT DISCHARGED FROM OT?

There are several reasons for discharge. The most positive outcome is to discharge because all goals are met. Other reasons for discharge include a plateau in recovery (no longer making progress), lack of compliance, lack of attendance in treatment, patient choosing to end services, and transition of services from one setting to another (eg, receiving outpatient services and qualifies to receive school-based services or transfer from acute to rehab). It is important to understand why a patient is being discharged from occupational therapy services, no matter what the setting.

Examples of appropriate re-consult:

■ A patient was discharged from OT in an acute care setting but before hospital discharge and, while admitted, their functional status changes.

■ If the patient is discharged from outpatient OT because all goals were met and it is determined during a follow-up appointment with a physician that there are more functional limitations or new functional limitations to be addressed.

Examples of inappropriate re-consult:

■ A patient was discharged from OT in an acute care setting after the patient and/or caregivers have been instructed on a home exercise program to help maintain his/her level of function during patient's hospitalization, and patient's level of function has not changed.

■ If the patient is discharged from OT from an outpatient setting secondary to lack of progress or lack of participation (unless a significant change improves participation and likelihood of improvement. For example, weight-bearing restrictions are lifted).

■ HOW DO I GET OT FOR MY PATIENTS?

An order must be written for an OT to consult with your patient for inpatient or outpatient services.

■ WHAT HAPPENS ONCE AN OT REFERRAL IS PLACED?

Inpatient: Once an order is received, the OT will do a chart review and call a member of the medical team to clarify any orders or precautions as needed. It is very helpful for precautions to be written on the prescription to forego any delays in initiation of services. Once the chart review is complete, the OT will meet with the patient and begin the evaluation process. Once the evaluation is complete, the therapist will write a report and place it in the medical chart (pending the setting, it may be electronic or paper chart). The therapist will include a plan of care, recommended frequency, possible consult recommendations, and possible discharge planning recommendations. The OT or OTA will then initiate the treatment plan as outlined in the evaluation report.

Outpatient: This prescription may be handed to the patient and/or caregiver to provide to the OT at the evaluation, or in some cases, may be entered into the electronic medical record for the OT to view at the evaluation if in the same facility. Whenever possible, the therapist will do a chart review prior to the evaluation. If no records are available to therapist, the beginning of the evaluation will consist of an interview with the patient and/or caregiver to determine the history and progress. If there is insufficient information obtained during this interview process, the OT may stop the evaluation process to call a member of the patient's medical team to obtain any necessary medical information. Once the evaluation is complete, the therapist will then write up an evaluation report including evaluation findings, plan of care, and recommendations. Pending on the setting, the OT may send a summary of their findings, a full report, or a notification that a report is available to the referring physician. On the basis of insurance, the treatment plan may be initiated immediately, or the patient may need to wait until insurance approval before initiation of treatment.

■ **WHAT IS THE FREQUENCY OF OT?**

Frequencies are determined on a variety of factors. There are some physicians who prefer to prescribe a certain number of visits, while other physicians allow the therapist to use their best discretion. The frequency is also, often times now, dictated by insurance. There may be protocols based on diagnosis or it may be from evidence-based practice recommendations. This is a good opportunity to talk with the OT to determine the best plan of care.

For more information about occupational therapy:

Visit the national association's Web site at *www.aota.org* or the specific state's association Web sites (ie, Illinois Occupational Therapy Association Web site at *www.ilota.org*).

■ **REFERENCES**

   1. American Occupational Therapy Association; *www.aota.org*
   2. *http://money.cnn.com/magazines/moneymag/bestjobs/2009/snapshots/14.html*

7

Speech-Language Pathology

Martin B. Brodsky

■ WHAT IS A SPEECH-LANGUAGE PATHOLOGIST?

Speech-language pathologists, or SLPs, are professionals who assess, diagnose, and treat individuals who have speech-language, voice, and swallowing disorders. At a minimum, SLPs have a Master's degree in communication disorders, a clinical fellowship following graduate school, and pass a national certification examination administered by the Educational Testing Service. Satisfactory completion of these 3 steps will earn an SLP the Certificate of Clinical Competence in Speech-Language Pathology (CCC-SLP) granted by the American Speech-Language-Hearing Association (ASHA), the professional, scientific, and credentialing organization for audiologists, speech-language pathologists, and speech-language and hearing scientists. Earned credit through continuing education activities, combined with annual membership dues, will maintain this certification. Additionally, SLPs may be required to have state licensure, a requisite of which is ASHA certification.

■ IN WHAT SETTINGS DO SPEECH-LANGUAGE PATHOLOGISTS WORK?

By the end of 2009, there were over 120,700 ASHA-certified SLPs. With the capability of assessing, diagnosing, and treating patients from birth through senescence, SLPs may be found to work with any patient who is experiencing or is suspected to have communication and/or swallowing difficulties. Patients will range from children with developmental delays to adults who are intubated requiring mechanical ventilation, and to individuals who have stroke, progressive disease, and/or head and neck cancer. SLP professionals can be found in various settings, including public and private schools, private practice clinics, hospitals, rehabilitation facilities, extended care facilities/nursing homes, community clinics, and academic departments. You may also see SLPs conducting research in any of the above-named settings, and in positions of leadership in state and federal government agencies.

■ WHAT TYPES OF DISORDERS ARE APPROPRIATE FOR REFERRALS?

The types of disorders SLPs treat vary depending on the age of the patient and the nature of the disorder. SLPs *habilitate*, or treat patients to develop skills that were either not present or dysfunctional from birth. Likewise, SLPs also *rehabilitate*, or treat patients who have lost function in speech, language, voice, and swallowing as a result of a neurological injury (eg, stroke, traumatic brain injury), progressive disease (eg, Parkinson's disease, multiple sclerosis), orofacial and myofunctional disorders (eg, cleft lip/palate, tongue thrust), or head and neck cancer.

Within each of the broad classifications of communication and swallowing disorders are many types of dysfunction. It is important to characterize and distinguish the types of disorders within each of these classifications for a more complete understanding. Following are brief explanations for common disorders.

SPEECH DISORDERS

APRAXIA OF SPEECH/VERBAL APRAXIA

This is a motor speech disorder affecting the planning for speech acts. A person with apraxia of speech fails to consistently execute speech correctly, due to problems unrelated to muscle weakness and changes in reflexes. This speech disorder is independent of movement, sensation, or language deficits. The primary characteristic is the inability to transition within and between segments of sounds resulting in extended durations of consonants and vowels. Distortions are perceived as sound substitutions and stress changes that may be changed within words, phrases, and sentences, with consistency of location within utterances and invariable in type.

ARTICULATION/PHONOLOGICAL PROCESSES

These disorders are generally associated with young children; however they are frequently seen in persons with aphasia and some degenerative diseases. They manifest themselves as difficulty in correctly producing specific sounds (eg, sound omissions, lisps), or sound patterns (eg, substituting "t" for "k," a process called "fronting" in which sounds made in the back of the mouth are made in the front of the mouth).

DYSARTHRIA

A muscular weakness and dyscoordination that results in reduced clarity of sounds, breaks in pitch, changes in nasality/voice resonance, alterations to the rhythm of speech, or disruption in the ability to produce air (ie, breathing) for voice. Often, dysarthria is described as slurred or slow speech that may be difficult to understand.

STUTTERING/FLUENCY

A disorder, in the absence of weakness, resulting in a disruption in the production of sounds. This problem can be characterized by repetition or prolongation of sounds, syllables, or words. Other disruptions may include an increase in word or sentence starters such as "umm . . ." or "uh. . . ."

LANGUAGE DISORDERS
LANGUAGE-BASED LEARNING DISABILITIES
These are disabilities specific to reading, writing, and spelling, having little to do with intelligence. Many language disorders are reflected in spoken and listening disorders as well as these literacy deficits. Dysfunctions in these areas may result in difficulties in reading or spoken comprehension (eg, following directions), expression of written thought, and writing letters/numbers (eg, naming).

APHASIA
An acquired disorder from a neurological event that results in disordered uses of language in *all* of the following areas of language: (1) auditory comprehension, (2) reading comprehension, (3) spoken expression, and (4) written expression. Among the most common difficulties are reduced ability to follow conversation and directions (spoken or written), difficulty in identifying and/or naming objects, problems retrieving the correct words to express thought (spoken or written), and difficulty in coherent/cohesive writing.

RIGHT HEMISPHERE/TRAUMATIC BRAIN INJURY/COGNITIVE-LINGUISTIC IMPAIRMENTS
This is an acquired communication disorder from stroke, brain injury, or progressive disease (eg, dementia) that may lead to any combination of impairments of memory, awareness/attention, visual–perceptual skills, problem solving/reasoning, thought organization, and use of language in social situations (ie, pragmatics).

VOICE AND VOICE DISORDERS
DYSPHONIA
Simply stated, dysphonia involves an abnormality in the sound of the voice. Changes to the quality of voice (including resonance) may be the result of anatomical changes (eg, tracheotomy, laryngectomy, growths on the vocal folds such as nodules or polyps), neurological changes (eg, vocal fold paresis/paralysis), or other health issues affecting vocal fold tissue (eg, immunological issues). Sometimes, physical bases do not explain dysphonia, which is, instead, related to muscle use patterns. Examples of voice changes with dysphonia include hoarseness, "rough voice" and tremor or "shaky" voice.

RESONANCE
This term addresses the quality of an individual's voice in terms of how the pharynx, nasal cavity, and oral cavity shape the sound vibrations produced by the vocal folds in the larynx. *Nasality* is a term used to describe, specifically, how the velum allows air to escape (or not) during speech. A *hypernasal* voice is one that sounds like someone is "talking through his/her nose" (ie, more air is escaping through the

nose than normal). A *hyponasal* voice is one that sounds like someone is "all stopped up," a common quality of one's voice when someone has a cold.

INTUBATION AND TRACHEOSTOMY

Although a patient with a tracheostomy tube is not considered to have a voice disorder, a patient with a tracheostomy does require SLP services. These patients may be able to phonate (ie, produce voice) with the proper adjustments to these types of indwelling respiratory devices. In cases in which patients are not able to phonate, an SLP can assist with patient-to-caregiver communication by providing assistive devices.

LARYNGECTOMY

Patients with parts of the larynx or the entire larynx removed will need SLP services for potential voice and swallowing disorders. An SLP will provide pre- and post-operative assessment and counseling for voice and swallowing restoration, and the therapy required to improve the patient's functional outcomes in these domains. An SLP will assist in maximizing use of voice that may still remain or alternatively provide a different source for voice (ie, alaryngeal speech).

SWALLOWING DISORDERS

Dysphagia is the term used to refer to the symptom of difficulty related to swallowing (ie, "The patient complains of dysphagia.") and a patient's diagnosis of having a swallowing disorder. Many clinicians divide swallowing into 3 phases: (1) oral phase, (2) pharyngeal phase, and (3) esophageal phase. Although these phases serve the purpose of describing the location of the bolus of liquid or food, it is difficult to use "phases" to describe the precise location of the problem producing dysphagia. There is a large amount of overlap and interdependence between the different physiologic components of swallowing, thus, making it difficult to distinguish these phases. For purposes of explanation below, use of term "phases" refers to the *location of the bolus.*

FEEDING DISORDERS

This domain is an "adjunct" area for SLPs. Strictly speaking, *feeding* refers to how an individual functions to get food or drink "from the table to his/her mouth." Attention to the physical movements of this act are largely assessed and treated by an occupational therapist (OT). In concert with the OT, the SLP addresses cognitive-behavioral aspects of feeding. These aspects typically include reducing the amount of distractions during mealtimes (generally used with patients who have difficulties with focus/attention/concentration), the speed of feeding, the amount of food placed on the fork or spoon, the volume of drink ingested, and the manner of liquid transport (ie, spoon, cup, or straw).

ORAL DYSPHAGIA

The oral phase can be subdivided into 2 functions: (1) oral preparatory phase and (2) oral propulsive phase. The manner in which the bolus is prepared for swallowing is highly dependent upon the type of food or liquid ingested. Liquids, for example, are not masticated.

During the oral preparatory phase, saliva is secreted, the bolus is manipulated (and masticated with solid food), and the food and/or drink mixed with saliva. This phase softens and lubricates solid boluses in preparation for transport from the oral cavity and through the pharynx and esophagus. Disorders in this phase may include difficulties with control and manipulation of the bolus, secretion of saliva, cleft lip/palate, and muscle strength for mastication.

During the oral propulsive phase, the now-prepared food and/or drink is placed on the blade of the tongue for transport posteriorly into the pharynx. Disorders in this phase may include difficulties with bolus control and with initiation of the propulsive sequence. The vocal folds close and breathing ceases during this phase in many individuals, this behavior often regarded as protective by clinicians and researchers. The cessation of breathing is in preparation for the movement of the bolus toward the pharynx, while the airway is still open and vulnerable to bolus entry.

PHARYNGEAL DYSPHAGIA

During the "pharyngeal phase" many physiologic events occur in rapid succession. The velum closes to prevent the bolus from entering the nasopharynx before the bolus is transported posteriorly from the oral cavity. The oral tongue and tongue base, in concert with the posterior pharyngeal wall, act as the primary forces behind the bolus, pushing it through the pharynx and into the esophagus. During tongue base retraction and pharyngeal contraction, the upper airway closes to prevent bolus entry into the larynx, the pharynx shortens for efficient bolus transport, and the pharyngoesophageal segment (an area in the pharynx that contains the upper esophageal sphincter) opens allowing the passage of the bolus into the esophagus. Once the bolus has been pushed through the pharynx and into the esophagus, the system returns to rest by closing the pharyngoesophageal segment, reopening the airway, relaxing the tongue, reopening the velum, and restoring normal breathing. Disorders of the pharyngeal phase include delayed initiation of the pharyngeal swallow, insufficient retraction of the velum, reduced tongue base retraction, reduced hyolaryngeal excursion, reduced pharyngeal contraction, and reduced pharyngoesophageal segment opening. These dysfunctions may result in pharyngeal residue, laryngeal penetration (entrance of the bolus into the airway while remaining superior to the vocal folds), and/or aspiration (movement of the bolus inferiorly through the vocal folds and into the lower airways).

ESOPHAGEAL DYSPHAGIA

SLPs do not assess, diagnose, or treat esophageal disorders. However, with the assistance of a physician, SLPs are able to screen for difficulties with esophageal clearance, making appropriate recommendations for further testing related to esophageal motility and other esophageal disorders, for which patients may be referred to gastroenterology, otolaryngology, and/or radiology services.

■ HOW ARE SPEECH-LANGUAGE, VOICE, AND SWALLOWING DISORDERS ASSESSED AND TREATED?

As with any type of therapy or treatment program, prognosis is highly dependent on the nature of the disorder, the severity of the disorder, an individual's cognitive functioning, cooperation and tenacity, support system, and ability to generalize SLP-trained behaviors to new contexts.

ASSESSMENT AND TREATMENT OF SPEECH DISORDERS

Speech disorders are assessed through multiple approaches. In most cases, testing of the cranial nerves associated with speech (ie, V, VII, IX, X, and XII), along with an oral motor examination, are standard. Once cranial nerve testing is completed, an articulation and/or phonological inventory may be taken, depending on the case. Such assessments can range from the sound level (production of individual sounds) to elicited and narrative speech to determine the level of breakdown. For example, a patient might be able to produce a sound or group of sounds correctly in isolation or single syllable words, but have difficulty producing the same sounds in multiple syllable words or in conversational speech. When assessing individuals with dysarthria, a motor speech disorder, the SLP must take into account all subsystems of speech (ie, respiration, phonation, articulation, prosody, and resonance) and how they affect intelligibility and verbal expression. Treatment time may be short or long, depending on the severity of difficulties, and will target individual sounds, short phrases, sentences, and finally conversational speech. Each level of treatment will focus on transfer and maintenance from the earlier levels. Assistive devices such as communication boards may be able to assist the patient who is unintelligible, but still able to use language. Although "perfect" speech is the ideal goal, intelligible speech to express wants and needs efficiently may be an endpoint in therapy.

ASSESSMENT AND TREATMENT OF LANGUAGE DISORDERS

Language disorders span many different domains, among them morphology (meaningful word units, ie, root words, prefixes, suffixes), semantics (word meaning), and syntax (construction of phrases, clauses, sentences, paragraphs, stories). Additional areas of language include naming, comprehension (written or spoken), expression (written or spoken), calculations, and pragmatics (how language is used). Added into this broad area of language is executive function, or cognitive-linguistic impairments. Topics in this area include awareness, attention, and concentration; memory; initiation of appropriate actions (or inhibition of inappropriate actions); planning; problem solving; reasoning; and cognitive flexibility. Depending on the need, these evaluations might take a gestalt approach, reviewing many areas of language and/or cognitive-linguistic impairments within the same evaluation, or they may have a more directed approach to address specific needs. Treatment periods are often lengthy, but depend on the severity of the impairment. Focuses in therapy may be situational (eg, scripted for specific situations) or adaptive (ie, broad application to many different contexts). As with speech, assistive devices such as communication boards may assist in providing the opportunity for patients to express wants and needs. These devices are especially helpful when patients are mechanically ventilated or have unintelligible speech. Treatment decisions and goals will largely depend on each patient's comfort level, physical, and overall cognitive abilities.

ASSESSMENT AND TREATMENT OF VOICE

Voice is assessed in many different ways. Laryngoscopy, or viewing of the vocal folds will allow the professional to assess functional and/ or anatomical changes to the larynx that might be affecting voice. Stroboscopy, a type of laryngoscopy whereby a pulsed light allows for a sampled viewing of the vocal folds in motion, is one manner to assess vocal fold function. Other types of evaluations might include respiratory plethysmography, acoustic assessments (eg, pitch/frequency, volume/ loudness, and acoustic surrogates of voice quality), and inventories completed by the patient. Most voice therapy has a short duration and is designed to improve changes in vocal behaviors (ie, reduce abusive and maladaptive behaviors) and possibly lifestyle to improve the condition producing voice problems.

Voice assessment in patients with laryngeal cancer is similar to that described above. Treatment for these types of patients may be more involved and includes pre- and post-surgical assessments with counseling. In patients who have impaired voice or the vocal folds are removed, alaryngeal speech may be an option. Examples of alaryngeal speech include training for use of a prosthesis, an electrolarynx, and esophageal speech. Use of each of these techniques will depend on the surgery and remaining anatomy, use of additional medical and/or oncological therapies (eg, radiation therapy, chemotherapy), and patient goals. Most SLP treatments for patients with laryngectomy have a short duration; however, there may be frequent clinical follow-up appointments. Extent of treatments (ie, surgery, radiation, chemotherapy), impairments in cognitive functioning, and patient compliance may increase the amount of therapy time.

ASSESSMENT AND TREATMENT OF DYSPHAGIA

There are 2 types of assessments typically completed by SLPs for dysphagia—clinical and instrumental. The clinical swallowing examination, often referred to as a "bedside swallowing evaluation" (BSE), is a noninstrumental evaluation. Often, it includes a detailed history of the patient's swallowing problems; a screening of the patient's cognitive functioning, including speech, language, and voice functions; a careful review of the motor and sensory functions of the patient's oral, pharyngeal, and laryngeal anatomy; and trial feedings when deemed appropriate. Two methods of instrumental examination are most common for the assessment of dysphagia—fiberoptic endoscopic evaluation of swallowing (FEES) and videofluoroscopic swallow study (VFSS). Whereas the BSE may not necessarily be conclusive, instrumental examinations are diagnostic and each provides greater detail of swallowing physiology and function than the BSE. However, there are considerations for each.

FEES uses a fiberoptic endoscope that is passed transnasally through the nasopharynx and into the upper pharynx past the velum to view swallowing function. This procedure may be used with or without a nasal decongestant and/or a topical anesthetic to ease passing of the endoscope. Once in place, the patient is asked to swallow various consistencies of liquids and food. The clinician is able to assess velum function, pharyngeal weakness, and pharyngeal sensory impairments during this assessment. Additionally, laryngeal penetration and aspiration may be viewed *before* the swallow is initiated and *after* the swallow is completed. Viewing pharyngeal and laryngeal function *during* the swallow is not possible because the light from the endoscope's light source bounces back into the lens of the endoscope during the pharyngeal swallow as the tongue base retracts, epiglottis inverts, and the pharynx contracts, effectively creating a "white-out period" when laryngeal structures cannot be seen and physiology cannot be assessed. Although this white-out period is a shortcoming of the procedure and FEES does not have a standardized scoring procedure, among the benefits of FEES are the ability to perform the procedure bedside without a time limit for completion of the examination and the use of real food.

The VFSS, sometimes called a modified barium swallow study (MBSS), allows for observation of the oral cavity, nasopharynx, oropharynx, larynx, pharynx, and esophagus to assess individual components of swallowing physiology. Patients arrive in the radiology department and are placed in the fluoroscope, typically, while seated or standing. Patients are then presented with varying volumes and consistencies of liquid barium and solid food coated with barium. Each swallow is observed and judgments of efficiency and physiology are made by the SLP. Most often, SLPs perform this evaluation collaboratively with a physician, most commonly a radiologist or physiatrist. Although much more physiologic function of the swallow can be observed using VFSS as compared to FEES, laryngeal penetration and aspiration *during* the swallow may be observed and compensatory strategies are directly viewed for their effectiveness, there are several clinical disadvantages of the procedure. Among the clinical disadvantages are radiation exposure leading to a limitation in observation time for swallowing physiology; consumption of foreign tastes, textures, substances (ie, barium); confined spaces for larger patients; and obstructed fluoroscopic views from positioning and hardware.

Treatment for dysphagia varies. Therapy may last from a few days to a few months, depending on severity. A home program is key to therapy in the outpatient setting. Impairments in cognitive functioning may increase the amount of therapy time.

■ SUMMARY

SLPs are professionals who are educated in the anatomy, neuroanatomy, physiology, and psychology of assessment and treatment for speech-language, voice, and swallowing disorders. Each of these areas provides important life functions, yet are often taken for granted. When disordered, these types of impairments may span the gamut from the mildest of difficulties to the most devastating of dysfunctions, possibly leading to medical and behavioral/mental disorders. A proper referral for SLP services for patients who experience these types of impairments may provide the improved function and improved quality of life your patient deserves.

■ SUGGESTED READING

SPEECH

Bernthal JE, Bankson NW, Flipsen P. *Articulation and Phonological Disorders.* 6th ed. Boston, MA: Allyn & Bacon; 2008.

Darley FL, Aronson AE, Brown JR. *Motor Speech Disorders.* Philadelphia, PA: W.B. Saunders; 1975.

Duffy JR. *Motor Speech Disorders: Substrates, Differential Diagnosis, and Management.* Maryland Heights, MO: Mosby Elsevier; 2005.

Guitar B. *Stuttering: An Integrated Approach to Its Nature and Treatment.* 3rd ed. Baltimore, MD: Lippincott Williams & Wilkins; 2005.

Hall PK, Jordan LS, Robin DA. *Developmental Apraxia of Speech: Theory and Clinical Practice.* 2nd ed. Austin, TX: Pro-Ed; 2007.

McNeil MR. ed. *Clinical Management of Sensorimotor Speech Disorders.* New York, NY: Thieme; 1997.

WEB SITES

The Childhood Apraxia of Speech Association of North America
  http://www.apraxia-kids.org/
International Fluency Association
  http://www.theifa.org/
National Stuttering Association
  http://www.nsastutter.org/

The Stuttering Foundation
  http://www.stuttersfa.org/

LANGUAGE

Fletcher P, MacWhinney B. eds. *The Handbook of Child Language.* Oxford, UK: Wiley-Blackwell; 1996.

Hurtig RR, Downey DA. *Augmentative and Alternative Communication in Acute Care Settings.* San Diego, CA: Plural Publishing, Inc; 2008.

Klein E, Mancinelli J. *Acquired Language Disorders: A Case-Based Approach.* San Diego, CA: Plural Publishing, Inc; 2009.

LaPointe LL. ed. *Aphasia and Related Neurogenic Language Disorders.* 3rd ed. New York, NY: Thieme Medical Publishers, Inc; 2004.

McCauley R, Fey ME. eds. *Treatment of Language Disorders in Children.* Baltimore, MD: Brookes Publishing; 2006.

Tompkins CA. *Right Hemisphere Communication Disorders: Theory and Management.* San Diego, CA: Singular Publishing Group, Inc; 1995.

WEB SITES

International Association for the Study of Child Language
  http://iascl.talkbank.org/
National Aphasia Association
  http://www.aphasia.org/

VOICE

Boone DR, McFarlane SC, Von Berg SL, Zraick RI. *The Voice and Voice Therapy.* 8th ed. Boston, MA: Allyn & Bacon; 2009.

Colton RH, Casper JK, Leonard RJ. *Understanding Voice Problems: A Physiological Perspective for Diagnosis and Treatment.* 3rd ed. Baltimore, MD: Lippincott Williams & Wilkins; 2005.

Dikeman KJ, Kazandjian MS. *Communication and Swallowing Management of Tracheostomized and Ventilator-Dependent Adults.* 2nd ed. Canada: Delmar Learning; 2003.

Stemple JC, Glaze L, Klaben B. *Clinical Voice Pathology: Theory and Management.* 4th ed. San Diego, CA: Plural Publishing, Inc; 2009.

Verdolini K, Rosen CA, Branski RC. eds. Classification Manual for Voice Disorders-I. Mahwah, NJ: Lawrence Erlbaum; 2006.

Ward EC, van As-Brooks CJ. eds. *Head and Neck Cancer: Treatment, Rehabilitation, and Outcomes.* San Diego, CA: Plural Publishing, Inc; 2007.

WEB SITES

Voice Foundation
  http://www.voicefoundation.org/

SWALLOWING

Arvedson JC, Brodsky L. *Pediatric Swallowing and Feeding: Assessment and Management.* 2nd ed. Albany, NY: Singular Publishing Group; 2002.

Goyal RK, Shaker R. *Oral Cavity, Pharynx and Esophagus;* 2003. http://www.nature.com/gimo/index.html. Accessed May.

Groher ME, Crary MA. eds. *Dysphagia: Clinical Management in Adults and Children.* Maryland Heights, MO: Mosby Elsevier; 2010.

Jones B. ed. *Normal and Abnormal Swallowing: Imaging in Diagnosis and Therapy.* 2nd ed. New York, NY: Springer; 2003.

Jones HN, Rosenbek JC. eds. *Dysphagia in Rare Conditions: An Encyclopedia.* San Diego, CA: Plural Publishing, Inc; 2010.

Langmore SE. ed. *Endoscopic Evaluation and Treatment of Swallowing Disorders.* New York, NY: Thieme; 2001.

Logemann JA. *Evaluation and Treatment of Swallowing Disorders.* 2nd ed. Austin, TX: Pro-Ed; 1998.

Perlman AL, Schulze-Delrieu K. eds. *Deglutition and Its Disorders: Anatomy, Physiology, Clinical Diagnosis, and Management.* San Diego, CA: Singular Publishing Group, Inc; 1997.

WEB SITES

Dysphagia Research Society
  http://dysphagiaresearch.org/

Specialty Board on Swallowing and Swallowing Disorders
  http://swallowingdisorders.org/

Speech-Language, Voice, and Swallowing Web Resources American Cleft Palate-Craniofacial Association
  http://www.acpa-cpf.org/

American Speech-Language-Hearing Association
  http://www.asha.org/

American Stroke Association
  http://www.strokeassociation.org

Brain Injury Association of America
  http://www.biausa.org/

FACES: The National Craniofacial Association
  http://www.faces-cranio.org/

Head and Neck Cancer Alliance
  http://www.ohancaw.com/

International Directory of Communication Disorders
  http://www.comdisinternational.com/

National Library of Medicine: Speech and Communication Disorders
  http://www.nlm.nih.gov/medlineplus/speechandcommunicationdisorders.html

National Institute on Deafness and Other Communication Disorders/NIH
  http://www.nidcd.nih.gov/

Rehabilitation Psychology

Maggi A. Budd and Christine L. Yantz

Physiatrists' goal is to restore a person with injury, illness, or disability to maximum functioning by treating the whole person rather than the medical issue alone (1). This is best accomplished through an interdisciplinary team that provides collaborative care (2). Rehabilitation psychologists, as a part of this team, facilitate effective, integrated care with specialized knowledge of psychosocial and psychophysiological processes in tandem with other disciplines. Collaborative medical care that includes mental health services has been shown to reduce treatment time and overall costs (3) as well as improve patient outcomes and satisfaction (4,5). Common psychological services in the rehabilitation setting include patient education and fostering self-management of chronic conditions, family and caregiver education and support, consultation with other care providers, program evaluation, and an array of psychotherapeutic interventions. This chapter outlines practical rehabilitation psychology applications to help rehabilitation teams better understand patients' experiences and best manage behavioral reactions and psychological processes during inpatient stays.

■ MODEL FOR REHABILITATION: INTERFACE BETWEEN PERSONAL, SOCIAL, AND ENVIRONMENTAL FACTORS

Rehabilitation psychology is founded on the premise that multiple causal pathways interact to produce physical and mental outcomes, and the whole person (eg, the various factors impacting outcomes) has to be treated (2,6); even outcomes from the best surgical treatments will be affected by nonsurgical factors.

Kurt Lewin's classic psychological theory (7) that describes the cause of observable human behavior has been used in the context of rehabilitation (2). The formula $B = f (P \times O \times E)$ translates into behavior (B) is a function of the person (P), the organic or biologic (O), and the environment (E). This formula encompasses the total situation that has to be taken into account for behavioral change to occur. For example, an individual's tendency to react (P) coupled with a family's adjustment and/or support or financial assets (E) within the context of physical problems (O) can have a tremendous positive or negative impact on the patient's behaviors and compliance with rehabilitation recommendations (B).

Lewin's model supports the mission and essence of rehabilitation with convergence of multiple levels and expertise in the assessment, conceptualization, and treatment for each patient. This globalistic way of approaching a patient in rehabilitation is key to understanding all the potential factors that contribute to outcomes so that all patient needs can be addressed.

ASSESSMENT

Rehabilitation psychologists perform assessments to identify barriers to full participation in rehabilitation programs and possible obstacles for generalizing skills into the patient's home environment (Table 8.1). Psychological assessments are also helpful to determine what other services and supervision needs can be expected after discharge. Psychological assessments on an inpatient service are generally brief (ie, approximately 60 min) compared with outpatient services (ie, several hours). However, both can address issues such as poor adjustment, inadequate pain management, cognitive or emotional issues, or concurrent substance dependence (8).

Cognitive assessment (ie, neuropsychological assessment) is particularly important as cognitive impairments often substantially affect the rehabilitation adherence and functional outcomes (9). This is achieved by a psychologist examining brain–behavior relationships through quantitative tests of cognitive abilities across several domains. Collectively, data are then interpreted in the context of each patient's unique history.

TABLE 8.1 ■ Components of brief psychological assessments for inpatient rehabilitation.

- Clinical interview
  - Medical, psychiatric, social history
  - Substance use history
  - Estimate of premorbid functioning
- Behavioral observations, orientation, mental health screening
  - Depressive symptoms
  - Anxious symptoms
  - Hallucinations and/or delusions
  - Suicidality
- Current pain status (including expectations, fluctuations, and treatments)
- Cognitive screening
  - Attention
  - Learning and memory
  - Executive functioning (eg, planning, organizing, initiating, inhibiting)
  - Language
  - Visuospatial processing

INTERVENTIONS TO PROMOTE COLLABORATIVE CARE
RAPPORT

Rehabilitation is most effective when it is patient centered and with a high degree of patient collaboration (2,10). Studies of psychotherapy outcomes have shown that strong relationships between clinician and patient account for as much success as the specific therapeutic intervention (11). Qualities of effective clinical relationships include a team mentality (ie, that the clinician is "on the patient's side"), clinician empathy (warmth, compassion, and understanding), and collaboration on goals (12).

Satisfactory communication between patient and doctor is essential for a collaborative relationship (Table 8.2). Patients expect to have their concerns attended to and investigated with interest and thoroughness. Any perception otherwise can leave a patient feeling unsafe and threatened, which can manifest into anger, distrust, or noncompliance. When confronted with a dissatisfied patient, it is important that the treatment providers keep their response in check (eg, feeling defensive, insulted, or disappointed) and be careful not to reciprocate with anger or withdrawal (13). In these situations, an understanding, nonjudgmental response is most helpful. For example, "You seem angry, can you tell me more about it?" followed by listening to their response. Soliciting the patient's perspective on solving problems that arise is also often helpful. A typical exchange of this type may take an additional 50 seconds (13), which is likely a minor cost compared with major gains in trust and mutual satisfaction.

PATIENT REACTIONS AND TEAM RESPONSES TO POTENTIAL BARRIERS

Patient reactions to injury are not always predictable (14), so interventions must be tailored to each individual patient and within that individual's life context. Individuals entering rehabilitation can have a number of stressors that can affect outcome: fear of continual decline, anxiety and/or shame about new dependency, unfamiliar environment, difficulty understanding hospital procedures and health care policies, and loss of future plans or dreams. There is no universal

TABLE 8.2 ■ Components of respectful doctor–patient interactions.

- Make eye contact at patient's level (eg, sit down)
- Adjust speaking pace, complexity, and volume based on individuals' needs
- Ask for patient's input, including questions or suggestions
- Expect some patients to require slower than typical interactions for accurate comprehension
- Check patient's understanding of discussed information by asking for a summary
- Encourage the patient's active role in recovery by praising observed milestones and/or activity

response to crisis or disability (15) or identified discrete stages for adjustment (16). However, there are shared elements and common rules for rehabilitation patients in which broad interventions can be applied (15, Table 8.3). Foremost, interventions are most effective when the collective team has similar understanding of the case, agrees with treatment recommendations, and applies techniques consistently.

PSYCHOLOGICAL SYMPTOMS

The prevalence rate of emotional symptoms is not higher in rehabilitation populations than that in other medical populations (17), but medical populations overall have higher rates of emotional symptoms than the general population (18). Rehabilitation psychologists can help identify psychological factors and apply appropriate interventions to accentuate assets and ameliorate negative effects on recovery. Table 8.4 lists some common psychological reactions to disability that could be barriers to rehabilitation, things to consider relating to these reactions, and suggested interventions.

TABLE 8.3 ■ Suggestions to manage problem behaviors.

Behaviors	Approaches to Better Manage	Example of Management
Frequent or excessive Pt demands *Recognize that coping skills may be limited and that these behaviors repel others at a time when the Pt is in most need of attention.*	• Avoid judging or blaming the Pt and maintain an objective viewpoint • Identify the need being expressed and how the environment may be reinforcing it • Establish alternative contingencies • Listen and offer reassurance; suggest other activities	• Pt rings call bell very often • Nurse consistently comes when call bell used, but not at other times • Nurse and Pt agree on scheduled times for nurse to check on Pt and reasons to use call bell otherwise • After brief discussion, Pt expresses loneliness when nurse leaves; Pt and staff agree that Pt should call friends or family instead

Partial information from Refs. (13,15).

TABLE 8.3 ■ *(Continued)*

Behaviors	Approaches to Better Manage	Example of Management
Anger *Avoid becoming defensive*	• Listen to the complaint • Elicit an explanation or experience that surrounds the anger • Empathize • If appropriate, apologize or problem solve	• Pt describes anger at being asked to participate in PT despite pain • "How had you hoped that I could help you?" • "Pain can make people want to rest and avoid movement, even when exercise is the way we know to lessen the pain." • Discuss plan to schedule pain medications prior to PT
Agitation	• Use a calm, firm voice • Reduce environmental stimulation (private room, low lights, limit visitors). Play soft music • Avoid under- and overstimulation; use timeouts/distraction as necessary • Contract with agreeable goals and consequences • Schedule tasks when most rested • Talk about their interests	• Pt is restless and irritable most of the time, particularly when in the gym • Therapist plans to hold therapy in private, quiet space • Team discuss goals and plan with patient upfront • Calmly refer to and remind about agreed upon goals to encourage task completion Refer to agreed upon goals, calmly, to encourage task completion
Apathy or silence	• Check for hearing or language barriers • Assess mood • Explain the need for collaboration for full benefits • Collaborate on modest and reachable goals, create graph to chart progress	• Pt appears apathetic and does not agree or disagree with stated team goals • Elicit Pt's input • "Just like you, the team has the same goal of restoring a good amount of functioning." • Chart, reinforce activity

(Continued)

TABLE 8.3 ▦ *(Continued)*

Behaviors	Approaches to Better Manage	Example of Management
Suspiciousness	• Assess mental status and presence of delusions • Ignore accusations • Be factual and consistent across team members • Write down factual information and place in Pt's view	• Pt believes the medical team wants to keep him sick because the team wants job security • May be due to delirium or premorbid psychotic disorder; each needs to be assessed • Refer to written information regarding rationale of treatment routinely and consistently
Decreased participation	• Check Pt's understanding • Learn about personal reinforcers • Highlight and chart progress to motivate	• Pt terminates each treatment session early with varying excuses (eg, fatigue, pain, expecting a visitor) • Elicit input/understanding • Use reinforcers (praise, rest breaks, pep talks)
Impulsivity	• Elicit Pt's feedback on the factors contributing to the behavior • Focus on positive behaviors with praise • Consistently (across team members and time) tell Pt behaviors that are unacceptable	• Despite education about precautions, Pt gets out of bed on her own • Use praise ("Thank you for using the call bell and waiting when you wanted to get up") • "Stay in bed until there is help, for safety"
Verbal outbursts	• Teach and rehearse a "pause factor": stop, think and organize thoughts before responding	• Pt becomes angry at an aide and reacts with name calling • He later expresses regret and becomes apologetic • Reinforce his interest in behavior change • Practice taking pauses

TABLE 8.4 ■ Psychological issues and suggested intervention strategies.

Psychological Issues	Things to Consider	Intervention Suggestions
Noncompliance	Consider Pt readiness to change	Discern performance ability from inability
	Explore cultural expectations	Discuss reasons for discrepancy in goals and actions
	Assess for psychological issues (depression or anxiety)	Have Pt state potential negative consequences and the probability for these outcomes
		Clarify the context of noncompliance (eg, how others respond and identify usual and potential consequences)
Depression/Low mood	*Could reflect appropriate recognition of a problem*	Listen actively to lessen feelings of isolation/loneliness and learn what contributes to the distress
	The patient may feel isolated and alone or guilty	Correct misinformation regarding fears or guilt
	The patient may not fully understand medical status	Highlight assets and progress Focus on the positive aspects of the situation
Anxiety (generalized)	Mild episodes are normal	Teach smooth, deep breathing and educate about stress response
	Intense, frequent, or prolonged anxiety can be problematic	Add predictable routines to the schedule
	Can be due to lack of understanding of medical status or lack of control/predictability	Offer unhurried explanations of medical status and upcoming events
		Plan activities incompatible with anxiety (play games/watch movies)

Partial information from Ref. (18).

(Continued)

TABLE 8.4 ■ *(Continued)*

Psychological Issues	Things to Consider	Intervention Suggestions
Anxiety (specific)	Anxiety is a learned fear response that is experienced under conditions associated with unpleasantness	Brainstorm Pt-specific relaxation techniques (music; imagery of positive outcome with feared stimuli; deep breathing; mantras)
		Educate that specific anxiety responses can be unlearned
Conversion reactions	Expression of psychological stress in a physical way	Treat with regular rehab with explicit expectations that Pt will be "healed" in X sessions with Y therapy
		Consult with rehabilitation psychologist to ensure stressors can be addressed
		Coordinate treatment team so that positive expectations and praise of progress are consistent

COGNITIVE PROBLEMS

At times, cognitive problems can be the main barrier to optimal patient–team collaboration and engagement in rehabilitation services. Table 8.5 lists some deficits that frequently present during rehabilitation and some strategies to improve functioning.

PHYSICAL FACTORS

Rehabilitation psychologists help teams not only with interventions relating to adjustment or cognitive problems but also with interventions that involve physical issues such as pain or sexuality. Rehabilitation psychologists often integrate both psychological and physical factors that may affect a patient's ability to fully engage in rehabilitation and offer suggestions when physical symptoms may affect a person's rehabilitation (Table 8.6). Pain can affect cognitive abilities, emotional coping, and/or social relationships, and pain contributes considerably to additional loss of function and related disability (19); treatment will be compromised if either psychological or physical factors are neglected (20). Psychosocial

TABLE 8.5 ■ Cognitive issues and strategies to improve functioning.

Deficit	Strategies
Orientation or confusion or advanced dementia	Create familiarity and predictability in the environment, routines, and caretakers
	Place calendar, clock, and familiar pictures in the environment
	Have treatment goals written and placed for regular viewing
	Talk in a slow, calm, soothing manner, and ensure you have Pt's attention
	Do not expect information to be retained and understood
	Reasoning will not be helpful
Attention	Reduce environmental distractions
	Concentrate on one task at a time
	Discourage conversation during therapy exercises
	Organize therapy tasks hierarchically with repeated activation
Initiation	Check comprehension
	Structure and routinize activities
	Divide complex tasks into discrete steps
	Create a chart of progress
	Reinforce efforts and small successes
Memory	Use a calendar for future reminders, and log daily events for historical reminders
	Provide written information and cues often
	Use alarms or cues for designated tasks (eg, meds, cooking)
	Involve and educate family early in the process
Communication	Use brief, direct sentences with few words
	Response choices can be used to express answers if nonverbal
Speed of processing	Adjust expectations to reduce frustration
	Structure and fully prepare for tasks to improve efficiency
	Expect and schedule additional time
	Increase pauses between sentences to permit comprehension

(Continued)

TABLE 8.5 ■ *(Continued)*

Deficit	Strategies
Visuospatial	Position environment to ensure safety
	Ensure appropriate supervision for mobility tasks
Unawareness	Educate Pt about how impairments may affect daily functioning
	Ask Pt for expectation prior to task, then compare expectation to performance
	Remind of progress by listing specific improvements
	Chart improvements as tangible feedback

TABLE 8.6 ■ Things to consider when physical factors affect rehabilitation.

Physical Factors	Things to Consider
Chronic pain	Schedule longer-acting medications to permit patients to focus on "other" things rather than PRN
	Educate about possible poor correlation between pain and pathology and benefits of activity and dangers of inactivity
	Educate about acute pain and chronic pain
	Acknowledge both physical (eg, it is uncomfortable) and psychological experiences (eg, frustration)
	Assess resting and procedural pain
	Rule out undermedication and consider aspects that may reduce effectiveness (eg, history of addiction)
	Encourage behavioral pain management (relaxation training, imagery, hypnosis, distraction, etc.)
Oversedation	Reduce or discontinue benzodiazepines, narcotics, or other sedative medications
Poor sleep	Open shades and discourage naps during the day
	Ask about sleep habits before hospitalization
	Encourage daytime activities; discourage daytime napping
	Use eye masks or ear plugs if applicable at night
	Limit late meals and caffeine intake
	Use soft music or relaxation strategies to reduce autonomic arousal
	Assess for depression or anxiety

TABLE 8.6 ■ *(Continued)*

Physical Factors	Things to Consider
	Be aware of the physical dependence possibility from frequent use of prescribed sleep aids and/or rebound insomnia
Inadequate food intake	Increase socialization during meal times to increase intake
	Educate about nutrition's role in healing and recovery
	Assess for depression and dental issues
Fatigue and related agitation	Space therapy times to reduce fatigue
	When possible, schedule challenging therapies in half-h blocks
	Limit visitations and environmental stimulation
	Assess for sleep quality, depression, or anxiety problems
Substance use and abuse	Avoid blaming or punishing
	Focus on education and dialog of options for behavior change
	Fill the behavioral void by replacing bad habits (smoking while in the car) with new ones (singing songs on the radio; taking a "walk break" instead of smoke break)
Sexual problems	Use the PLISSIT model (Permission, Limited Information, Specific Suggestions, and Intensive Therapy) (23)
	Address at least the first 2 during rehabilitation: raise the topic and offer a few basic facts
	Provide referrals for further suggestions or counseling if the Pt wishes

factors related to pain have been found to be better predictors of return to work than medical aspects of the patient and demands of the job (21). Educating patients about factual medical benefits of activity and harm of inactivity is imperative for patients in acute rehabilitation. Otherwise, the impact of *acute* pain can go along a "psychological cascade," with progressively more (*persistent*) interference on one's physical and cognitive functioning and ultimately one's life satisfaction or identity (see Ref. [22] for elaboration).

■ SUMMARY

Given the complexity of each patient in the acute rehabilitation setting, rehabilitation psychologists can play a unique role in the treatment team. This chapter provides a brief framework for rehabilitation teams to better understand, assess, and treat patients to encourage collaborative care and optimize functional outcomes.

■ **REFERENCES**

1. American Academy of Physical Medicine and Rehabilitation (AAPM&R). http://www.aapmr.org/condtreat/what.htm.

2. Wright BA. *Physical Disability: A Psychological Approach*. New York, NY: Harper & Row; 1983.

3. van Orden MA, Hoffman T, Haffman J, et al. Collaborative mental health care versus care as usual in a primary care setting: a randomized controlled trial. *Psychiatr Serv*. 2009;60:74–79.

4. Blumenthal JA, Sherwood A, Babyak MA, et al. Effects of exercise and stress management training on markers of cardiovascular risk in patients with ischemic heart disease: a randomized controlled trial. *JAMA*. 2005; 293(13);1626–1634.

5. Bruns D, Disorbio JM. Assessment of biopsychosocial risk factors for medical treatment: a collaborative approach. *J Clin Psychol Med Settings*. 2009;16;127–147.

6. Havelka M, Lucanin JD, Lucanin D. Biopsychosocial model—The integrated approach to health and disease. *Coll Antropol*. 2009;33(1);303–310.

7. Lewin K. Field theory and experiment in social psychology: concepts and methods. *Am J Soc*. 1939;44(6);868–896.

8. Wegener ST, Kortte KB, Hill-Briggs F, et al. Psychologic assessment and intervention in rehabilitation. In: Braddom RL, ed. *Physical Medicine and Rehabilitation*. 3rd ed. Philadelphia, PA: Elsevier; 2006:63–91.

9. Bosworth HB, Oddone EZ, Weinberger M. *Patient Treatment Adherence: Concepts, Interventions, and Measurement*. Mahwah, NJ: Taylor and Francis; 2005.

10. Lopez MA, Mermelstein RJ. A cognitive-behavioral program to improve geriatric rehabilitation outcome. *Geront*. 1995;35(5);696–700.

11. Wampold BE. *The Great Psychotherapy Debate: Models, Methods, and Findings*. Mahwah, NJ: Erlbaum; 2001.

12. Norcross JC, Hill CE. Compendium of empirically supported therapy relationships. In: Koocher GP, Norcross JC, Hill SS, eds. *Psychologists' Desk Reference*. Oxford, UK: Oxford University Press, 2005.

13. Beckman HB. Difficult patients. In: Feldman MD, Christensen JF, eds. *Behavioral Medicine in Primary Care: A Practical Guide*. 2nd ed. New York, NY: Lange Medical Books/McGraw-Hill; 2003.

14. Wortman CB, Silver RC. The myths of coping with loss. *J Consult Clin Psych*. 1989;57(3):349–357.

15. Greif E, Matarazzo RG. *Behavioral Approaches to Rehabilitation*. New York, NY: Springer; 1982.

16. Rodin G, Voshart K. Depression in the medically ill: an overview. *Am J Psychiatry*. 1986;143(6):696–705.

17. Weissman MM, Meyers JK. Affective disorders in a US urban community, the use of research diagnostic criteria in an epidemiological survey. *Arch Gen Psychiatry*. 1978;35(11):1304–1311.

18. Rusin MJ, Johngsma AE. *The Rehabilitation Psychology Treatment Planner.* New York, NY: John Wiley & Sons; 2001.
19. Stanos S, Tyburski M, Harden R. Management of chronic pain. In: Braddom RL, ed. *Physical Medicine and Rehabilitation.* 3rd ed. Philadelphia, PA: Elsevier, 2006:951–988.
20. Turk DC, Monarch ES. Biopsychosocial perspective on chronic pain. In: Turk DC, Gatchel RJ, eds. *Psychological Approaches to Pain Management: A Practitioner's Handbook.* New York, NY: Guilford Press; 2002: 3–29.
21. Blyth FM, March LM, Nicholas MK, Cousins, MJ. Chronic pain, work performance and litigation. *Pain.* 2003;103;41–47.
22. Morley SJ, Eccleston C. The object of fear in pain. In: Asmundson JG, Vlaeyen J, Crombez G, eds. *Understanding and Treating Fear of Pain.* Oxford University Press; 2004:163–188.
23. Annon J. *The Behavioral Treatment of Sexual Problems.* Vol. 1. Honolulu, HI: Enabling Systems, Inc; 1974.

9

Rehabilitation Nursing

Sue Carol Verrillo

■ INTRODUCTION

Acute inpatient rehabilitation nursing is a specialty, just like ICU nursing. Instead of juggling vasoactive drips and watching monitors and hemodynamic parameters that characterize the world of ICU nursing, the rehabilitation nurse is just as concerned about how the patient is assimilating adaptive strategies to a permanent impairment, integrating coping mechanisms into their daily routines to achieve as full and productive a life as possible and maximizing their functionality. The rehabilitation team is just as specialized and skilled as the ICU team but in a different skill set. The unique role of the rehabilitation nurse is to act as team coordinator to keep all members focused and on the same page to achieve the aforementioned goals for the patient, because outside of the 3 hours of therapy a day, the rest of the patient's day is under the supervision of the nursing staff. This chapter discusses some of the key individual components of the rehabilitation nurse's role in an acute inpatient rehabilitation program.

■ CORE MEASURES

Rehabilitation nursing is much more comprehensive than simply administering medications or doing bladder scans. Today's rehabilitation nurse needs to be cognizant of clinical benchmarks, best practices, core measures and so on. How will stakeholders be apprised of the quality of the program, and how will defects be addressed through quality improvement initiatives? What benchmarks will be maintained, and how will the hash marks be moved forward? These are all questions that need nursing/patient data collected and analyzed to identify and differentiate among system barriers, process issues, and communication/teamwork defects.

Typical core measures usually include Functional Independence Measure (FIM UDS) change, 90-day mortality, 90-day rehospitalization, "bounce-backs" to acute care hospital within 72 hours of admission to the rehabilitation unit, and number of falls per month.

The FIM takes specific training of the nursing staff in order for the assessed measures to be accurate and for staff to apply the algorithms uniformly from shift to shift. Nursing shift report needs to include falls, urinal spills, episodes of incontinence and how many spills during the shift, how much the patient assisted in bathing and dressing the upper body and lower body, and how much help was needed in transferring (ie, minimal, moderate, maximum assist, contact guard, or supervision, and making sure everyone is using the same definition). These points are then included on the comprehensive data reported for each patient, resulting in accurate FIM reports.

Ninety-day mortality and rehospitalization monitor the appropriateness of the admission into the acute inpatient rehabilitation program. A rate higher than region or nation would indicate that the preadmission evaluation of the patient needs to be reviewed and perhaps admission criteria into the acute inpatient rehabilitation program need to be reviewed. A much stronger pulse of a program is a monthly review of all "bounce-backs" to an acute care hospital within 72 hours of admission to the acute inpatient rehabilitation program. This review will immediately identify program defects, necessitating discussion between nursing and leadership regarding how to correct the defect. The investment on nursing staff administrative time to review charts and carving out time to discuss the findings with the medical leadership benefits the overall health of the program.

■ TEAMWORK AND COMMUNICATION

Nursing works most closely with the attending physicians and the resident physicians in rehabilitation units. Both health care providers have a major impact on each other's efficiency, effectiveness, and workflow. A hallmark that could set a program apart from competitors is communication. An effective communication tool can be a written document (sign-out) available on a common source (usually electronic) and updated daily by each team member. This document could greatly improve patient safety and communication between the disciplines and possibly decrease length of stay by informing colleagues of the patient's progress (or lack thereof), which otherwise might be missed. Essential test results, treatment plans, or outstanding "to do" lists are examples of things that could be passed on from shift to shift.

Communication skills can also be learned through teamwork and communication workshops. Some communication skill examples include using the SBAR (situation, background, assessment, recommendation [see Appendix 19]) framework for taking/giving reports to other units, using the 2 attempt rule before going up the chain of command, or using the DESC script for interpersonal conflict cases.

■ CLINICAL ISSUES
PAIN MANAGEMENT

Pain management is a challenge in an inpatient rehabilitation setting, for multiple reasons. Some patient's pain might never have been adequately controlled. Other patients could have had controlled pain but when their exercise/therapy time is tripled from 1 hour or less a day to 3 hours a day, their pain increases with the increased demand on their body. Another subset of patients could have an added anxiety component to their pain that needs to be identified and addressed through the services of neuropsychology or pain management. The literature is starting to address the issues of persistent pain and how to screen for this specific and troublesome patient care issue in older adults (1).

Nursing should be doing patient pain assessments every 4 hours and reassessments within 2 hours of administering oral pain medication. Nursing staff have the best overall picture of how much short-acting pain medicine the patient is using, whether or not a long-acting agent needs to be added or increased, the effectiveness of the pain relieving agent, and any untoward effects. Effectively tracking pain and response to treatment is critical for optimizing pain management and is crucial information for the prescribing practitioner.

BOWEL AND BLADDER TRAINING

Bowel and bladder training is essential in any rehabilitation effort. The more proactive nursing is to schedule time for bowel and bladder training, the better the results (2). It is just as important to schedule this time as it is to schedule physical therapy or occupational therapy. The more consistent nurses are from shift to shift to toilet the patient on the same schedule, the better the outcome. Nurses can minimize or prevent urinary tract infections by toileting every 3 to 4 hours, watching intake/output and lab values and verifying that the patient is emptying their bladder completely through follow-up post void residual bladder scans (3). The rehabilitation nurse has to assess if bowel incontinence is a newly acquired deficit in self-care or a chronic/permanent deficit. Does bowel training involve an ostomy or is there an underlying infection like Clostridium difficile (C.diff)? After thorough assessment, a plan needs to emerge to help the patient adapt to this self-care need, in order to assist them in regaining some measure of control over their body. It takes a sensitive, listening, and empathetic nurse to help the patient work through these issues during their short stay. The nurse needs to be part teacher, part coach, and part salesperson to gain the patient's trust and cooperation to initially participate in a bowel regimen and eventually independently maintain it. Again communication from shift to shift and standardized care are the keys to helping the patient regain as much of this functionality as possible. Nursing also needs to schedule this time on an equal basis with other therapy times.

Nursing needs to be vigilant about assessing for C. diff, watching lab results, documenting numbers of and characteristics of each stool, and reporting this information to the health care provider. Good hand hygiene and minimizing the sharing of equipment, like shower chairs, is essential in eradicating outbreaks of nosocomial infections.

Awareness of the effects of prescribed medications on bowel function is critical. Some medications cause constipation, and others can cause diarrhea; the nurse should be able to differentiate between an untoward medication effect and an allergic reaction. The patient and family will need to be educated when the best bowel program is achieved and how they will need to continue at home.

SKIN

A majority of patients come to acute inpatient rehabilitation after some sort of surgery or trauma. Various incision sites, drains, and catheters have to be managed and scheduled into the daily care regimen. In addition to these, pressure ulcers should be monitored, assessed, and a treatment plan developed with the input of physicians and wound care specialists. One study indicated that the most common parameters for predicting the occurrence of pressure ulcers are men with moist, edematous skin, with a previous episode of centralized circulation dysfunction that resulted in mottled or reddened skin (4).

The wound care team must work closely with the nursing staff, particularly on complicated or infected wounds. Wound measurements (length × width × depth) and the color of the wound base should be documented. The nursing staff usually communicates the degree of effectiveness of the wound care regimen to health care providers and makes recommendations for changes, if needed. Nursing also works in conjunction with therapy to verify that the patient has the correct wheelchair cushion for pressure relief, reinforces pressure relieving techniques, and schedules treatments like pulse lavage. Individual patients might also need a specialized pressure relieving mattress overlay or specialty beds to assist in the management of their wounds. Close to discharge, nursing has to assess what modalities the patient will need at home and arrange for the inclusion of this equipment at home. Nursing and wound care work in conjunction with nutritionists, the patient, and their family to maximize their nutrition to facilitate healing. The final step is patient and family teaching to continue needed therapies at home.

Surgical incisions are also addressed by rehabilitation nurses. These can present within a wide spectrum of healing. Some incisions are simple, needing only minimal care. Other incisions can become problematic, necessitating rehospitalization for a washout and a full course of IV antibiotics. Rehabilitation nurses need to be vigilant in identifying as early as possible any signs or symptoms of infection. Early intervention can mean the difference between staying on the rehabilitation unit with oral antibiotics or having to terminate rehabilitation for acute care management. As previously mentioned, communication needs to be clear and specific regarding the progress or lack of progress in the patient's wound healing.

MOBILITY

Physical therapists and nurses have to work closely to treat mobility difficulties in order to maximize the patient's progress without compromising their safety. Rehabilitation nurses should have hands-on training on adaptive equipment like beasy boards, patient lift devices, as well as transfer techniques and other specific plans for mobility (5). The benefit of this training comes in the off hours, when nursing can reinforce the skills the patient has learned in their therapy sessions.

Therefore, nursing not only needs to be instructed in proper techniques for any transfers but also needs the instructions for adapting to specific limitations in mobility that any particular patient might have or include the use of adaptive equipment, such as a splint used for shoulder subluxation, an AFO for foot drop, or use of multipodus boots at night. Nursing and therapy must work collaboratively to determine when the patient shows signs of being ready to challenge their deficit or impairment. These patients are the ones that benefit from co-treat sessions. For example, nursing could even move a stroke patient with neglect to a room with a furniture orientation, which forces the patient to attend to their neglected side.

One of the biggest challenges rehabilitation nurses face is encouraging the patient to practice newly acquired skills for balance, gait, and ambulation while being aware of and staying within their individual safety parameters. The literature has reported that the higher the patient's level of impulsivity and the lower their safety awareness or situational awareness then the higher their fall rate. It is a constant effort to maintain safety while practicing newly acquired skills (6).

FALLS, SITTERS, AND RESTRAINTS
Part of the complexity of decreasing fall rates can be addressed through technology, but state-of-the art technology can only be as effective as its consistent use by the staff. If the bed alarms are not turned on or sounding alarms investigated promptly, then technology doesn't matter. Part of the goals in rehabilitation is to increase the functionality and independence, but increasing independence might put the patient at a higher fall risk (7). Hourly rounding is important to address the 3 most cited reasons for falls: toileting, pain, and positioning. The literature suggests that it is important to identify the fall risk factors present for each patient and reduce them as much as possible or eliminate them (8). A risk assessment on each patient should identify extrinsic and intrinsic factors, as well as environmental factors (9). The most commonly restrained patients are those who had had a stroke (10). Increasing cognitive impairment and slower ambulation speed place patients at higher risk of falls regardless of any fall reduction initiatives (11).

OTHER
The rehabilitation nurse has to consult closely with the dietician and ancillary support team to monitor nutrition status via laboratory values, trending intake/output, weights, and response to therapy. Nutritional management can be further complicated by impaired swallowing and the presence of a gastrostomy (PEG) tube.

When a PEG is present, nursing needs to report the volume of residual feeding in the stomach each shift and how well the patient is tolerating the tube feed and work to transition the patient from continuous feeds to cyclic feeds to bolus feeds, if possible. Nursing must keep a watchful eye on the hydration status of the patient, as this is often overlooked. The main means of monitoring hydration are by trending renal laboratory values, checking skin turgor daily, and following 24-hour intake/output trends and blood pressures.

■ CONCLUSION

Rehabilitation nursing is complex, in that, the care a rehabilitation nurse gives is multidisciplinary. The rehabilitation nurse collaborates, consults, communicates, and advocates to maximize patient, clinical, and financial outcomes. Priorities have to be reassessed throughout any given shift and essential data shared with all appropriate members of the team.

■ REFERENCES

1. McLennon SM. Evidence-based guideline: persistent pain management. *J Gerontol Nurs.* 2007;5–14.

2. Roe B, Milne J, Ostaszkiewicz J, Wallace S. Systematic reviews of bladder training and voiding programmes in adults: a synopsis of findings on theory and methods using metastudy techniques. *J Adv Nurs.* 2006;57:3–14.

3. Ostaszkiewicz J. Incomplete bladder emptying in frail older adults: a clinical conundrum. *Int J Urol Nurs.* 2007;1:87–91.

4. Compton F, Hoffman F, Hortig T, et al. Pressure ulcer predictors in ICU patients: nursing skin assessment versus objective parameters. *J Wound Care.* 2008;17:417–424.

5. Nelson A, Harwood KJ, Tracey CA, Dunn KL. Myths and facts about safe patient handling in rehabilitation. *Rehabil Nurs.* 2008;33:10–17.

6. Kneafsey, R. A systematic review of nursing contributions to mobility rehabilitation: examining the quality and content of the evidence. *JCI.* 2007;16: 325–340.

7. Gilewski MJ, Roberts P, Hirata J. Discriminating high fall risk on an inpatient rehabilitation unit. *Rehabil Nurs.* 2007;32:234–240.

8. Nazarko L. Falls part 1: causes and consequences. *BJHCA.* 2008;2:381–384.

9. Hignett S, Masud T. A review of environmental hazards associated with in-patient falls. *Ergonomics.* 2006;49:605–616.

10. Gallinagh R, Nevin R, McIlory D, et al. The use of physical restraints as a safety measure in the care of older people in four rehabilitation wards: findings from an exploratory study. *Int J Nurs Stud.* 2002;39:147–156.

11. Rabadi MH, Rabadi FM, Peterson M. An analysis of falls occurring in patients with stroke on an acute rehabilitation unit. *Rehabil Nurs.* 2008;33:104–109.

10

Anticoagulation/Venous Thromboembolism

Robert Samuel Mayer

■ INTRODUCTION

Venous thromboembolism (VTE) refers to deep venous thrombosis (DVT) and pulmonary embolism (PE). In the United States, the annual incidence of VTE is estimated to exceed 600 000 with nearly 300 000 fatalities (1), making it the most common preventable cause of hospital-related death (2). Indeed, in 2001, the U.S. Agency for Healthcare Research and Quality found that appropriate use of VTE prophylaxis was the most highly rated safe practice among 79 safe practices evaluated for impact and effectiveness. (http://www.ahrq .gov/clinic/ptsafety/). Unfortunately, only 50% of VTE events found at autopsy were diagnosed clinically before death. Hence, prevention and early diagnosis and treatment are critical (3).

RISK FACTORS

Risk factors for VTE are major trauma, immobility, paresis, malignancy, previous VTE, increasing age, pregnancy and postpartum period, acute infection, heart failure, respiratory failure, obesity, and smoking (4). The vast majority of rehabilitation inpatients fit into at least one of these categories. Thus, it is incumbent upon physiatrists to be adept in the prevention, early diagnosis, and treatment of VTE.

PREVENTION

Only 33% of inpatients in US hospitals receive appropriate VTE prophylaxis (5). The American College of Chest Physicians (ACCP) has established the most widely used guidelines (6). These guidelines have been developed on evidence-based medicine but are not without controversy. Below are some alternative diagnosis-specific guidelines. Most vary little from the ACCP guidelines.

ORTHOPEDIC SURGERY

The American Academy of Orthopedic Surgery (AAOS) has published alternative guidelines, which reflect the concern among some orthopedic surgeons over the risk of postoperative hematomas in joint replacement patients placed on low molecular weight heparins (LMWH) (7). The main difference between the ACCP and AAOS guidelines is that the AAOS guidelines allow for the optional use of high-dose aspirin in total knee replacements, whereas the ACCP guidelines advise against this practice.

COMPLEX MEDICAL
In a meta-analysis of hospitalized internal medicine patients, LMWH and unfractionated heparin (UFH) 5000 units subcutaneously 3 times daily were found to be equally efficacious in preventing DVT with similar risks of bleeding (8). The effect on the incidence of PE in that study could not be determined due to inadequate sample size. In neurosurgical patients, a meta-analysis of 18 studies indicated that LMWH could prevent VTE in patients without a contraindication to its use, whereas intermittent compression devices (ICDs) could also prevent VTE when there was a contraindication. Furthermore, UFH had a higher risk of VTE complications (9).

TRAUMATIC BRAIN INJURY
A survey of NIDRR Brain Injury Model Systems revealed no clear consensus about VTE prophylaxis; only 56% of centers routinely used anticoagulants prophylactically (10). The same study reported an incidence of fatal PE of 0.42 per practice year, emphasizing the need for guidelines (10).

SPINAL CORD INJURY
Guidelines have been released for the prevention of VTE in cervical spinal cord injury (SCI) (11). The use of LMWH prophylaxis in SCI patients undergoing acute rehabilitation resulted in a drop in the incidence of VTE from 21% to 7.9% compared with the use of low-dose UFH (12).

CANCER
The National Comprehensive Cancer Center Network released guidelines in 2007 recommending anticoagulation for VTE prophylaxis in all hospitalized cancer patients under active therapy who do not have contraindications (13).

INTERMITTENT COMPRESSION DEVICES
ICDs have some effectiveness in preventing DVTs when used alone compared with no intervention and should be used when there are contraindications to anticoagulation. The use of ICDs was substantially less effective than pharmacologic prophylaxis but did add additional benefit when used in combination with anticoagulation (14). In stroke

patients, no benefit to the use of mechanical prophylaxis has been demonstrated (15).

INFERIOR VENA CAVA FILTERS

Inferior vena cava filters (IVCFs) can be used to prevent a DVT from propagating to a PE in patients with contraindications to anticoagulation. However, there is no demonstrated benefit to using them as a primary prophylaxis (16).

PREVENTION SAVES LIVES

The rigorous implementation of ACCP guidelines can result in a dramatic decrease in the incidence of VTE. In one study, the application of the ACCP guidelines in an academic hospital rehabilitation unit resulted in a 6-fold decrease in VTE events (17).

■ DIAGNOSIS

Diagnosis of VTE is notoriously difficult. Up to 70% of fatal PE is first diagnosed at autopsy (18). It is optimal to diagnose VTE at the stage of DVT, as PE frequently results in sudden death.

DIAGNOSING DVT

The gold standard for the diagnosis of lower limb DVT is venography. However, it is seldom used clinically outside the research setting as noninvasive testing, especially venous Doppler ultrasound (US), has such high positive and negative predictive values (PPVs and NPVs). It has an even higher NPV (99.5%) when duplex color technology is used (19). This has become the optimal test for diagnosing DVT in patients with symptoms, that is, unilateral lower limb swelling or sudden onset of calf pain.

WHAT ABOUT D-DIMER?

Some have advocated the use of D-dimer to screen symptomatic patients prior to ordering a US. This may have some utility in the outpatient setting in patients at low risk (20). However, in postoperative patients, it is of little benefit because the PPV is so low, and false positives are so frequent (21).

SURVEILLANCE DOPPLERS

On first glance, it might make sense to screen all high-risk patients for VTE with US upon admission to the rehabilitation unit. Indeed, in a survey of NIDRR Brain Injury Model Systems, 50% of facilities did so (10). However, this practice has been shown to be costly and ineffective (22). It is not recommended under the ACCP guidelines (6).

DIAGNOSING PE

Physicians need to maintain a high level of suspicion for PE, particularly in rehabilitation inpatients, who typically carry a high risk (23). One widely used system for stratifying diagnostic suspicion for PE is the Wells rule (Table 10.1). It has been revised into a simplified form, which carries similar validity in identifying patients with a high probability of PE upon further testing (24).

Basically, the presence of more than one of the following signs and symptoms should trigger a physician to order diagnostic testing for PE: clinical signs of DVT, tachycardia, immobilization in the last month, previous VTE, hemoptysis, malignancy, and an alternative diagnosis are less likely than PE.

DIAGNOSTIC TESTING FOR PE

Pulmonary angiography is the gold standard for diagnosing PE, but similar to venography, it is seldom used in clinical settings as noninvasive testing has nearly matched its sensitivity and specificity (19). Ventilation–perfusion scintographic studies (V/Q) can have diagnostically definitive results in most patients, but a subset of patients will have intermediate probability scans (25). Therefore, increasingly clinicians rely on spiral computerized tomography in patients who do not have a contraindication to this test (the primary contraindications being renal insufficiency or dye allergy) (19).

TABLE 10.1 ■ Scoring of the various elements in the original, modified, and simplified Wells rule.

	Original	**Modified**	**Simplified**
1. Clinical signs and symptoms DVT	3	2	1
2. Tachycardia (>100/min)	1.5	1	1
3. Immobilization or surgery in the previous 4 wk	1.5	1	1
4. Previous DVT/PE	1.5	1	1
5. Hemoptysis	1	1	1
6. Malignancy	1	1	1
7. An alternative diagnosis is less likely than PE	3	2	1
Cutoff for PE unlikely	≤4	≤2	≤1

Abbreviation: DVT, deep venous thrombosis; PE, pulmonary embolism. With permission from Ref. 24.

■ TREATMENT
Physiatrists are often the first physicians to initiate treatment of VTE in hospitalized patients. The advent of LMWH in the last decade has allowed the treatment of VTE with less intensive monitoring than UFH given intravenously. Dosages are weight based and far higher than prophylactic dosing. While baseline laboratory tests (CBC, aPTT, PT/INR, BMP) are advisable, there is no need to monitor aPTT as with UFH intravenously. This substantially simplifies care and reduces total cost (26).

AMERICAN COLLEGE OF PHYSICIANS (ACP)/AMERICAN ACADEMY OF FAMILY PHYSICIAN (AAFP) GUIDELINES
The joint guidelines from the ACP and the AAFP (27) recommend the preferential use of LMWH for DVT and find equal efficacy for the use of LMWH and UFH for PE. The exceptions are patients with renal insufficiency, who should be treated with UFH, and patients with contraindications to anticoagulation (eg, active bleeding, thrombocytopenia, hereditary bleeding disorder).

TREATMENT OF PATIENTS WITH CONTRAINDICATIONS TO ANTICOAGULATION
Patients who cannot be anticoagulated can be safely treated with IVCFs (16). These now are removable in cases where long-term use is not needed. It should be remembered that IVCFs do not treat DVT and indeed may worsen edema and pain; they frequently lead to postthrombotic syndrome. What they are intended to do is to prevent the propagation of DVT to PE. They are not recommended for prophylactic use (6). The ACP/AAFP guidelines recommend that most cases of DVT, and perhaps some cases of PE, can be safely treated in the outpatient setting (27). The implication for physiatrists is that most patients with acute DVT, and perhaps some with hemodynamically stable PE, can be managed on the rehabilitation unit without transfer to acute care.

BED REST AND COMPRESSION HOSE
Traditionally, physicians have recommended bed rest and the removal of compression devices for several days after DVT, for fear of propagation to PE. This appears to be bad advice, at least according to a retrospective study in Italy (28). DVT patients who were immobilized and did not receive compression devices actually had a higher risk of developing PE subsequently.

LONG-TERM MANAGEMENT
A systematic review of management of VTE (29) recommends 3 months of treatment with a vitamin K antagonist (Warfarin) for VTE in patients with transient risk factors (eg, postoperatively) and 12-month patients

with "unprovoked" VTE or those with ongoing risk (eg, tetraplegia). LMWH was found to be an equally efficacious alternative, especially in cancer patients. The use of below knee compression stockings after DVT reduces the incidence of postthrombotic syndrome by 50% (30).

ICD codes

■ 2010: 453.40—Acute venous embolism and thrombosis of unspecified deep vessels of lower extremity

■ 2010: 453.41—Acute venous embolism and thrombosis of deep vessels of proximal lower extremity

■ 2010: 453.42—Acute venous embolism and thrombosis of deep vessels of distal lower extremity (ie, the calf, lower leg NOS, peroneal, and tibia.)

■ 2010: 453.8—Other venous embolism and thrombosis of other specified veins (eg, upper extremity vein)

If DVT is documented as a postoperative complication or iatrogenic, first assign code 997.2, followed by

■ 451.11: Iatrogenic pulmonary embolism and infarction

■ 451.12: Septic pulmonary embolism (first code the underlying infection)

■ 451.19: Other pulmonary embolism and infarction

Deep Vein Thrombosis Sample Evaluation and Order Set

Jarrod David Friedman

DVT

Evaluation of the patient with acute or subacute limb edema.

Does the Patient Appear

A. Stable with regular breathing pattern, pulse regular and not tachycardic, and pulse oxygenation within normal limits. -> Start workup.

OR

B. Patient appears unstable; call your support team/code team.

Use Wells score/criteria: (detailed previously) then based on the scoring

If ≥2 DVT, likely a workup is indicated.

If <2 DVT, less likely workup dependent upon individual suspicion.

Remember that other causes are still possible and, subsequently, an appropriate evaluation for edema is necessary.

If the situation is not an emergency, consider the following steps.

Check Chart History for Risk Factors of DVT

Acute infection	Immobility (plane, car, cast, bed bound)	Multiple fracture	Paresis	Previous VTE
Heart failure	Malignancy	Obesity	Pregnancy	Respiratory failure
Increased age	Major trauma	Oral contra-ceptives	Postpartum period	Smoking

Check the Medication List

Is the patient on DVT prophylaxis currently? If yes, is it a therapeutic dose? If no, is there another method of prophylaxis being used, that is, compression stocking, pneumatic compression, and so on.

Check Most Recent Laboratory Test

(PTT, PT/INR, bleeding time, hemoglobin/hematocrit, platelets, albumin, protein)?
Is anything abnormal that increases DVT risk or risk of soft tissue edema (ie, low protein—peripheral edema or hypercoagulable state—DVT).

Physical Examination

- Is the edema focal to one limb? This increases likelihood of DVT.

- Is pain present in the involved limb? Is the pain more intense along deep or superficial veins suggestive of venous pathology or on other areas such as bony or muscle region suggestive of other causes.

- Check for pitting versus nonpitting edema and palpable cords.

- Measure calves: >3 cm difference is significant (measured 10 cm below tibial tuberosity)

- Is erythema or general warmth present in the involved limb? This could suggest cellulitis or thrombophlebitis.

- Check opposite limb for varicose or abnormal veins.

- Perform a heart and lung examination if not previously performed.

If after evaluating history, physical examination, and previous laboratory findings there is high suspicion for DVT:

1. Venous duplex ultrasound with or without color enhancement

2. If concerned about PE: Spiral CT scan or V/Q scan

Laboratory tests to consider:

CBC with differential, D-dimer, albumin, preablumin, liver function tests, electrolytes, BUN/creatinine, protein C, protein S antithrombin III, anticardiolipin AB.

Treatment:
Diagnosis: DVT
Precautions: Bed rest for first 24 to 48 hours or until fully anticoagulated.
Restrictions on activity depend on a multiplicity of factors: patient stability, extent and size of clot, patient history, comorbid diseases, and physician comfort level.
Nursing: Calf measurements Q Day.
Diet: Regular
Treatment:
Medications:
Initiate anticoagulation therapy:

1. Enoxaparin at a dose of 1 mg/kg subcutaneously every 12 hours. Until INR therapeutic.

2. Warfarin: Tailor dose to attain INR goal. Usually 2 to 2.5.

(Remember, traditionally it takes at least 3 days for full effect of an individual Coumadin dose to effect an increase in INR. Daily INR is a trend. Too frequent changes in dose might be counterproductive.)

If not a candidate for anticoagulation, then consider an Inferior Vena Cava filter.
Chronic course: Continue Coumadin for the recommended length of time depending on underlying diagnoses and risk factors. Follow-up US evaluation is customary in some institutions but not necessary.

Anticoagulation Overdose

Activity: depends upon degree of overdose and INR elevation; conservative method is bed rest hold therapy, fall precautions, and avoiding brushing teeth or shaving.
Treatment:

1. Discontinue anticoagulants.

2. When overdose involves:

a. Enoxaparin or low molecular weight heparin—Consider Protamine sulfate 1 mg IV for each 1 mg of Enoxaparin given. Repeat if bleeding is present or continues. If continued bleeding beyond 2 to 4 hours, consider Factor Xa level.

b. Warfarin

If moderate overdose with minor bleeding: Consider vitamin K 10 to 20 mg IV or SQ immediate and then in 12 hours. Repeat INR in 12 hours and adjust dose as needed.

If severe bleeding: Transfer off rehab unit to medical service. Vitamin K (10–20 mg with IV fluid over 1 hour) FFP 2 to 4 units, and possible 2 units PRBCs wide open.

Labs: CBC with platelets, PT/INR, PTT, bleeding time, blood type, and cross (if severe bleeding).

■ REFERENCES

1. Anderson FA, Zayaruzny M, Heit JA, Fidan D, Cohen AT. Estimated annual numbers of US acute-care hospital patients at risk for venous thromboembolism. *Am J Hematol.* 2007;82(9):777–782.
2. Michota FA. Bridging the gap between evidence and practice in venous thromboembolism prophylaxis: the quality improvement process. *J Gen Intern Med.* 2007;22(12):1762–1770.
3. Laporte S, Mismetti P, Decousus H, et al; RIETE Investigators. Clinical predictors for fatal pulmonary embolism in 15,520 patients with venous thromboembolism: findings from the registro informatizado de la enfermedad TromboEmbolica venosa (RIETE) registry. *Circulation.* 2008;117(13): 1711–1716.
4. Alikhan R, Cohen AT, Combe S, et al; MEDENOX study. Risk factors for venous thromboembolism in hospitalized patients with acute medical illness: analysis of the MEDENOX study. *Arch Intern Med.* 2004;164(9): 963–968.
5. Amin AN, Stemkowski S, Lin J, Yang G. Preventing venous thromboembolism in US hospitals: are surgical patients receiving appropriate prophylaxis? *Thromb Haemost.* 2008;99(4):796–797.
6. Geerts WH, Bergqvist D, Pineo GF, et al; American College of Chest Physicians. Prevention of venous thromboembolism: American College of Chest Physicians Evidence-Based Clinical Practice Guidelines (8th edition). *Chest.* 2008;133(6)(suppl):381S.
7. Parvizi J, Azzam K, Rothman RH. Deep venous thrombosis prophylaxis for total joint arthroplasty: American Academy of Orthopaedic Surgeons Guidelines. *J Arthroplasty.* 2008;23(7)(suppl):2–5.
8. Kanaan AO, Silva MA, Donovan JL, Roy T, Al-Homsi AS. Meta-analysis of venous thromboembolism prophylaxis in medically ill patients. *Clin Ther.* 2007;29(11):2395–2405.
9. Collen JF, Jackson JL, Shorr AF, Moores LK. Prevention of venous thromboembolism in neurosurgery: A metaanalysis. *Chest.* 2008;134(2):237–249.
10. Carlile MC, Yablon SA, Mysiw WJ, Frol AB, Lo D, Diaz-Arrastia R. Deep venous thrombosis management following traumatic brain injury: a practice survey of the traumatic brain injury model systems. *J Head Trauma Rehabil.* 2006;21(6):483–490.
11. Deep venous thrombosis and thromboembolism in patients with cervical spinal cord injuries. *Neurosurgery.* 2002;50(3)(suppl):S73–S80.
12. Green D, Sullivan S, Simpson J, Soltysik RC, Yarnold PR. Evolving risk for thromboembolism in spinal cord injury (SPIRATE study). *Am J Phys Med Rehabil.* 2005;84(6):420–422.
13. Khorana AA. The NCCN clinical practice guidelines on venous thromboembolic disease: strategies for improving VTE prophylaxis in hospitalized cancer patients. *Oncologist.* 2007;12(11):1361–1370.
14. Kakkos SK, Caprini JA, Geroulakos G, Nicolaides AN, Stansby GP, Reddy DJ. Combined intermittent pneumatic leg compression and pharmacological prophylaxis for prevention of venous thromboembolism in high-risk patients. *Cochrane Database Syst Rev.* 2008;(4):CD005258.
15. Mazzone C, Chiodo GF, Sandercock P, Miccio M, Salvi R. Physical methods for preventing deep vein thrombosis in stroke. *Cochrane Database Syst Rev.* 2004;(4):CD001922.

16. Austin MS, Parvizi J, Grossman S, Restrepo C, Klein GR, Rothman RH. The inferior vena cava filter is effective in preventing fatal pulmonary embolus after hip and knee arthroplasties. *J Arthroplasty.* 2007;22(3):343–348.

17. Mayer RS, Halpert DE, Streiff MB, Hobson DB, Berenholz SM. In: Implementation of evidence-based guidelines for venous thromboembolism prophylaxis leads to decreased incidence of venous thromboembolism among rehabilitation inpatients. Association of Academic Physiatrists; February; Colorado Springs, CO, USA; 2009.

18. Stein PD, Henry JW. Prevalence of acute pulmonary embolism among patients in a general hospital and at autopsy. *Chest.* 1995;108(4):978–981.

19. Michiels JJ, Gadisseur A, Van Der Planken M, et al. A critical appraisal of non-invasive diagnosis and exclusion of deep vein thrombosis and pulmonary embolism in outpatients with suspected deep vein thrombosis or pulmonary embolism: how many tests do we need? *Int Angiol.* 2005;24(1):27–39.

20. Kraaijenhagen RA, Piovella F, Bernardi E, et al. Simplification of the diagnostic management of suspected deep vein thrombosis. *Arch Intern Med.* 200222;162(8):907–911.

21. Rafee A, Herlikar D, Gilbert R, Stockwell RC, McLauchlan GJ. D-dimer in the diagnosis of deep vein thrombosis following total hip and knee replacement: a prospective study. *Ann R Coll Surg Engl.* 2008;90(2):123–126.

22. Schwarcz TH, Matthews MR, Hartford JM, et al. Surveillance venous duplex is not clinically useful after total joint arthroplasty when effective deep venous thrombosis prophylaxis is used. *Ann Vasc Surg.* 2004;18(2):193–198.

23. Muntz JE. Prevention of thromboembolic complications in the rehabilitation center: diagnostic and risk factor stratification tools. *Am J Phys Med Rehabil.* 2000;79(5)(suppl):S17–S21.

24. Gibson NS, Sohne M, Kruip MJ, et al. Further validation and simplification of the Wells clinical decision rule in pulmonary embolism. *Thromb Haemost.* 2008;99(1):229–234.

25. Sostman HD, Stein PD, Gottschalk A, Matta F, Hull R, Goodman L. Acute pulmonary embolism: sensitivity and specificity of ventilation-perfusion scintigraphy in PIOPED II study. *Radiology.* 2008;246(3):941–946.

26. Fanikos J. Guidelines and performance measures for the prevention and treatment of venous thromboembolism. *J Manag Care Pharm.* 2008;14(6)(suppl A):14–23.

27. Snow V, Qaseem A, Barry P, et al. Management of venous thromboembolism: a clinical practice guideline from the American College of Physicians and the American Academy of Family Physicians. *Ann Intern Med.* 2007;146(3):204–210.

28. Manganaro A, Ando G, Lembo D, Sutera Sardo L, Buda D. A retrospective analysis of hospitalized patients with documented deep-venous thrombosis and their risk of pulmonary embolism. *Angiology.* 2008;59(5):599–604.
29. Segal JB, Streiff MB, Hofmann LV, Thornton K, Bass EB. Management of venous thromboembolism: a systematic review for a practice guideline. *Ann Intern Med.* 2007;146(3):211–222.
30. Prandoni P, Lensing AW, Prins MH et al. Below-knee elastic compression stockings to prevent the post-thrombotic syndrome: a randomized, controlled trial. *Ann Intern Med.* 2004;141(4):249–256.

11

Assistive Technologies

Mark A. Young, Andrew Sears, Bryan O'Young, and Michael J. Young

■ INTRODUCTION

Assistive technology (AT) has come to play a critically important role in the rehabilitation and functional self-sufficiency of persons with disability. With the aging of the population, there is a growing demographic trend toward improved longevity of individuals with chronic disease and associated disabilities and impairments. While the "gracefully graying" and disabled population often experiences challenges to their quality of life resulting from sensory, motor, and cognitive restrictions, AT has the capacity to substantially improve quality of life, bolster self-esteem, and enhance vocational potential. As the number of individuals with disabilities who use computers (both for vocational and recreational purposes) continues to grow, the importance of computer-related accessible technology solutions has concomitantly grown as well.

■ CHAPTER OVERVIEW

This chapter is intended as a primer and familiarization guide. Its goal is to enable the rehabilitation clinician to optimize care of patients with disability through educated selection of various empowering AT solutions aimed at computer-based vocational re-entry. The chapter will provide a birds-eye overview of the most common physical impairments encountered and specific AT solutions that can be applied.

Specific categories of impairments that affect computer use directly to be discussed include

1. Hearing Impairments

2. Visual Impairments

3. Motor and Dexterity Impairments

For a more in-depth discussion of other forms of impairments including cognitive impairments and language and communication impairments, the reader is referred to other sources.

Although the scope of this chapter is a limited discussion of computer-associated and software-based assistive technologies, each section is preceded by a short discussion of general accessible technologies that are not necessarily computer related. In light of the vast number of technologies and fee-based add-on programs available, the authors have elected to limit their consideration of specific interventions to those that are complimentary and often freely bundled as part of existing versions of standard operating systems (OS) such as those manufactured by Microsoft and Apple. Since computers are an important tool for vocational re-entry and personal satisfaction, the central focus of this chapter is to highlight specific assistive technologies that increase the prognostic efficacy of vocational programs. Often times, the process may simply involve the clinician suggesting a specific "tweak and adjustment" made to standard OS to enable the activation of disability access utilities that are freely available on all computers. The technologies objectively surveyed will include those in the Windows and Apple OS.

■ ASSISTIVE TECHNOLOGY: NOMENCLATURE

AT is a general term referring to any assistive, adaptive, or rehabilitative device employed by persons with disabilities for the purpose of achieving independence. Assistive Technology Act 2004, defined officially by US Government Public Law as "Any item, piece of equipment or product (commercial or off the shelf), modified or customized used to increase or improve functional capabilities of people with disabilities," AT can improve both physical function as well as psychological status by promoting self-esteem and vocational independence (1).

AT can be a powerful tool to modify disablement and enable participation in activities of daily living, recreation, and vocational pursuits (2).

Individuals with disability are thought to benefit from AT in multiple dimensions: within their own body (eg, cochlear transplant to enhance hearing), in direct contact (scooter to improve mobility), and in the immediate environment (wheelchair lift adapted van) (3).

The term accessible technology has recently been introduced by the disability community as a "politically correct" more enabling alternative to AT, which emphasizes a person's abilities.

■ ASSISTIVE TECHNOLOGY: RELEVANCE TO PHYSIATRY

Since enhancing quality of life for people with disabilities is an overarching goal of physiatry, PM&R physicians must be well versed in AT options in order to better serve patients.

When physical limitations and impairments hamper basic activities of daily living and functional skill, the physiatrist must serve as a vital intermediary to suggest solutions.

HEALTH CONDITION, IMPAIRMENT, DISABILITY AND HANDICAP, AND THE ENABLING ROLE OF AT

When considering the role of AT in enhancing quality of life among people with disabilities, it is important to review several fundamental definitions:

A health condition is a disease, disorder, injury or trauma (eg, spinal cord injury, multiple sclerosis, or arthritis) that can result in some functional impairment.

Impairment is an absence or abnormality of body structure or function (eg, reduced strength, amputation, or decreased range of motion).

A disability is an activity limitation resulting from impairment (eg, reduced strength in an arm (impairment) can prevent a person from using a computer mouse and keyboard).

A handicap is an activity limitation (social or otherwise) resulting from an underlying disability. (eg, a woman who is unable to speak due to aphasia [disability from activity limitation in communication] and resulting in handicap [cannot meaningfully continue to work in a social setting that requires understanding and/or expressing speech]).

■ HEARING IMPAIRMENTS

Hearing impairments constitute a wide range of conditions ranging from mild hearing loss to deafness, and are often serendipitously discovered on the rehabilitation unit or in the outpatient PM&R setting. The incidence and prevalence of hearing impairment rises dramatically with age and its presence can often interfere with the rehabilitation process. Hearing impairments within the occupational setting that are unaddressed can lead to reduced work productivity and decreased efficiency. People who have hearing impairments might be able to hear some sound, but might not be able to understand spoken words. Among adult computer users in the United States, it is estimated that 1 in 5 (21%) have a hearing difficulty.

■ GENERAL OVERVIEW–HEARING

I. ASSISTIVE TECHNOLOGY FOR PEOPLE WITH HEARING IMPAIRMENT

Amplification devices have long been the mainstay for people who are hard of hearing.

Amplification devices include hearing aides, amplification telephones and other technologies.

It is important for the clinician to remember that situations often arise in which hearing aides are incapable of providing adequate hearing assistance in noisy environments including shopping malls, weddings, or sporting events. In such venues, hearing might be alternatively remedied by assistive listening devices such as induction loops, infrared, FM or personal amplification devices with directional microphones. With focused listening, these solutions often enhance the users' ability to optimize their experiences in movies, meetings, and seminars. An additional AT solution is TV monitor closed captioning. This device enables hearing impaired or deaf individuals to interact with computers by receiving information visually. With many of these add-on programs, it is possible to adjust sound options and volume.

II. ASSISTIVE TECHNOLOGY FOR PEOPLE WHO ARE DEAF
GENERAL OVERVIEW

Individuals who are deaf are often aided by flashing lights and vibrating signals to alert them about ringing phones, doorbells, smoke detectors, and alarm clocks. In addition, vibrating alarm watches and pagers exist. Teletypewriters (TTYs) or text telephones (TTs) also serve an important role. The standard communications protocol for the deaf or hard of hearing is called TT. TTY or TTs provide the deaf person access to outsiders with normal hearing when used in conjunction with a relay service. A deaf individual wishing to speak over the phone can use a "Voice Carry Over Relay Service" feature in the phone, which vocalizes outgoing messages and simultaneously displays incoming messages. Currently, there is now a "Video Relay Technology," which enables deaf people who communicate in sign language to place a call to outsiders via a Signer intermediary. With increasing frequency, individuals who are deaf are using text messaging capabilities, with devices such as the Blackberry, to communicate without the need for an intermediary.

III. AT FOR PEOPLE WITH MIXED SENSORY IMPAIRMENTS
(IE, DEAFNESS AND BLINDNESS)

Individuals with significant loss of vision and hearing are sometimes referred to as persons who are deaf–blind. Many of the technologies helpful to people with individual sensory impairments also apply to the deaf–blind population. Adaptations are often necessary. Telephone access can be optimized through the use of TTY's with large print capability. Refreshable Braille Displays are another useful technology. People with even partial residual hearing ability can employ amplification phones equipped with Braille markings on large buttons.

To alert people about particular environmental sounds that might occur in the workplace, alerting devices that use vibration, scent, or fan-driven air provide an environmental signal that the phone is ringing or a smoke detector is activated. Alarm clocks equipped with crystal and tactile markings as well as pillow alarms are also available.

Computer hardware coupled with software can successfully be deployed to translate television closed caption to TTY tones for reading on a Braille Output. Refreshable Braille displays for computers are an option for people who are blind and a necessity for people who are deaf blind.

■ ACCESSING COMPUTERS

SOLUTIONS FOR PERSONS WITH HEARING IMPAIRMENTS: THE WINDOWS ENVIRONMENT (WINDOWS VISTA)

The most recent version of Microsoft's Windows Operating System, Vista, comes equipped with an array of features capable of accommodating the hearing impaired or deaf end-user. These features can all be found in Vista's Ease of Access Center (pictured below), which can be found within the system control panel.

At the most basic level, Microsoft allows for the toggling of system sounds and volume to optimize the computing process. Beyond these options, Vista includes a Sound Sentry feature that replaces system sounds with visual, on-screen, alerts. Vista also allows the end-user to activate closed captioning for spoken dialogue. Manufacturer instructions on how to activate these features are below.

Turn on visual notifications for sounds (Sound Sentry)

To enable persons with hearing impairment to receive notifications for system sounds *visually* rather than *audibly*, the clinician can select **Turn on visual notifications for sounds (Sound Sentry)**, and then choose the visual warning's needed.

Mouse Actions	Keyboard Actions
1. To open the **Ease of Access Center,** select: • **Start.** • **Control Panel.** • **Ease of Access.** • **Ease of Access Center.**	To open the **Ease of Access Center,** press: • Windows logo key+U.
2. Under **Explore all settings,** select: • **Use text or visual alternatives for sounds.**	Under **Explore all settings,** select: • **Use text or visual alternatives for sounds** by pressing TAB, and then ENTER.
3. Under **Use visual cues instead of sounds,** select: • **Turn on visual notifications for sounds (Sound Sentry).**	Under **Use visual cues instead of sounds,** select: • **Turn on visual notifications for sounds (Sound Sentry)** by pressing ALT+R.

4. Under **Choose visual warning,** select one of the following options:
   - **None.**
   - **Flash active caption bar.**
   - **Flash active window.**
   - **Flash desktop.**
   - Select **Save.**

Under **Choose visual warning,** select one of the following options:
   - **None** by pressing ALT+N.
   - **Flash active caption bar** by pressing ALT+B.
   - **Flash active window** by pressing ALT+W.
   - **Flash desktop** by pressing ALT+K.
   - Select **Save** by pressing ALT+S.

SOLUTIONS FOR PERSONS WITH HEARING IMPAIRMENTS: THE APPLE OS (LEOPARD) ENVIRONMENT

Mac OS X v10.5 Leopard provides a variety of features designed to assist those who have difficulty in hearing computer speech or discerning sounds. Within the employment setting, this is an important accessibility feature as it could allow a deaf or hearing impaired employee to accomplish occupational tasks such as seeing an incoming e-mail alert.

VISUAL ALERT FEATURES

This feature within Apple OS (Leopard) enables the user to opt for a flashing screen cue instead of an audio cue when a system application issues an alert. Growl, a third-party notification system for Mac OS X, enables applications that support Growl to send deaf user notifications via e-mail or visual prompt, thereby bypassing the difficulties that default audio alerts present to deaf or hearing impaired end-users.

Notifications are a way for Apple applications to provide the deaf or hearing impaired user with new information (in written hearing impairment friendly format), without the hearing impaired user having to switch applications. Growl notifications can also be configured to appear as spoken notifications (useful to blind users), e-mail messages, or most commonly, on-screen alerts with or without accompanying sound effects (4).

ICHAT

For deaf employees in the workplace, the need for multiple means of communication is ever present. iChat is an internet-based text, audio and video conferencing application that enables employees to communicate with each other. iChat can be used with existing chat programs such as AIM (the largest instant messaging community in the United States), MobileMe, Google Talk, and Jabber. Using iChat, employees can communicate with fellow employees on either Mac or Windows PC in text, audio, or video chats.

Although iChat has been available on earlier versions of Mac OS, the Mac OS X Leopard version includes a number of enhanced features. These features include the ability to log in to multiple services simultaneously, manage multiple chats as tabs in a single window, forward SMS messages, and transfer files to a buddy during a chat session.

iChat incorporates a high-quality video frame rate, which optimizes communication for employees using sign language. It is also a helpful utility for hands-on video relay service at <u>HOVRS.com</u>. The finger and hand movements of others taking part in the chat can be readily seen.

CLOSED CAPTIONING
Within the Apple OS, deaf or hard of hearing persons can set QuickTime Player and DVD Player to display open and closed captioning. The clinician can help his/her patient by activating the captions feature in the System Preferences or the application's preferences, and have them displayed on screen.

TECHNOLOGY FOR PEOPLE WITH VISUAL IMPAIRMENT INCLUDING LOW VISION
GENERAL OVERVIEW
Technology Solutions for People with Low Vision.

For people with low vision, there are many magnification options including handheld optics, monocular glasses and binocular desks. For greater magnification, CCTV (closed circuit TV) may be employed to magnify and enhance images. CCTVs are readily available in a variety of formats including handheld cameras, self-contained units, and virtual reality style helmets.

Computer users with low vision may benefit from screen magnification programs, contrast enhancement applications, as well as cursor enhancement features. Screen color configurations can be altered to match the visual requirements of low vision patients. There are several screen magnification programs that offer an adjunctive speech component, which supplements the visible text with voice interpretation.

TECHNOLOGY SOLUTIONS FOR THE BLIND
Blind people often benefit from provision of synthetic speech software that reads text aloud. There are a variety of "read aloud" devices including watches, clocks, thermostats, thermometers, scales, calculators, microwave ovens, money identifiers, compasses, sphygmomanometers, toys, and dictionaries. Talking signs and talking glucometers are also available.

Additional solutions for the blind include items with Braille or tactile markings including thermostats, telephones, rulers, clocks, calendars, and ATM machines. Within the computer realm, QWERTY keyboards equipped with Braille output are available. Computer users can use screen reader programs. For people who prefer not to listen to computer synthesized voice output and would rather obtain Braille output, a refreshable Braille display offers an alternative. Refreshable Braille displays work by employing small retractable pins on a flat panel, which is sometimes attached to the keyboard. The message from the computer screen is sent to this Braille panel.

People who are blind can also benefit from books on tape and radio stations that broadcast aural readings of newspapers.

THE LOW VISION AND BLIND DIABETIC: TECHNOLOGIC SOLUTIONS
BLINDNESS: THE DETRIMENTAL EFFECT OF FAILING VISION ON EMPLOYMENT

Failing or completely absent vision or blindness is frequently encountered among diabetics.

Often in the acute rehabilitation setting as well as in the sub-acute and outpatient arena, these diabetic related visual impairments become obvious to the clinician. For those diabetic patients identified in the rehabilitation setting who do not have visual disturbances or other forms of diabetic secondary complications, the rehabilitation team can actually play an essential preventive and educational role in averting the long-term consequences of the disease.

The blind diabetic poses a special rehabilitation challenge because of the critically important goal of balancing optimal management of glycemic control (maintaining sugars at a normal level) while addressing the goal of improving functional status through upgrade of essential activities of daily living.

Blind diabetics who live alone often encounter problems reading their standard glucose meters and drawing up insulin. Often this may lead to worsening of complications down the line.

REHABILITATION OF THE BLIND DIABETIC: THE ROLE OF THE "TALKING GLUCOMETER"

The role of AT has evolved mightily in enhancing quality of life for people with disabilities, including those with visual deficits resulting from blindness. It is estimated that diabetic patients with visual impairment have approximately 75% reliability in monitoring and managing their sugars. For those who do *not* have access to helpers such as nurses, caregivers, relatives or volunteers to monitor sugars, a newly introduced "talking glucometer" can provide essential assistance.

The recent introduction of "talking glucometers"—a blood glucose monitoring device that "speaks out" the blood glucose levels, and which verbalizes other data such as the time, date, and historical sugar levels, has revolutionized the lives of people with disabilities.

TECHNOLOGIC SOLUTIONS TO ENABLE BLIND & LOW VISION PATIENT'S TO USE COMPUTERS
SPEECH TECHNOLOGY

The most recent version of Mac OS X includes a text-to-speech (TTS) system (known as Alex), which is helpful to blind persons enabling natural intonation even when set at quick speaking rates. This program works with all applications that support Apple speech synthesis. One of the advantages of the MAC OS X TTS system is its ability to analyze text one paragraph at a time and is thought to interpret the context more accurately. The Alex program will speak a sentence differently depending on its precise location in the text and based on concepts found in previous sentences. This is in contrast to most TTS systems, which analyze and synthesize text one sentence at a time and are not context sensitive.

Another advantage to Alex is its ability to enhance the users' understanding of the flow and nuance of human speech, since its voice more closely resembles human speech rather than computeresque speech. With Alex reciting a long passage, there is a "breath capability" built-in to the speech synthesizer so that it sounds more natural. The synthesizer inserts a breath based on a variety of factors including appropriateness, time duration since last breath, the structure and form of the text that is being read, and the amount of time required for Alex to finish speaking.

The Windows OS also includes a dynamic TTS system, Narrator, which is highly customizable.

Make the keyboard easier to use

■ Press keyboard shortcuts one key at a time (Sticky Keys).

■ Hear a tone when you press CAPS LOCK, NUM LOCK, or SCROLL LOCK (Toggle Keys).

■ Ignore or slow down brief or repeated keystrokes (Filter Keys).

■ Turn on bounce keys.

■ Turn on repeat keys and slow keys.

■ Underline keyboard shortcuts and access keys.

■ Choose a Dvorak keyboard layout.

■ Adjust cursor blink rate.

■ Adjust character repeat rate.

■ Find keyboard shortcuts.

Make the mouse easier to use

■ Change the color and size of mouse pointers.

■ Control the mouse pointer with the keyboard (mouse keys).

■ Activate a window by hovering over it with the mouse.

■ Change what the mouse pointer looks like.

■ SpeechWare: a prosthesis for speech and motor impairment (5).

Summary: SpeechWare 2.0 is a customizable speech prosthesis for people with communications as well as motor disabilities. It runs on an Apple Macintosh computer and provides user empowerment over synthesized and digitized speech, telephone and print communications, and household environmental control. The advantage of a ProsthesisWare approach is that it permits customization for each person's cognitive and physical capabilities and does not depend on neurological plasticity. The disadvantage is that ProsthesisWare requires new technical, programming, and support infrastructures to be established in the rehabilitation industry.

■ Change mouse button settings.

Use the computer without a mouse or keyboard

■ Type without using the keyboard (on-screen keyboard).

■ Start speech recognition.

MOTOR AND DEXTERITY IMPAIRMENTS
GENERAL OVERVIEW
A new and evolving generation of AT has facilitated the use of computers by people with motor disabilities. Modified keyboard size and mouse alternatives are available. Within the Windows and Apple OS, there are multiple adaptations. To improve typing accuracy, word prediction software reduces keystroke errors by guessing the next word and presenting a list of alternatives. Artificial intelligence enables the software to learn the vocabulary most often uses.

Although voice recognition technology is often a viable alternative, many people with residual function prefer to use whatever residual function exists. Ergonomic configuration of the workstation can optimize access as well. Patients with quadriplegia, stoke, ALS, amputations or CP may benefit from environmental control units. Examples include doors that open with electronic openers and electronic locks. Other examples include coffee makers, lights, call buttons, and TV sets that can be controlled by switch control. Computer access can be optimized by simple switch access or by using on-screen keyboard. For people with NO hand use at all, a chin mouse, a radio signal generated by a headset, an eye gaze unit, or a mouth stick might represent reasonable alternatives.

AT SOLUTIONS TO ENHANCE COMPUTER USE AMONG PERSONS WITH MOTOR AND DEXTERITY IMPAIRMENTS
Persons in the workplace or newly disabled individuals with motor or dexterity impediments often encounter difficulty using a standard keyboard or mouse or trackpad. Among adult computer users in the United States, it is

estimated that 1 in 4 (26%) have dexterity difficulties. Dexterity and coordination difficulty and impairment can be caused by a number of neurological and musculoskeletal conditions including stroke, carpal tunnel, arthritis, stroke, cerebral palsy, Parkinson's disease, multiple sclerosis, loss of limbs or digits, spinal cord injuries, and repetitive stress injury, among others. For a comprehensive survey of Health Conditions that induce impairments that affect computer use, the reader is referred to Sears textbook, *The Human Computer Interaction Handbook* (6).

Individuals with dexterity difficulties and impairments may benefit from the following AT solutions.

■ Speech recognition systems, also called voice recognition programs, allow people to give commands and enter data using their voices rather than a mouse or keyboard.

■ On-screen keyboard programs provide an image of a standard or modified keyboard on the computer screen. The user selects the keys with an alternative device such as a mouse, touch screen, trackball, joystick, switch, or eye gaze system.

■ Keyboard filters can include typing aids, such as word prediction utilities and add-on spelling checkers. These products reduce the required number of keystrokes. Keyboard filters enable users to quickly access the letters they need and to avoid inadvertently selecting keys they don't want.

■ Touch screens are devices placed on the computer monitor (or built into it) that allow direct selection or activation of the computer by touching the screen.

■ Alternative input devices (including alternative keyboards, electronic pointing devices, sip-and-puff systems, wands and sticks, joysticks, and trackballs) allow individuals to control their computers through means other than a standard keyboard or pointing device.

DEXTERITY IMPAIRMENTS: ALTERNATIVE FORMS OF INPUT
"HANDS-ON VERSUS HANDS-FREE"
Hands-on

■ Keyboard

■ Mouse

■ Joystick

■ Trackball

■ Touch pads

■ Touch screen

Hands-free

■ Sips and puffs

■ Head movement

- Eye movement
- Touch screen
- Foot movement

SOFTWARE-BASED (OPERATING SYSTEM) ADAPTATIONS
Filter-Key Feature

- Ignores or "blocks" repeated keystrokes
- Ignore rapid or extraneous keystrokes or slow down repeat rates
- Appropriate for tremors, stiffness, poor coordination, for example, Parkinsonism
- Enable the users to quickly access the letters they need
- Avoid inadvertently selecting keys they do not need

Key guard

- A simple frame that fits over the keyboard, with a cutout over each key to guide the user's fingers, helping reduce errant keystrokes
- Appropriate for any type of poor coordination

Spell Prediction Software

- As each key is typed, the list changes accordingly and predicts the current word (word completion) the user is trying to enter
- Improves typing speed by offering a list of words based on what keys the user has already typed
- Also predicts the next word (word prediction) and offers "abbreviation expansion" and speech output
- Checks the spelling for the word
- Reduces number of keys typed and improves accuracy of the word

■ CONCLUSION

ASSISTIVE TECHNOLOGY ACCESS: THE ROLE OF THE CARING PHYSICIAN

Physiatrists can play an important role in the care of people with disabilities by identifying particular disabilities likely to benefit from AT provision, and by forging collaborative partnerships with patients by assisting patients in integrating AT into their lives.

■ REFERENCES

1. Young MA, Levi S, Tumanon RC, Desei M, Sokal JO. Independence for people with disabilities: a physician's primer on assistive technology. *Md Med.* Summer 2000;1(3):28–32.

2. Stiens SA. Personhood, disablement, and mobility technology. In: Gray DB, Quatrano LA, Lieberman M, eds. *Designing and Using Assistive Technology: The Human Perspective*; 1998:29–49.
3. Boninger ML, Choi H, Johnson K, Young MA, Stiens SA, Sears A. Assistive technologies: catalysts for adaptive function. In: O'Young BJ, Young MA, Stiens SA, eds. PM&R Secrets. 3rd ed. Philadelphia, PA: Mosby Elsevier Press; 2008.
4. *http://atmac.org/growl-useful-notifications-that-you-control/*
5. Chute DL, Quillen S. Computing applications to assist persons with disabilities, 1992. In: Proceedings of the Johns Hopkins National Search for. February 1-5, 1992:124–126. doi:10.1109/CAAPWD.1992.217426.
6. Sears A, Young M, Feng J. *Physical Disabilities and Computing Techonologies: An Analysis of Impairments*. In: The Human-Computer Interaction Handbook: Fundamentals, Evolving Technologies and Emerging Applications (2nd ed.). Sears A, Jacko J, eds. Florida: CRC Press, 2007:829–852.

Bladder Management

SriKrishna Chandran and
Marlís González-Fernández

■ **INTRODUCTION**

Voiding dysfunction is a common sequela following many neurologic processes. It can be classified based on presenting symptoms and confirmed using urodynamic testing. Untreated, a neurogenic bladder can lead to a variety of complications including urinary tract infections, renal calculi, renal failure, poor therapy participation, and poor reintegration into society. The proper diagnosis and management of a neurogenic bladder is paramount to rehabilitation.

■ **ANATOMY OF THE URINARY TRACT**

The urinary system is divided into an upper and lower urinary tract. The upper urinary tract consists of the kidneys and ureters. The lower urinary tract consists of the bladder and the urethra (1).

UPPER URINARY TRACT

The kidney can be further subdivided into 2 portions: the renal parenchyma and the renal pelvis. The function of the renal parenchyma is to secrete, concentrate, and excrete urine into the renal pelvis. At the ureteropelvic junction, the renal pelvis narrows to become the ureter (1,2). From here, the ureter functions as a conduit for urine to flow into the bladder. There are 3 areas of physiologic narrowing along the ureter: the ureteropelvic junction, the crossing point of the iliac artery, and the ureterovesical junction. These areas are of clinical importance when considering postrenal obstruction (1,2). The ureteropelvic junction is the point where the ureter opens to the bladder. It allows urine to flow into the bladder while effectively creating a 1-way valve preventing urine reflux into the ureter. The ureteropelvic junction accomplishes this task by traversing obliquely between the muscular and submucosal layers of the bladder. In times of high intravesical pressures, these layers pinch the ureter, preventing urine reflux. Periods of sustained, high intravesical pressures can result in a physiologic postrenal obstruction (1–3).

LOWER URINARY TRACT

The bladder can be divided into the detrusor and trigone (3,4). The detrusor is a syncytium of smooth muscle fibers that interweave each other. As these fibers approach the bladder neck, they form 3 distinct layers arranged in a circular fashion. This arrangement allows them to act as a functional sphincter. The trigone extends from the ureteral orifices to the bladder neck on the inferior base of the bladder (1,2).

The urethra differs in both women and men. In women, the urethra is shorter and contains an inner longitudinal and outer semicircular layer of smooth muscle. In men, the urethra is surrounded by the corpus spongiosum (1).

URETHRAL SPHINCTERS

The urethra has 2 sphincters: the internal and the external sphincter. The internal sphincter is not a true anatomic sphincter. Rather, it is formed from the circular arrangement of bladder smooth muscle fibers. The voluntary, external sphincter differs in both men and women. In men, the striated muscle fibers run from the base of the bladder to the membranous urethra. In women, the striated muscle fibers circle the upper two-thirds of the urethra (2).

URINE TRANSPORT

Urine is propelled from the kidneys to the bladder by the proximal tubular filtration pressure and the peristalsis of the calices, renal pelvis, and ureter. Ureteral dilation may impede efficient peristalsis which, overtime, may lead to hydronephrosis (3,4).

■ NEUROANATOMY AND NEUROPHYSIOLOGY OF THE URINARY SYSTEM

Urine retention and micturition is the result of a complex interplay of cerebral, parasympathetic, sympathetic, and somatic signals to the bladder, urinary sphincters, and urethra. It can be described in terms of an efferent and afferent system (2).

EFFERENT SYSTEM

The **parasympathetic** efferent nervous supply functions to promote micturition. Parasympathetic impulses begin in the intermediolateral grey matter of the second, third, and fourth sacral segments (S2–S4). They exit the cord as preganglionic fibers in the ventral roots and travel within the **pelvic nerve.** These preganglionic fibers synapse adjacent to or within the detrusor muscle stimulating muscle contraction by releasing acetylcholine (1–3).

The **sympathetic** efferent nervous supply functions to promote urine retention. Sympathetic impulses begin in the intermediolateral grey matter of the 11th thoracic segment extending to the second lumbar segment (T11–L2). They exit the cord and quickly synapse on the lumbar sympathetic paravertebral ganglia (5,6). Postganglionic fibers travel within the hypogastric nerve and synapse on α- and β-adrenergic receptors within the bladder and urethra where they release norepinephrine (4–6). α- and β-adrenergic receptors are strategically placed in the bladder and urethra (4). Stimulation of β-receptors causes smooth muscle relaxation within the superior portion of the bladder. Stimulation of α-receptors in the base of the bladder and prostatic urethra causes smooth muscle contraction (4). Together, this allows for increased bladder distention and sphincter constriction allowing for increased urine retention (5–8).

SOMATIC
Somatic efferent nervous supply travels from the first through the fourth sacral segments (S1–S4) within the **pudendal nerve,** ultimately synapsing on the external sphincter. Activation of the external sphincter promotes contraction and thus, voluntary urine retention.

AFFERENT SYSTEM
The main function of afferent system is to receive sensory input from the bladder to stimulate a voiding response. There are 2 types of afferent fibers: myelinated αδ-fibers and unmyelinated C-fibers (4). The myelinated αδ-fibers are the predominant fibers involved in voiding and respond to bladder distention. Unmyelinated C-fibers are activated by cold or chemical irritation of the bladder wall. Unmyelinated C-fibers are commonly termed "silent C-fibers" under normal circumstances because they do not respond to bladder distention (3,4,9).

CENTRAL NERVOUS SYSTEM INPUT
The central pontine micturition center modulates micturition. Through its connections with the spinal cord, it may send either excitatory or inhibitory impulses to coordinate detrusor contraction and sphincter relaxation. This enables normal urination.

■ VOIDING PHYSIOLOGY
Micturition is completely under voluntary control. The detrusor response to stretch can be inhibited just as detrusor contraction can be voluntarily initiated. Micturition consists of 2 phases: a filling (storage) phase and an emptying (voiding) phase (3,4).

FILLING (STORAGE) PHASE

The filling phase is predominantly controlled by the action of the sympathetic nervous system. During filling, there is very little rise in intravesical pressure due to bladder distention (4). This is coupled with an increase in urethral sphincter contraction. Normal end filling pressures are between 0 and 6 cm H_2O (3,4). When they reach levels greater than 15 cm H_2O, the elastic properties of detrusor are exceeded (3,4). The resulting discomfort, under normal circumstances, cannot be tolerated (3,4).

EMPTYING (VOIDING) PHASE

The emptying phase is predominately controlled by the action of the parasympathetic nervous system. The loss of sympathetic input to the urethral sphincter causes urethral relaxation. This is followed by the parasympathetically mediated detrusor contraction. The urethral sphincter remains open during voiding and there is no increase in intraabdominal pressure.

■ PATHOPHYSIOLOGICAL RESPONSE TO BRAIN AND SPINAL CORD INJURY

A number of pathophysiological changes have been noted in response to spinal cord injury. Denervation hypersensitivity refers to the increased smooth muscle response to a given concentration of neurotransmitters that occurs following spinal cord injury (4). The distribution of α- and β-receptors is also noted to be different. Some studies have suggested that following spinal cord injury, the relative concentration of β-receptors is decreased in the superior portion of the bladder leading to decreased bladder compliance (4). Detrusor Sphincter Dyssynergia (DSD) refers to the simultaneous contraction of the urinary sphincter and contraction of the detrusor that occurs when the pontine micturition center or its connections with the spinal cord are disrupted. Suprapontine lesions may result in detrusor hyperreflexia without DSD.

■ NEUROLOGIC HISTORY AND PHYSICAL EXAM

A thorough history is important to the diagnosis of a neurogenic bladder to differentiate between urinary retention and incontinence. Signs of retention include decreased stream, intermittent stream, sense of incomplete urination, and straining. Signs of urinary incontinence include frequency, urgency, and a feeling of wetness.

A thorough history also includes a complete review of systems as well as past medical history. Reversible causes of retention/incontinence in the elderly can be summarized by the mnemonic: DIAPPERS (10).

D-Delirium

I-Infection

A-Atrophic vaginitis, urethritis

P-Pharmaceuticals

P-Psychological

E-Endocrine

R-Reduced mobility

S-Stool impaction

Portions of the physiatric history of particular importance in the diagnosis and management of neurogenic bladder include: hand function, dressing skills, sitting balance, the ability to perform transfers, and the ability to ambulate (4).

A thorough neurologic exam must be completed with attention paid to motor or sensory deficits and signs of hyperreflexia.

■ URODYNAMIC TESTING
Urodynamics evaluate the function of the lower urinary tract. One commonly used method of urodynamic testing is the waterfill urodynamic study. It evaluates urine storage, transport, and voiding by examining intravesical, urethral sphincter, and intraabdominal pressures in addition to urine flow rate (Figure 12.1) (3).

Important pharmacologic Interventions for bladder management are summarized in Table 12.1 (11).

■ SURGICAL INTERVENTIONS
In adults with severe neurogenic bladder, surgical management is sometimes necessary. Indications for surgical intervention include severe detrusor hyperreflexia, bladder wall compliance, continued upper tract deterioration despite aggressive pharmacotherapy, behavioral treatment, or modalities. Surgical interventions include augmentation cystoplasty, artificial sphincter placement, subarachnoid block, sphincterotomy, cordectomy, and anterior or anteroposterior rhizotomy (3).

■ BEHAVIORAL MODIFICATIONS
Patients with urinary incontinence may benefit from a scheduled voiding regimen (timed voiding). Bladder training can be accomplished by progressively increasing the time between voids by 10 to 15 minutes every 2 to 5 days until a reasonable interval between voiding is obtained. In other cases, diapers may be used as a backup to other modifications (3).

Condom catheters may be used in men with urinary incontinence. While they need only be changed daily, they do increase the risk of penile skin breakdown, catheter related infection, and may fall off.

Alternatively, clean intermittent catheterization may be used. Important principles include the restriction of fluids to 2 liters daily and frequent catheterizations to maintain bladder volumes below 500 mL (3).

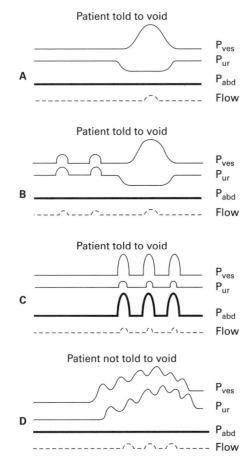

FIGURE 12.1 ■ Schematic representation of various voiding patterns. **A,** Normal. **B,** Uninhibited contractions occur with filling. The sphincter is attempting to inhibit contractions. Patient has a normal voiding phase. **C,** No bladder contractions. Rises in bladder pressure result from rises in abdominal pressure (ie, Valsalva voiding). **D,** Uninhibited contractions occur with simultaneous sphincter contractions (ie, detrusor sphincter dyssynergia).

P_{abd}, intraabdominal pressure; P_{ur}, urethral sphincter pressure; P_{ves}, intravesical pressure.

TABLE 12.1 ■ Pharmacologic interventions for bladder management.

Agent	Indication	Mechanism of Action	Starting Dose	Side Effects	Comments
Tolterodine	Urge incontinence	Anticholinergic. Competitive antagonist of muscarinic receptors.	Regular release: 2 mg PO q 12 h Long acting: 2 mg PO daily	Dry eyes, dry mouth, disorientation, headache, dizziness, constipation	Dose adjustment may be needed in pts. Taking CYP 3A4 inhibitors. Contraindications: Gastric retention, urinary retention, angle closure glaucoma
Oxybutynin	Urge incontinence	Antispasmotic. Anticholinergic.	Regular release: 5 mg PO 2–3 times/dLong acting: 5 mg PO daily Transdermal: 3.9 mg/d patch q 3–4 days	Dry eyes, dry mouth, disorientation, headache, dizziness, constipation	Transdermal patch may contain conducting metal. Contraindications: Gastric retention, urinary retention, angle closure glaucoma
Imipramine	Urge Incontinence	Tricyclic antidepressant	25 mg PO at bedtime	Agitation, anxiety, confusion, QT prolongation	Contraindications: Anticholinergic action. Concurrent or recent use of MAO inhibitors
Tamsulosin	Sphincter spasticity	α1-adrenergic blocker	0.4 mg PO daily	Hypotension, orthostasis dizziness, somnolence, weakness	Contraindications: Severe sulfonamide allergy

When possible, indwelling urinary catheters should be avoided due to risk of meatal ulceration and a high incidence of urinary tract infections. Patients with urinary catheters may have asymptomatic bacteriuria that should not be treated unless a stone forming organism is identified (most commonly Proteus sp. but also Serratia sp. and Klebsiella sp.) (12).

In patients with stress incontinence, Kegel exercises to strengthen the pelvic, floor muscles may be beneficial (3).

In patients with urinary retention, the addition of the Crede maneuver or Valsalva to increase intraabdominal pressure may allow bladder emptying. Bladder tapping to trigger bladder contraction may also be used. Patients using these maneuvers in conjunction with catheterization should aim to discontinue catheterizations when regular and complete bladder emptying (<100 mL) is reached (3). It is important to note that these methods should be limited to individuals with lower motor neuron lesions, those who are status postsphincterotomy, or those who have decreased urethral sphincter activity. Maneuvers to increase intraabdominal pressures in those with DSD or increased sphincter tone often worsen symptoms (3).

■ COMPLICATIONS

Complications of a neurogenic bladder include urinary tract infections, vesicoureteral reflux, hydronephrosis, renal calculi, renal deterioration, and bladder cancer.

■ SUGGESTED READING

McKinley, WO, Jackson, AB, Cardenas, DD, DeVivo, MJ. Long-term medical complications after traumatic spinal cord injury: a regional model systems analysis. *Arch Phys Med Rehabil.* 1999;80:1402.

■ REFERENCES

1. Agur AMR, Lee MD, Grant JCB. *Grant's Atlas of Anatomy.* 10th ed. Baltimore, MD: Lippincott Williams & Wilkins; 1999: 184–188.
2. Standring S. *Grays Anatomy: The Anatomical Basis of Clinical Practice.* 39th ed. Edinburgh, UK: Elsevier; 2005:1269–1294.
3. Delisa J, Gans B. *Rehabilitation Medicine: Principles and Practice.* 3rd ed. Philadelphia, PA: Lippincott-Raven; 1999:1073–1094.
4. Kirshblum S, Campagnolo D, DeLisa J. *Spinal Cord Medicine.* Philadelphia, PA: Lippincott Williams & Wilkins; 2002:181–203.
5. Fletcher TF, Bradley WE. Neuroanatomy of the bladder-urethra. *J Urol.* 1978;119:153–160.
6. Benson GS, McConnell JA, Wood JG. Adrenergic innervation of the human bladder body. *J Urol.* 1979;122:189–191.

7. Elbadawi A. Autonomic muscular innervation of the vesical outlet and its role in micturation. In: Hinman F Jr, ed. *Benign Prostatic Hypertrophy.* New York: Springer-Verlag; 1983:330–348.

8. Brunstock G. The changing face of autonomic neurotransmission. *Acta Physiol Scand.* 1986;126:67–91.

9. De Groat WC. Mechanism underlying the recovery of lower urinary tract function following spinal cord injury. *Paraplegia* 1995;33:493–505.

10. Resnick NM, Yalla SV. Management of urinary incontinence in the elderly. *N Engl J Med.* 1985;313:800–805.

11. UptoDate (Lexi-Comp) [computer program]. Lexi-Comp; July 17, 2010.

12. Favazza T, Midha M, Martin J, Grob M. Factors influencing bladder stone formation in spinal cord injury. *J Spinal Cord Med.* 2004;27(3):252–254.

13

Bowel Management (Neurogenic)

Katherine Dawn Travnicek

Neurogenic bowel (NBw) refers to the loss of normal bowel function due to the loss of direct somatic sensory or motor control with or without impaired sympathetic and parasympathetic innervation. Spinal cord injury (SCI) is most frequently associated with NBw, but there are multiple neurological conditions that can cause this impairment. These include stroke, amyotrophic lateral sclerosis, traumatic brain injury, multiple sclerosis, pelvic surgery, vaginal delivery, polyneuropathies, diabetes, conus or cauda equina lesions, muscular dystrophy, and even chronic straining. Patients can experience a variety of problems such as paralytic ileus, constipation, diarrhea, incontinence, gastric ulcers, gastroesophageal reflux disease, autonomic dysreflexia, and nausea to name a few. Bowel dysfunction can greatly affect a patient's quality of life as social incontinence is depressing and humiliating. After a complete work up and diagnosis, establishing an effective bowel program that prevents these complications can allow patients to be socially and vocationally active.

Normal defecation requires intact intrinsic enteric nervous system (ENS) and extrinsic somatic and autonomic innervation, which include sympathetic and parasympathetic systems. The ENS extends from esophagus to anus and coordinates colonic wall movement, which mixes and advances stool from segment to segment. It consists of 2 layers, the submucosal Meissner's plexus and the intramuscular myenteric Auerbach's plexus. Except in neuropathies, the ENS remains intact, even without autonomic and somatic innervation, and can be used for bowel habit training. The extrinsic colonic innervation consists of the autonomic and somatic systems. When stimulated, the sympathetic nervous system promotes fecal storage by enhancing anal tone and inhibiting colonic contractions via the superior and inferior mesenteric (T9-T12) and hypogastric (T12-L3) nerves. The parasympathetic system enhances colonic motility from the esophagus to colonic splenic flexure via the vagus nerve. The pelvic nerve (also called the nervi ergentes or inferior splanchnics) carries parasympathetic fibers from S2-S4 spinal cord levels to the descending colon and rectum. The vagus, pelvic, and hypogastric nerves carry the afferent and efferent fibers, which complete the reflex arcs and modulate peristalsis.

Finally, the external anal sphincter (EAS) and pelvic floor are somatically innervated by the pudendal nerve (S2-S4) (1–3).

Normal colon physiology has 4 stages: storage, propulsion, continence, and defecation. Storage occurs as long as colonic pressure is less than that of the anal sphincter. Propulsion is coordinated by the ENS, chemically by neurotransmitters and hormones and myogenically. When the intestinal wall is stretched and dilated, the myenteric plexus causes the muscles above the dilation to constrict and muscles below to relax to allow propulsion. Vagal, gastrocolic, rectocolic, and spinal cord mediated reflexes via the pelvic nerve also increase motility and propulsive peristalsis. Continence is maintained by the anal sphincter mechanism. Sympathetically mediated tonic contraction of the internal anal sphincter (IAS) occurs while the puborectalis and EAS normal resting state is in tonic contraction. Of note, IAS tone is inhibited with rectal dilation by stool or digital stimulation. Defecation occurs by voluntary controlled contraction of abdominal musculature and relaxation of EAS and puborectalis muscles. The urge to defecate is due to stretching of the rectum and puborectalis, and one can retain stool by EAS voluntary contraction (1,2).

NBw diagnosis is done by physical exam and divided into reflexic, upper motor neuron (UMN), and areflexic, lower motor neuron (LMN) bowel. UMN bowel is typically due to neurological lesions in and above the conus medullaris, while LMN is due to lesions below conus, such as cauda equina syndrome. The key physical exam components include a rectal exam and all sacral reflexes such as anal tone and anocutaneous and bulbocavernosus reflexes. UMN diagnosis requires an intact reflex arc of the rectosigmoid and pelvic floor. These patients have normal or increased anal sphincter tone, intact anocutaneous reflexes (anal wink), and bulbocavernosus reflexes. LMN or areflexic bowel patients have reduced to no anal tone, absent anal wink, and bulbocavernosus reflexes, and the anus appears flattened due to tone loss (2). These are important distinctions to make as the bowel program and treatment plans are very different.

Any patient who has risk factors for developing NBw and gastrointestinal (GI) complaints should have a comprehensive and systematic history, physical exam, and any additional diagnostic testing. The patient history should include the following elements: new and chronic medical conditions, recent surgeries or vaginal deliveries, premorbid and current bowel function, frequency, timing, stool consistency, medication use, accidents, and whether they have a current scheduled bowel program. What are the patient's symptoms such as abdominal distention, early satiety, nausea, difficult or unplanned evacuations, rectal bleeding, diarrhea, and pain? How does this affect patient's ability to perform activities of daily living, to do leisure activities, and carry out work responsibilities? What is their nutrition—daily fluid intake, constipating foods/meds, lactose intolerance, amount of daily fiber, calories, and meal frequency? (1–4).

A full functional history to evaluate the patient's activity level, knowledge, cognition, and ability to perform bowel care should be obtained to determine the individual's ability to complete care independently, at a modified independent level, or by directing a caregiver safely and effectively. This assessment should include the following elements: ability to learn and to direct others, sitting tolerance and balance, upper extremity strength and proprioception, coordination, spasticity, transfer skills, actual and potential risks to skin, anthropometric measurements, home accessibility, and equipment needs (1–4).

A physical examination should include the following: a thorough neurological exam, a complete abdominal assessment, including palpation along the course of the colon, a rectal exam, and all sacral reflexes (anal tone, anal wink, bulbocavernosus reflexes). An ASIA exam should be performed in traumatic SCI patients. Stool testing for occult blood should begin at age 50. After a complete physical exam, a UMN or LMN NBw diagnosis can be made (1,2).

After taking the history, conducting physical exam, diagnosing the type of NBw, and considering the patient's overall functional status, an individualized, patient-centered bowel program should be designed. The program should provide predictable and effective elimination to reduce evacuation problems and GI complaints and prevent medical complications, and it must be reviewed and revised as needed throughout the continuum of care (1,4). Differences in bowel programs will be primarily due to the cause (reflexic UMN bowel vs areflexic LMN bowel) as well as patient preference. An effective program must include all of the following components: the type, dose, and timing of a rectal stimulant; goal consistency of stool; frequency of bowel care; optimal scheduling; optimal positioning; and appropriate fluid, fiber, and caloric intake. In LMN bowel, the reflex arcs are not intact. The goal stool consistency is firm formed, which can be manually evacuated easily. Patients are taught to assume side lying or upright position and perform gentle Valsalva with manual evacuation to be done once or twice daily (1–3). UMN NBw care programs differ in that these patients have bowel reflex arcs, on which a chemical stimulant will work, and need to have soft-formed stools (1–3). They assume the same position, place the stimulant on the rectal mucosa, and wait for it to activate. Some patients will need to use assistive techniques or repeat the stimulation until evacuation occurs.

NBw management in the home and community needs close attention as well. Appropriate bowel care adaptive equipment should be prescribed based on the patient's functional status, need for a caregiver, and environment. Adequate social and emotional support should be available to help individuals manage actual or potential disabilities and handicaps associated with NBw. All aspects of a patient's bowel program should be easily simulated in the patient's home and other common settings. Patient and caregiver knowledge of, performance of, and confidence in the NBw management program should also be assessed (3,4).

To evaluate effectiveness, the following variables should be documented with all NBw programs: GI symptoms, incontinence, evacuation frequency, time of day, position, stool color, consistency, amount, mechanical stimulation techniques, pharmacological regimen, any adverse side effects, time from rectal stimulation until completed defecation, total time for completion of bowel care, diet, fluid intake, and level of activity. When a patient reports strict adherence to one's bowel program but complains of continuing incontinence, GI symptoms, or other problems, one should consider all aspects of the program mentioned above for changes. Current guidelines recommend that a bowel regimen be completed 3 to 5 bowel care cycles before changes are made, unless the patient is having medical complications. Be sure to change only one element at a time to ensure effectiveness (3,4).

Finally, patient education on the rationale, goals, and techniques of bowel management is vital for adherence and independence. A formal education program must be comprehensive and well organized and involves the following topics: anatomy; basic bowel physiology and causes of NBw; long-term management of bowel dysfunction; safe use of assistive devices; the importance of timing, positioning, and regularity; and preventing complications such as diarrhea, impaction, hemorrhoids, rectal prolapse, obstruction and perforation, diverticula, colon cancer, and autonomic dysreflexia in SCI patients. The content and timing of such programs will depend on medical stability, readiness to learn, and other related factors (3,4).

■ REFERENCES

1. Braddom RL. *Physical Medicine and Rehabilitation*. 3rd ed.
2. Delisa JA. *Physical Medicine and Rehabilitation: Principles and Practice*. 4th ed. Vol. 2. 2005:1641-1649.
3. Paralyzed Veterans of America. Neurogenic Bowel Management in Adults with Spinal Cord Injury.
4. *http://www.guideline.gov/summary/summary.aspx?doc_id=850*

14

Burn Injuries Rehabilitation

Lauren T. Shapiro

■ **INITIAL RESUSCITATION AND ASSESSMENT OF INJURY**
ACUTE MANAGEMENT

The primary survey of an individual with a major burn is carried out as soon as the patient is brought to a safe place. The cervical spine should be stabilized if there is any suspicion for a neck injury. The airway should be assessed and the presence of any singed facial hair or carbon particles in the nose or sputum should be noted, as these signs suggest an inhalation injury. Early intubation should be considered in those with likely inhalation injuries, as it may be difficult to intubate them later as airway edema develops. 100% oxygen should be administered with close monitoring of pulse oximetry. Two large-bore intravenous lines should be established, preferably at sites away from burned areas. If a patient is profoundly hypotensive on initial assessment, he/she should be assessed for cardiac abnormalities and for blood loss. The patient's level of responsiveness should be assessed using the Glasgow Coma Scale, and a thorough examination for concomitant injuries should be carried out. Environmental control is necessary to prevent hypothermia. Circumferential burns are usually treated with emergent escharotomies to prevent compartment syndrome and, when involving the trunk, to allow adequate chest movement for breathing.

ASSESSING THE SEVERITY OF BURNS
BURN DEPTH

Superficial burns, like most sunburns, involve only the epidermis. They may be quite painful but heal on their own. Partial-thickness burns involve both the epidermis and dermis. They may be superficial or deep. Superficial partial-thickness burns should blanch with pressure and should also heal on their own. Deep partial-thickness burns extend down to the subdermal tissue. They are associated with hypertrophic scarring and often require grafting. Lastly, full-thickness burns involve the epidermis, dermis, and subdermal tissue and may be less painful than more superficial burns due to damaged nerve endings. These burns also damage the sweat glands and can result in the impaired ability to regulate body temperature. Young children and the elderly are at risk for deeper burns due to their relatively thin dermal layers.

TOTAL BODY SURFACE AREA

The percent of the total body surface area (TBSA) burned in adults can be determined using the Wallace rule of nines. The head and arm each represent 9% TBSA, and each leg represents 18% TBSA. The anterior and posterior trunk each represent 18% TBSA. The perineum represents the remaining 1%. The Lund and Browder chart is used to determine percent TBSA in children, as it is necessary to account for age-related differences in head and body proportions. Superficial burns are not included in the calculation of % TBSA.

FLUID RESUSCITATION

Fluid resuscitation is required in the initial management of major burns. The Parkland formula (4 mL/kg per % TBSA) is commonly used to approximate the volume of Lactated Ringer's required during the first 24 hours following a burn. The rate of fluid administration should be adjusted as needed to maintain a normal urine output of at least 30 cc/hr.

CONCOMITANT INJURIES

Peripheral nerve injuries are common after severe burns and will be further described later. Brain injuries may occur in patients who have had a period of hypoxia, which may occur due to smoke inhalation or a cardiac arrest. Brain and spinal cord injuries may result from electrical injuries, and such damage may not be apparent on imaging studies. Amputations may be seen following electrical injuries as well.

■ NUTRITION

Severe burn injuries are associated with a hypermetabolic state. Patients will have increased caloric needs, and consultation by a nutritionist is recommended to ensure these needs are met. High-protein diets are usually administered. Vitamin C and zinc supplementation may also be given to facilitate wound healing. Oxandrolone is an anabolic steroid that is sometimes used in the acute hospital to promote weight gain and improve muscle protein synthesis.

■ WOUND AND SKIN CARE
TOPICAL ANTIMICROBIAL AGENTS

Topical antibacterial agents are applied after the burn wound is cleaned and dead tissue is debrided to prevent wound infection. Silver dressings are commonly used for this purpose.

DEBRIDEMENT

Debridement refers to the removal of dead tissue and is performed to prevent infection and to allow for definitive wound coverage. Surgical debridement is often performed, but it can be accomplished by mechanical means as well. Hydrotherapy with a handheld shower sprayer is commonly used to help remove dressings and dead tissue. Enzymatic debriding agents may also be used for smaller areas.

GRAFTING

Full-thickness and deep partial-thickness burns are unlikely to heal on their own and thus usually require excision and grafting. Temporary wound coverage with an allograft or xenograft may be performed, but these will eventually be rejected. Split-thickness autografts can be used to cover large areas. The grafted site is usually immobilized for 3 to 5 days postprocedure. Dermal replacement products, such as the Integra Dermal Regeneration Template, may be used for coverage in patients with large burns who lack sufficient donor sites. After placement of a dermal substitute, immobilization for 5 to 7 days is typical.

PROTECTION OF THE SKIN

Vigilance is required to protect healing or healed skin after burn injury. Newly formed skin remains very fragile and vulnerable to even mild trauma. Healed burns may lack moisture, and the use of emollients is recommended to prevent cracks and skin breakdown. It is also recommended that healed or healing skin be protected from the sun. When avoidance of sun exposure is not possible, use of sunscreen should be encouraged.

PRESSURE SORES

Patients with burn injuries are also at risk for pressure sores. The occiput is particularly vulnerable to skin breakdown in these patients. Caution is required with the use of bulky dressings and splints to prevent excessive pressure on the skin. The use of pressure-reducing devices may help prevent sores from developing and may be especially beneficial when used in the operating room during prolonged procedures.

■ POSITIONING AND RANGE OF MOTION
POSITIONING

Following burn injuries, patients will often assume a flexed and adducted position, which is usually the most comfortable position for them, but it predisposes them to contracture. Patients' positioning needs will depend on the location of their burn(s), but the typical positions used to prevent contracture in patients with burns are listed below.

■ Neck: neutral or slight extension

■ Shoulders: 90° of abduction, 20° of forward flexion

- Elbows: extension and supination
- Wrists: slight extension
- Hands: MCP joints 60° to 90° of flexion; PIP and DIP joints in full extension, thumb in abduction and opposition
- Hips: extension, neutral rotation, 15° to 20° of abduction
- Knees: full extension
- Ankles: neutral to slight dorsiflexion

SPLINTING

Splinting may be used to maintain the aforementioned positions in non-compliant patients, to reduce the potential for rupture of exposed tendons and to protect exposed joints. Oral devices that stretch the tissues around the mouth are commonly employed in facial burns to facilitate speech and eating. Resting hand splints are commonly used in hand burns to prevent claw hand deformity.

RANGE OF MOTION EXERCISES

Patients with burns should perform range of motion (ROM) exercises (Table 14.1). Stretching should be performed in the direction opposite the contractile force. When active ROM exercises cannot be performed by the patient, passive ROM should be performed for them. Consider applying a moisturizing cream to the involved skin prior to ROM exercises.

■ PAIN MANAGEMENT
BACKGROUND AND BREAKTHROUGH PAIN

Background pain is relatively constant pain that is present when the patient is at rest and not undergoing any procedures. This is best treated with the use of longer-acting regularly scheduled pain medications, such as long-acting oxycodone, methadone, or long-acting morphine. Patients may also experience breakthrough pain, which may occur

TABLE 14.1 ■ Recommended orders for burn patients in rehabilitation settings.

- Physical and occupational therapy for ROM, positioning, scar management, mobility, activities of daily living, etc.
- Psychology consult for adjustment issues
- Nutrition consult
- Wound care, including dressing changes and the use of emollient several times daily
- Pain medication, including a long-acting opioid for background pain control and short-acting opioid scheduled prior to dressing changes and therapy sessions and given prn for breakthrough pain

spontaneously or be induced by movement, and which is usually treated with short-acting pain medications. If breakthrough pain tends to occur toward the end of a dosing interval for the agent being used for background pain, consider shortening that dosing interval.

PROCEDURAL PAIN
Procedural pain is often the most intense pain among patients with burns and is associated with significant anxiety and distress. Causes of such pain include wound debridement, dressing changes, and therapy sessions. The pain is often described as having a burning or stinging quality and can persist for hours following a procedure. Short-acting opioids are often used in the treatment of procedural pain and should be given a sufficient amount of time before a planned procedure to take effect. Benzodiazepines may help reduce pain and anxiety during dressing changes in patients with burns, but distraction and behavioral techniques may also be effective.

TINGLING AND ITCHING
As patients' burns start to heal, they may experience an itching or tingling sensation. Pruritus can be very severe and may impair quality of life among burn survivors. Antihistamines and tricyclic antidepressants may be helpful in controlling itching. Massage and transcutaneous electrical nerve stimulation are also sometimes used to treat pruritus following burn injury.

■ **COMPLICATIONS OF BURNS**
HYPERTROPHIC SCARRING
Hypertrophic scars are red, firm, raised areas within a healed burn that can result in poor cosmesis and in contractures when they cross a joint. They can take several months to develop following a burn injury. Children and individuals with heavily pigmented skin are at increased risk for scarring.

Scar management may include compression, initially with elastic bandages or tubular elastic bandages (Tubigrip). When burns are near healed, patients may be fitted with custom pressure garments, which they should be instructed to wear for 23 hours daily for up to 1 year. They should be refitted with new garments approximately every 3 months. Compression therapy in the form of pressure garments or a face mask may also be used for facial scars. Although compression therapy is commonly used following burn injuries, further research is required to determine its efficacy in scar management.

CONTRACTURES
Contractures are also common following burn injuries, especially in those burns that cross a major joint. Other risk factors for contractures

include larger burns, prolonged hospitalizations, and inhalation injury. The shoulder and elbow are commonly affected joints. Therapy and positioning techniques are employed to help prevent contractures, but when they do occur treatment may include surgical contracture release or serial casting.

HETEROTOPIC OSSIFICATION
Heterotopic ossification (HO) is uncommon following burn injuries but when present, can cause significant impairment. The elbow is the most commonly affected joint, and here, ectopic bone may cause compression of the ulnar nerve. Signs and symptoms include decreased range of motion and pain. Radiographs may appear normal initially. Surgical excision can be considered if HO severely impairs function. Surgery is usually not performed until the heterotopic bone has matured, which may take a year or longer following injury.

NEUROPATHY
Neuropathy is a common complication following burn injury. Risk factors for polyneuropathy after a burn include age greater than 40 years, prolonged intensive care stays, and large burn size. Mononeuropathies are more common in patients with electrical injuries and those with a history of alcohol abuse. Careful attention to positioning should be given following burn injury to avoid pressure at common sites of nerve compression, including the fibular head.

■ PSYCHOLOGICAL ISSUES
PREMORBID PSYCHOLOGICAL ISSUES
The incidence of mental illness and personality disorders is higher in burn patients than that in the general population. Preexisting depression and substance abuse are prevalent among these patients. Suicide attempts and assaults are not uncommon causes of burn injuries.

DELIRIUM
Delirium is common among patients hospitalized with burns and is associated with an increased risk of death. Causes may include metabolic disturbance, alcohol withdrawal, sensory deprivation, and infection. Male patients, patients with larger burns, and those with a history of substance abuse are at increased risk for delirium.

ANXIETY AND DEPRESSION
The majority of burn survivors experience at least mild depression. Symptoms of anxiety and depression usually improve with time. Some have suggested that these symptoms are increased among those with facial and hand burns.

POSTTRAUMATIC STRESS DISORDER

Posttraumatic stress disorder (PTSD) is common following burn injuries. Symptoms include hyperarousal and reexperiencing the trauma, as in flashbacks. Risk factors for PTSD after burn injury include severe pain and large burn size.

BODY IMAGE

Disfigurement secondary to burns commonly affects one's body image, which may affect one's self-esteem and socialization. Body image may be more severely affected among women and those with larger burns.

■ BIBLIOGRAPHY

1. Edgar D, Brereton M. Rehabilitation after burn injury. *BMJ*. 2004; 329:343–345.
2. Esselman PC. Burn rehabilitation: an overview. *Arch Phys Med Rehabil*. 2007;88(suppl 2):S3–S6.
3. Esselman PC, Moore ML. Issues in burn rehabilitation. In: Braddom RL, ed. *Physical Medicine and Rehabilitation*. 3rd ed. Philadelphia, PA: Saunders Elsevier; 2007:1399–1413.
4. Esselman PC, Thombs BD, Magyar-Russell G, et al. Burn rehabilitation state of the science. *Am J Phys Med Rehabil*. 2006; 85(4):383–413.
5. Gordon MD, Gottschlich MM, Helvig EI, et al. Review of evidenced-based practice for the prevention of pressure sores in burn patients. *J Burn Care Rehabil*. 2004;25(5):388–410.
6. Helm PA, Kowalske K, Head M. Burn rehabilitation. In: DeLisa JA, Gans BM, Walsh NE, eds. *Physical Medicine & Rehabilitation: Principles and Practice*. 4th ed. Philadelphia, PA: Lippincott Williams & Wilkins; 2005: 1867–1889.
7. Hettiaratchy S, Papini R. Initial management of major burn: I—overview. *BMJ*. 2004;328:1555–1557.
8. Hettiaratchy S, Papini R. Initial management of major burn: II—assessment and resuscitation. *BMJ*. 2004;329:101–103.
9. Kowalske K, Holavanahalli R, Helm P. Neuropathy after burn injury. *J Burn Care Rehabil*. 2001;22(5):353–357.
10. Patterson DR, Everett JJ, Bombardier CH, et al. Psychological effects of severe burn injuries. *Psychol Bull*. 1993;113(2):362–378.
11. Schneider JC. Burns. In: Frontera WR, Silver JK, Rizzo TD, eds. *Essentials of Physical Medicine and Rehabilitation*. 2nd ed. Philadelphia, PA: Saunders Elsevier; 2008:609–613.
12. Schneider JC, Holavanahalli R, Helm P, et al. Contractures in burn injury: defining the problem. *J Burn Care Rehabil*. 2006;27(4):508–514.
13. Summer GJ, Puntillo KA, Miaskowski C, et al. Burn injury pain: the continuing challenge. *J Pain*. 2007;8(7):533–548.
14. Thombs BD, Notes LD, Lawrence JW, et al. From survival to socialization: a longitudinal study of body image in survivors of severe burn injury. *J Psychosom Res*. 2008;64:205–212.

15

Cancer Rehabilitation

Robert Samuel Mayer

■ **INTRODUCTION**

The National Cancer Institute Dictionary of Cancer Terms defines rehabilitation as "a process to restore mental and/or physical abilities lost to injury or disease, in order to function in a normal or near-normal way" (1). Rehabilitation is critical to improving quality of life for cancer survivors and maintaining dignity for those with terminal illness. Rehabilitation requires several components to be successful.

Rehabilitation should be individualized to the patient's needs, desires, and situation. Rehabilitation that fails to respect a patient's wishes will fail altogether. Most problems in rehabilitation occur when there are differences in the team's goals and those of the patient. Goals should be meaningful, measurable, and achievable. Health care providers must balance realism with hope in counseling patients about their goals. Rehabilitation is not something done *to* an individual; it must be done *with* the individual. Rehabilitation is largely an educational process for the patient and family members.

■ **INTERDISCIPLINARY TEAM APPROACH**

Team members must demonstrate a high degree of communication skills, humility, and commitment.

ACTIVE PARTICIPATION OF THE PATIENT

Rehabilitation is not something done *to* an individual; it must be done *with* the individual. Rehabilitation is largely an educational process for the patient and family members.

DISABILITY

The World Health Organization has recently published an International Classification of Functioning, Disability and Health (ICF), which is meant to supplement the International Classification of Diseases (ICD-10) (2). It lays out a series of definitions that are crucial to understanding the role of rehabilitation in improving quality of life (3).

■ EPIDEMIOLOGY OF CANCER DISABILITY

Due to the tremendous progress of prevention, early detection, and treatment of cancer in the last quarter century, there has been a decline in mortality rates from cancer. However, the number of cancer survivors continues to grow, as more people are living longer with cancer due to the new advances in surgery and medical and radiation oncology (3). The result is that increasing numbers of patients face more years with cancer-related disability (4). Data from the National Health Interview Survey 2002 indicate that 11.3% of patients with cancer have difficulty with activities of daily living (ADLs) compared with 3.8% of people without cancer in the United States (5).

■ PHASES OF CANCER REHABILITATION

Cancer management requires vigilance and a comprehensive and preventive approach to illness and disability. To accomplish this, a systematic approach to patient evaluation throughout all the phases of the disease process is necessary.

INITIAL STAGING PHASE

Anxiety and disruption of routines may present the greatest challenges. Education is a primary role for rehabilitation providers.

PRIMARY TREATMENT PHASE

Symptoms of fatigue, nausea, pain, and sleep disruption may be the most significant problems. Acute supportive care and symptom management become the primary responsibilities.

POSTTREATMENT RECOVERY

At this phase, pain, anxiety, depression, and treatment side effects such as edema, neuropathy, and weakness may limit participation in work, leisure, and family activities. Care should focus on resumption of a normal, healthy lifestyle.

RECURRENCE

At this stage, metastasis may cause significant neuromusculoskeletal, cardiopulmonary, or gastrointestinal impairments. Rehabilitation focuses on mobility, ADLs, endurance, bowel and bladder management, and education of both the patient and the family.

END OF LIFE

In terminal illness, focus should always be placed on quality-of-life issues. The patient may need to deal with issues of dependency, and caregiver burden is high. Symptom management is critical, as is psychosocial support.

■ IMPAIRMENTS

Cancer, even when localized to–or arising from–one organ system, causes the loss of bodily function across many organ systems in individuals. The physician must obtain a comprehensive review of systems when evaluating a cancer patient, as this will help identify impairments to be addressed by the treatment team. Delineating these impairments in individuals is the first step toward ameliorating them; this lies at the core of cancer rehabilitation (6).

PAIN

Virtually every cancer patient experiences pain during the course of the illness; it can often become debilitating (7,8). The etiology of pain in cancer patients is myriad, frequently having multifactorial causation. The pain may be visceral (arising from internal organs), somatic (from soft tissue, muscles, and/or bones), or neuropathic (from the central or peripheral nervous system) (9). Visceral pain tends to be poorly localized. It is often described as "deep" and "cramping." Somatic pain, on the other hand, is usually well localized. It is often characterized as "sharp" or "stabbing" and is frequently worsened by weight bearing or movement. There is often point tenderness on examination. Neuropathic pain tends to radiate along dermatomal or peripheral nerve distributions. Patients frequently describe "burning" or "pins and needles." The pain tends to be unrelenting. There may be associated allodynia (pain with light stroking).

Sadly, pain is often inadequately treated in cancer patients. As many as 50% to 80% of nonhospice cancer patients receive inadequate analgesia (10). Yet pain can be well controlled in over three quarters of cancer patients using multimodal treatment, according to one study of 2118 patients (11). Treatments can include opioids (12), adjuvant medications (13), complementary therapy (14), physical modalities and exercise (15), behavior management (16), injections (17), implantable opiate pumps (18), radiation therapy (19), and surgery (20).

FATIGUE

Cancer-related fatigue (CRF) is defined as "overwhelming and sustained exhaustion and decreased capacity for physical and mental work . . . not relieved by rest" (21,22). In addition, fatigue has been shown to impact negatively on one's economic, social, and emotional status (23). As many as 75% of cancer patients (24) have CRF. Exercise has been shown to mitigate fatigue (25).

DELIRIUM AND COGNITIVE DYSFUNCTION

The incidence of delirium in studies of advanced cancer patients ranges from 20% to 86% (26). Delirium may be reversible in 50% of the cases with proper identification and management (22). Delirium in cancer usually has multifactorial etiology. Direct involvement of the central nervous system by primary or metastatic tumors, especially with resultant cerebral edema, is the most readily apparent cause. However, distant tumor cytokine production may also play a role (27). Medication side effects also contribute, and necessary modifications should be considered.

MOOD DISORDERS
Patients may experience a variety of normal fears throughout their treatment course, including fears of disability, loss of societal roles, loss of control, loss of desirability, abandonment, and death. Although most patients cope well, a significant number do experience serious mood disorders. The average estimates of the prevalence of depression among cancer patients are from 15% to 25% (28). The importance of correctly diagnosing and treating depression is underlined by research, which shows that depression is associated with poor compliance with medical care, longer hospitalizations, and higher mortality rates in patients with chronic illnesses (29).

HEMIPLEGIA
Tumors affecting brain tissue are either primary or metastatic in origin, with metastatic lesions comprising roughly 50% of all intracranial tumors (30). Brain tumors vary widely in aggressiveness and prognosis. To what extent tumor type or location has an impact on rehabilitation outcomes is not clear. However, one study found a tendency for greater gains for meningiomas and patients with left hemispheric lesions. Brain tumor patients receiving inpatient acute rehabilitation show similar gains between those with metastatic origin and primary brain tumor (31). Brain tumor patients have been found in some studies to have shorter lengths of stay on acute rehabilitation units as compared with other noncancerous brain disorders (30), possibly as a result of higher initial levels of functional independence on admission, fewer behavioral issues, better social support, and expedited discharge planning due to cancer-related prognostic factors. In a study of patients with brain tumor undergoing acute rehabilitation, the most common neurologic deficits included impaired cognition (80%), weakness (78%), and visual–perceptual dysfunction (53%) (31).

PARAPLEGIA/TETRAPLEGIA
Cancer-related spinal cord injury (SCI) incidence may actually exceed that from trauma and represents the most frequent type of nontraumatic SCI (30). Spinal metastases occur more commonly in the thoracic spine (70%), followed by the lumbosacral (20%) and cervical (10%) spine, and most often originate from primary tumors of breast (15%), lungs (10%), and prostate (10%). Lymphoma, myeloma, and primaries of unknown origin also metastasize to the spine, each accounting for around 10% of cases. Ninety-five percent of metastatic spine involvement is extradural, arising from a vertebral body (32). Primary tumors of the spinal cord such as

meningiomas, neurofibromas, and gliomas are relatively rare. Spinal cord metastases produce a clinical syndrome characterized initially by pain in 90% of cases, followed by weakness, sensory loss, and sphincter dysfunction. Weakness is present in 74% to 76% of patients, autonomic dysfunction in 52% to 57%, and sensory loss in 51% to 53% (33). Positive results have been demonstrated following rehabilitation for individuals with disability from spinal cord tumors, with significant functional gains measured after inpatient rehabilitation (34,35).

BONE TUMORS, AMPUTATION, BONY METASTASES

In 2007, about 2370 new cases of cancer of the bones and joints were diagnosed, accounting for less than 0.2% of all cancers. Soft tissue and bony sarcomas are managed with amputation or limb-sparing procedures. Limb salvage procedures are increasing in frequency and are associated with long-term survival, local recurrence rates, and quality of life equivalent to those of amputations, largely made possible by improved surgical techniques that preserve unaffected tissue, advances in endoprosthetic design and durability, soft tissue reconstructive procedures, and radiation and chemotherapy effectiveness in controlling local and distal spread (36). Bone metastases are a frequent source of cancer-related physical impairment that requires the active involvement of the rehabilitation team. Challenges for the treating team arise when metastatic bone lesions produce severe pain that limits function or imposes risks of fracture during therapeutic exercise or mobility. Depending on the severity and location of the lesion, mobility restrictions can range from non-weight bearing to weight bearing as tolerated. Cancer patients suffering from pathological fractures and associated functional deficits have been shown to make significant gains when admitted to an inpatient rehabilitation hospital unit (37).

SOFT TISSUE IMPAIRMENTS ASSOCIATED WITH CANCER DIAGNOSES

Cancer and/or its treatments can cause significant soft-tissue abnormalities. One of the most frequently observed is lymphedema, extremity swelling that results from disruption of the lymphatics following axillary or groin dissection. The prevalence of this in breast cancer patients has been reported to be between 15% and 30% (38). Although the prevalence of limb edema is high following standard treatment, the treatment options for managing this have improved. The use of manual lymph drainage and compression garments is effective in controlling edema. When applied early in the course of treatment, before the development of significant volume increase (eg, >250 cc increase in the arm), lymphedema can almost be reversed (39). Radiation therapy can have long-term sequelae include fibrosis and contracture, eventually resulting in loss of muscle mass. The use of pentoxifylline in the treatment of this problem has shown promise (40). Allogeneic bone marrow transplantation has prolonged life for many with hematologic malignancies. One of the complications of this procedure has been the rejection of the host by the transplanted, immuno-competent engrafted cells, called graft vs host disease. The immunological reaction is often quite brisk, resulting in organ damage (fibrosis) to lung, liver, and notably skin and soft tissue. In the chronic form of graft vs host disease, limb edema, peau d'orange, fasciitis, and enthesitis can occur resulting in significant loss of joint motion. There may be subsequent muscle atrophy secondary to disuse and associated loss of upper and lower extremity mobility (41).

■ ACTIVITY LIMITATIONS

With their multitudes of possible impairments, it is not surprising that many individuals with cancer have significant limitations in their activities. These limitations include reduced mobility and limited ability to perform ADLs.

ACTIVITIES OF DAILY LIVING

Basic ADLs include feeding, dressing, hygiene, and toileting. Impairments of upper limb function play an obvious role in limiting performance of ADLs, but other impairments also can impede these functions. Cognition is critical to sequencing, awareness, and carry over in the performance of ADLs. Pain and fatigue can also limit the individual's ability to complete these tasks. Lower limb impairments can limit standing and transferring, making dressing, hygiene, and toileting difficult. When individuals become disabled enough to require assistance with these skills, the burden generally falls on caregivers. In one study of 483 cancer patients at varying stages of their disease course, 18.9% had unmet needs in their ADLs due to lack of a suitable caregiver (42). In advanced stage cancer patients, the percentage of caregivers with a high level of psychological distress varies from 41% to 62% directly depending upon the functional status of the patient (43). Rehabilitation efforts, particularly with the involvement of occupational therapy, can significantly reduce this burden on caregivers and enhance the quality of life for cancer patients with disabling impairments. To improve feeding independence among cancer patients with upper limb neurologic dysfunction, Chinese researchers used positioning, feeding aid supports, and upper limb supports and significantly improved function over a 3-week treatment intervention (44).

EXERCISE FOR CANCER PATIENTS

Exercise is one of the most effective strategies for symptoms associated with cancer fatigue, sleep disruption, and abnormalities of mood, physical function, and quality of life (45). A meta-analysis (46) suggests that for adults with a variety of cancer diagnoses and receiving a variety of exercise interventions, exercise improves physical function, QoL, cardiorespiratory fitness and decreases CRF. Contraindications for exercise include:

thrombocytopenia (<50 000 no resistive exercise; <20 000 only ADLs and light activity); *anemia:* Hb <8 g ADLs only, <10 g light exercise as tolerated; *bony metastatic disease*: 25% to 50% cortical involvement in long bone, partial weight-bearing, avoid lifting, 0% to 25% full weight-bearing, but no high impact sports.

■ PARTICIPATION RESTRICTIONS
Participation is the role an individual plays in a society. These roles can include family and social relationships, vocational and avocational pursuits, and often require modes of transportation to accomplish. Cancer patients are often restricted in many of these functions.

FAMILY AND SOCIAL RELATIONSHIPS
Cancer can often draw a family together; however, just as often it leads to significant distress for families. Support groups can be helpful, yet fewer than half of patients receive information about them, even in a large tertiary oncology center (47). There are also significant economic burdens on families (48).

VOCATIONAL REHABILITATION
Work disability following cancer diagnosis is a common occurrence. Short and colleagues (49) conducted phone interviews of 1433 cancer survivors at 1 to 5 years after diagnosis. More than half had quit work during their first year after cancer diagnosis, but fortunately 3 quarters of those returned to work subsequently. A projected 13% had indefinite work disability. Fortunately, US laws in recent years have provided more protection to the cancer survivor returning to work. These include the Americans with Disabilities Act, Family and Medical Leave Act, and the Health Information and Portability Act (50). Nevertheless, a great deal of barriers still stands in the way of gainful employment for cancer survivors with disability. These include ignorance of both employers and cancer survivors of their rights, discrimination, and limits on preexisting conditions in health insurance benefits (49).

PARTICIPATION IN RECREATION
Recreation is much more than fun and games; it is critical to physical and mental well-being. Fatigue, pain, weakness, depression, and other impairments will limit cancer survivors' participation in avocational pursuits. Health care providers and family members should encourage recreational activity for those with cancer. The benefits include improvements in fitness, musculoskeletal problems, immune system function, cognition, and sleep. One study looked at 97 European youngsters attending a summer camp for adolescents living with cancer and diabetes (51). Significant improvements were seen in self-esteem, self-efficacy, and anxiety. Adults benefit as well. For example, Tai Chi

Chuan, an Asian mind–body practice, has been shown to have beneficial effects on cancer survivors in 11 small studies (52).

TRANSPORTATION
Cancer patients may be limited in their ability to drive, fly, or take public transportation. They may not have caregivers available to help with transporting them. This can become a major barrier to cancer treatment, which often involves frequent medical visits. Some patients forgo recommended treatments because of lack of adequate transportation (53). Thus, it behooves physicians to explore with cancer patients any limits to their ability to get transportation.

Cancer Rehabilitation
Sample Order Set
Dorianne Rachelle Feldman

Diagnosis:	List specific **oncologic diagnosis**
Impairment:	**medically complex**
Condition:	Stable
Allergies:	List known drug or other allergies
Precautions:	Fall precautions
	No venipuncture, or VS measurement in involved limb, if PICC line present, or if lymphedema, mastectomy with axillary dissection
	Aspiration precautions, if appropriate
	Weight-bearing precautions, if appropriate
	Spine precautions, if appropriate
	Bleeding precautions
Isolation:	**Dependent on hospital infection policies**
	Neutropenic patients: (*No* rectal medications or temperature monitoring, or enemas)
	Contact precautions (depending on organism)
Vital Signs:	q8 hours or per routine for unit including pulse oximetry
	Set parameters to notify the house officer depending on diagnosis
Activity:	Out of bed with assistance until cleared by therapy
Diet:	Regular vs modified consistency with or without supervision.
	(Pureed/mechanical soft/soft/thin/liquidshoney thick, nectar, thin) Tube feedings, if applicable. Consult nutrition for enteral or parenteral feeding assistance.
IV Access:	Medi-Port access for blood draws and for chemotherapy if being given concurrently; while on rehabilitation unit; maintenance orders per hospital policy)
	PICC or central line maintenance orders (per hospital policy based on type of PICC or central line)

Hydration: Intravenous fluids, as needed with or without electrolyte repletion Include water flush order to ensure proper hydration for those receiving enteral nutrition.

Volume Status: Ins and outs as needed dependent on diagnosis.

Weight: Measure weight daily or weekly

Tracheostomy Care: **If applicable**
Suctioning per unit frequency (typically q4 or less)
Supplemental oxygen as needed

Bowel: Record stool output daily
Colace 100 mg BID
Senna 2 tabs QPM
Dulcolax suppository QHS as needed if bowel involvement
Do not give any agent rectally, if neutropenic
Ostomy nurse consult and ostomy care, if applicable

Bladder: Time void q4 hours while awake if genitourinary tract involvement
Bladder scan post void and record amount
Bladder scan q6 hours if no void
Straight catheter for volume greater than 350 mL
Nephrostomy tube care, if applicable

Skin: Check skin daily for skin breakdown, pressure areas
Inspect surgical incision site, if applicable daily
If dependent with bed mobility, reposition q2 hours.

DVT Prophylaxis: Lovenox 40 mg SQ Q Day or Heparin 5000 units q8 or q12 depending on VTE risk assessment

Pain Management: **Somatic examples:**
Tylenol 650 mg po q4 hours prn vs Tylenol po 1000 mg TID
And/or Ibuprofen 600 mg po TID with meals prn vs standing dose
And/or Ultram 50 mg to 100 mg po q6 hours prn
Narcotics can be ordered as needed in either po or IV formulation
Neuropathic examples:
Pregabalin: Start in most at 50 mg po BID
Neurontin: Start in very sensitive 100 mg QHS to 100 mg po TID and titrate gradually q3 days
Amitriptyline: Start at 25 mg po QHS or Q Day
Nortriptyline: Start at 10 to 25mg po QHS or Q Day
Duloxetine (Cymbalta®): Start at 30 mg po QHS or Q Day
Physical therapy: 1 to 2 h/d
ROM, strengthening, bed mobility, sitting balance, transfers, standing balance, ambulation, stair ambulation, community ambulation, balance, endurance
Initiation of specialized lymphedema treatment, if appropriate

Occupational
Therapy: 1 to 2 h/d
Upper extremity neuromuscular re-training if applicable, feeding, grooming, bathing, dressing, toileting, transfers, functional cognitive skills, visual–perceptual skills, household skills, adaptive equipment, positioning, wheelchair evaluation

Speech: 1 to 2 h/d
Cognitive linguistic and communication skills (after laryngectomy, speaking valve usage)
Dysphagia
Compensatory strategies, augmentative communication as needed

Psychology: Mood, adjustment, cognition.
Neuropsychological testing, as appropriate.

Vocational
Rehabilitation: May be appropriate as an outpatient once stable.

Social Work: Discharge planning and family organization and communication.

Medications:

- **Continue Baseline medications**

- **Agitation Medications examples**
  Trazodone (Desyrel®) 25 mg po q8 hours prn and 100 mg QHS
  And/or quetiapine (Seroquel®) 25 mg po q8 hours prn and 50 mg QHS
  And/or Valproic acid (Depakote®) 250 mg po BID
  And/or Lorazepam (Ativan®) 1 to 2mg IM/IV/PO q6 to q8 hours prn severe agitation
  And/or Haloperidol (Haldol®) 0.5 to 10 mg IM/IV/PO q1 to q4 prn agitation

- **Sleep Medications-examples**
  Trazodone (Desyrel®) Start at 25 to 50 mg po QHS
  Zolpidem (Ambien®) 5 to 10 mg po QHS
  Diphenhydramine (Benadryl®) Start at 25 mg po QHS

- **Depression Medications-examples**
  Serotonin selective re-uptake inhibitors (eg, Sertraline (Zoloft®) 100 mg po QHS, Escitalopram (Lexapro®) 10 to 20 mg po QHS)

- **Seizure Prophylaxis and/or Management**
  Valproic acid (Depakote®) 250 mg po BID (need to check level, need free level if hypoalbuminemic)
  Or Carbamazepine (Tegretol®) 200 mg po BID
  Or Levetiracetam (Keppra®) 500 mg po BID
  Or Phenytoin (Dilantin®) 100 mg po TID (maintenance not initiation dosing)
  (Check Phenytoin level; free and bound and titrate as needed)

- **Spasticity Medications**
  Dantrolene (Dantrium®) 25 mg to 100 mg po BID (monitor liver function)
  Baclofen (Lioresal®) Start at 5 mg po BID and titrate by 5 mg
      at each dosing interval q3 days (as tolerated)
  Diazepam (Valium®) 5 mg po daily to TID
  Tizanidine (Zanaflex®) Start 2 to 4 mg po daily and increase by
      2 to 4 mg increments q6 to 8 hours as needed.

Labs: Baseline CBC, CMP, Albumin or Pre-Albumin, Mg, Phos, and PT, Inr,
  APTT pending diagnosis
  Baseline EKG

Length of Stay: 7 to 21 days

Other Considerations:

Outpatient Specialized Lymphedema Treatment:
Patients should be seen preoperatively for prehabilitation
(education as to postoperative considerations, routine exercises to prevent
adhesive capsulitis) and **postoperatively** for treatment.

Manual Lymph Drainage (MLD)
Gentle manual massage technique that uses lymphatic pathways to
improve lymph flow and empty fluid-filled areas.

Compression Therapy
Multilayer low-stretch bandages are applied to the limb to prevent refill-
ing of the evacuated fluid providing compression with each layer. In later
phases of treatment, compression garments are worn during the day.

> **Decongestive Exercises**
> Specific lymphedema exercises while wearing compression bandages
> to improve the muscle pumping action.

> **Skin and Nail Care**
> Since infections can be a serious complication of lymphedema, patients
> are instructed in meticulous hygiene to eliminate bacterial and fungal
> growth to reduce the chance of infection.

> **Home Management**
> Training in bandaging and other home management basics is provided
> to ensure continued success after completion of the program. It
> is extremely important that patients understand the importance
> of compliance, as this is crucial to the overall efficacy of swelling
> management.

■ OUTPATIENT MEN'S AND WOMEN'S HEALTH REHABILITATION FOR PELVIC FLOOR MUSCLE DYSFUNCTION

Therapy evaluation includes biomechanical and/or musculoskeletal assessment, education for client and/or caregiver, strengthening particularly of core
muscles, myofascial and soft tissue techniques for pain relief abdominal, rectal, and vaginal, electrical stimulation and ultrasound, surface EMG for bio-
feedback to improve pelvic floor muscle functioning with and without the use
of vaginal dilators and/or rectal probes.

GOALS

1. Maintain medical stability and prevent medical complications, including thromboembolism, pneumonia, seizures, urinary tract infections, uncontrolled pain, contractures, and skin breakdown.

2. Optimize nutritional status.

3. Attain bowel and bladder continence or independence with management of ostomy or nephrostomy systems and self-catheterization and/or bowel program.

4. Achieve safe and independent function including mobility and activities of daily living (feeding, grooming, bathing dressing, toileting, transfers, locomotion (wheelchair or gait with appropriate assistive device), bed mobility, household skills, functional cognition, and visual–perceptual skills).

5. Establish effective cognitive and communication strategies.

6. Patient and caregiver education, training, and discharge planning.

■ REFERENCES

1. Directory of cancer terms [homepage on the Internet]. Behtesda, MD: National Cancer Institute; 2006. *www.cancer.gov/Templates/db_alpha. aspx?CdrlD=441257*. Accessed November 12, 2006.

2. National Cancer Policy board, Institute of Medicine. In: Hewitt M, Greenfield S, Stovall E. eds. *From Cancer Patient to Cancer survivor: Lost in Transition*. Committee on cancer survivorship: Improving care and quality of life; November 15, 2005; Washington, DC: National Academies Press; 2006.

3. World Health Organization. 54th World Health Assembly. In: *International Classification of Functioning, Disability and Health*; Geneva, Switzerland: United Nations World Health Organization; May 22, 2001:1–25.

4. Boult C, Altmann M, Gilbertson D, Yu C, Kane RL. Decreasing disability in the 21st century: the future effects of controling six fatal and non-fatal conditions. *Am J Public Health*. 1996;86(10):1388–1393.

5. Lethbridge-Cejku M, Schiller JS, Bernadel L. Summary health statistics for U.S. adults: National Health Interview Survey, 2002. *Vital Health Stat 10*. July 2004;(222):1–151.

6. Mayer RS, Silver K, Gerber NL. Rehabilitation of individuals with cancer. In: Abeloff MD, Armitage JO, Niederhuber JE, Kastan MB, McKenna WG, eds. *Abeloff's Clinical Oncology*. 4th ed. Philadephia, PA: Churchill Livingston/ Elsevier; 2008;579–590.

7. Cherney NI, Portenoy RK. The management of cancer pain. *CA Cancer J Clin*. 2000;44(5):262–303.

8. Ventrafridda V, Ripamonti C, De Conno F. Symptom prevalence and control during cancer patients' last days of life. *J Palliat Care*. 1990;6:7–11.

9. Chang HM. Pain and its management in patients with cancer. *Cancer Invest*. 2004;22(5):799–809.

10. von Roenn JH, Cleeland CS, Gonin R, Hatfiled AK, Pandya KJ. Physician attitudes and practice in cancer pain management: a survey from the eastern cooperative oncology group. *Ann Int Med.* 1993;119(2):121–126.

11. Zech DF, Grond S, Lynch J, Hertel D, Lehmann KA. Validation of World Health Organization guidelines for cancer pain relief: a 10 year prospective study. *Pain.* 1995;63:65–76.

12. Marinangeli F, Cicozzi A, Leonardis M, et al. Use of strong opioids in advanced cancer: a randomized trial. *J Pain Symptom Manage.* 2004;27(5):409–416.

13. Lucas LK, Lipman AG. Recent advances in pharmacotherapy for cancer pain management. *Cancer Pract.* 2002;10(suppl):S14–S20.

14. Weiger WA, Smith M, Boon H, Richardson MA, Kaptchuk TJ, Eisenberg DM. Advising patients who seek complimentary and alternative medical therapies for cancer. *Ann Int Med.* 2002;137:889–903.

15. Silver J, Mayer RS. Barriers to pain management in the rehabilitation of the surgical oncology patient. *J Surg Oncol.* 2007;95(5):427–435.

16. Turck DC, Monarch ES, Williams AD. Cancer patients in pain: considerations for assessing the whole person. *Hematol Oncol Clin N Am.* 2002;16:511–525.

17. Burton AW, Rajagopal A, Shah HN, et al. Epidural and intrathecal analgesia is effective in treating refractory cancer pain. *Pain Med.* 2004;5(3):239–247.

18. Smith TJ, Staats PS, Deer T, Stearns LJ, et al. Randomized clinical trial of an implantable drug delivery system compared with comprehensive medical management for refractory cancer pain: impact on pain, drug-related toxicity, and survival. *J Clin Onc.* 2002;20(19):4040–4049.

19. Vallieres I, Aubin M, Blondeau L, Simard S, Giguere A. Effectiveness of a clinical intervention in improving pain control in outpatients with cancer treated by radiation therapy. *Int J Rad Onc.* 2006;66(1):234–237.

20. Meyerson BA. Neurosurgical approaches to pain treatment. *Acta Anesthesiol Scand.* 2001;45:1108–1113.

21. Cella D, Peterman A, Passik S, Jacobsen P, Breitbart W. Progress toward guidelines for the management of fatigue. *Oncology (Williston Park).* 1998;12(11A):369–377.

22. Gagnon B, Allard P, Masse B, DeSerres M. Delirium in terminal cancer: a prospective study using daily screening, early diagnosis, and continuous monitoring. *J Pain Symptom Manage.* 2000;19(6):412–426.

23. Curt GA, Breitbart W, Cella D, et al. Impact of cancer-related fatigue on the lives of patients: new findings from the fatigue coalition. *Oncologist.* 2000;5(5):353–360.

24. Vogelzang NJ, Breitbart W, Cella D, et al. Patient, caregiver, and oncologist perceptions of cancer-related fatigue: results of a tripart assessment survey. The fatigue coalition. *Semin Hematol.* 1997;34(3)(suppl 2):4–12.

25. Mock V, Frangakis C, Davidson NE, et al. Exercise manages fatigue during breast cancer treatment: a randomized controlled trial. *Psychooncology.* 2005;14(6):464–477.

26. Centeno C, Sanz A, Bruera E. Delirium in advanced cancer patients. *Palliat Med.* 2004;18(3):184–194.

27. Dunlop RJ, Campbell CW. Cytokines and advanced cancer. *J Pain Symptom Manage.* 2000;20(3):214–232.

28. McDaniel JS, Musselman DI, Porter MR, Reed DA, Nemeroff CB. Depression in patients with cancer. Diagnosis, biology, and treatment. *Arch Gen Psychiatry*. 1995;52:89–99.

29. Koenig HG, Shelp F, Goli V, Cohen HJ, Blazer DG. Survival and health-care utilization in elderly medical inpatients with major depression. *J Am Geriatr Soc*. 1989;37:599–606.

30. Kirshblum S, O'Dell MW, Ho C, Barr K. Rehabilitation of persons with central nervous system tumors. *Cancer*. 2001;92(4)(suppl):1029–1038.

31. O'Dell MW, Barr K, Spanier D, Warnick RE. Functional outcome of inpatient rehabilitation in persons with brain tumors. *Arch Phys Med Rehabil*. 1998;79(12):1530–1534.

32. Vargo MM, Gerber LH. Rehabilitation for patients with cancer diagnoses. In: DeLisa J, Gans B, eds. *Physical Medicine and Rehabilitation: Principles and Practices*. 4th ed. Lippincott Williams & Wilkins; 2005;1771–1794, Hagerstown, MD.

33. Gilbert RW, Kim JH, Posner JB. Epidural spinal cord compression from metastatic tumor: diagnosis and treatment. *Ann Neurol*. 1978;3(1):40–51.

34. Eriks IE, Angenot EL, Lankhorst GJ. Epidural metastatic spinal cord compression: functional outcome and survival after inpatient rehabilitation. *Spinal Cord*. 2004;42(4):235–239.

35. McKinley WO, Huang ME, Tewksbury MA. Neoplastic vs. traumatic spinal cord injury: an inpatient rehabilitation comparison. *Am J Phys Med Rehabil*. 2000;79(2):138–144.

36. Lane JM, Christ GH, Khan SN, Backus SI. Rehabilitation for limb salvage patients: kinesiological parameters and psychological assessment. *Cancer*. 2001;92(4)(suppl): 1013–1019.

37. Bunting RW, Shea B. Bone metastasis and rehabilitation. *Cancer*. 2001;92(4)(suppl):1020–1028.

38. Kwan W, Jackson J, Weir LM, Dingee C, McGregor G,Olivotto IA. Chronic arm morbidity after curative breast cancer treatment: prevalence and impact on quality of life. *J Clinical Oncology*. 2002;20:4242–4248.

39. Ramos SM, O'Donnell LS, Knight G. Edema volume, not timing, is the key to success in lymphedema treatment. *Am J Surg*. 1999;178(4):311–315.

40. Okunieff P, Augustine E, Hicks JE, et al. Pentoxifylline in the treatment of radiation-induced fibrosis. *J Clin Oncol*. 2004;22(11):2207–2213.

41. Gillis TA, Donovan ES. Rehabilitation following bone marrow transplantation. *Cancer*. 2001;92(4)(suppl):998–1007.

42. Siegel K, Raveis VH, Houts P, Mor V. Caregiver burden and unmet patient needs. *Cancer*. 1991;68(5):1131–1140.

43. Dumont S, Turgeon J, Allard P, Gagnon P, Charbonneau C, Vezina L. Caring for a loved one with advanced cancer: determinants of psychological distress in family caregivers. *J Palliat Med*. 2006;9(4):912–921.

44. Lee WT, Chan HF, Wong E. Improvement of feeding independence in end-stage cancer patients under palliative care—a prospective, uncontrolled study. *Support Care Cancer*. 2005;13(12):1051–1056.

45. Burnham TR, Wilcox A. Effects of exercise on physiological and psychological variables in cancer survivors. *Med Sci Sports Exerc*. 2002;34(12):1863–1867.

46. Holtzman J, Schmitz K, Babes G, Kane RL, Duval S, Wilt TJ, et al. Effectiveness of behavioral interventions to modify physical activity behaviors in general populations and cancer patients and survivors. *Evid Rep Technol Assess* (Summ). June 2004;(102):1–8.

47. Guidry JJ, Aday LA, Zhang D, Winn RJ. The role of informal and formal social support networks for patients with cancer. *Cancer Pract*. 1997;5(4):241–246.

48. Yun YH, Rhee YS, Kang IO, et al. Economic burdens and quality of life of family caregivers of cancer patients. *Oncology*. 2005;68(2-3):107–114.

49. Short PF, Vargo MM. Responding to employment concerns of cancer survivors. *J Clin Oncol*. 2006;24(32):5138–5141.

50. Hoffman B. Cancer survivors' employment and insurance rights: A primer for oncologists. *Oncology (Williston Park)*. 1999;13(6): 841,6;discussion: 846, 849, 852.

51. Torok S, Kokonyei G, Karolyi L, Ittzes A, Tomcsanyi T. Outcome effectiveness of therapeutic recreation camping program for adolescents living with cancer and diabetes. *J Adolesc Health*. 2006;39(3):445–447.

52. Mansky P, Sannes T, Wallerstedt D, et al. Tai chi chuan: Mind-body practice or exercise intervention? Studying the benefit for cancer survivors. *Integr Cancer Ther*. 2006;5(3):192–201.

53. Guidry JJ, Aday LA, Zhang D, Winn RJ. Transportation as a barrier to cancer treatment. *Cancer Pract*. 1997;5(6):361–366.

16

Cardiac Rehabilitation

Erik Stanton Brand and Kerry J. Stewart

■ INTRODUCTION

Cardiac disease is the leading cause of mortality in men and women worldwide and accounts for 40% of deaths in the industrialized world (1). Cardiac rehabilitation reduces mortality by 28% (2) and improves quality of life including functional capacity, psychosocial function, exercise, and symptom tolerance (3). Multifactorial cardiac rehabilitation services are recommended in patients after a significant cardiac event. Unfortunately, only 25% to 30% and 10% to 20% of eligible men and women, respectively, participate in such programs (4).

■ ELIGIBILITY

The Centers for Medicare and Medicaid Services (CMS) provide insurance coverage for cardiac rehabilitation of patients with 6 diagnoses:

1. myocardial infarction (MI) within the preceding 12 months

2. stable angina pectoris

3. coronary artery bypass surgery

4. heart valve repair/replacement

5. percutaneous transluminal coronary angioplasty or stenting

6. heart (or heart–lung) transplant (5)

Appropriate indications for cardiac rehabilitation programs also include stable heart failure (6), but this diagnosis is not currently reimbursed by CMS. CMS guidelines allow 18 weeks in which to complete a maximum of 36 cardiac rehabilitation sessions. Additional sessions may be approved at the discretion of the local coverage determination contractor but may not exceed 72 sessions within 36 weeks (5). Although CMS is a dominant payer for cardiac rehabilitation and many other payers base their reimbursement on CMS rulings, the coverage parameters may vary by provider.

■ PROGRESSIVE EXERCISE TRAINING PRINCIPLES AND BENEFITS

Physiologic adaptation to exercise is known as the conditioning effect. Adaptation is triggered when the demands of an activity exceed that to which the body was previously conditioned, creating a state of overload. Overload triggers changes in the structure and function of specific bodily systems that were stressed, causing them to adapt to better perform that activity. This process occurs with a change in exercise parameters such as an increase in resistance, repetitions, or sets or a decrease in rest between exercises.

TYPES OF EXERCISE

Progressive exercise training in cardiac rehabilitation should include a combination of aerobic and resistance exercises to improve endurance and strength.

AEROBIC (ENDURANCE) TRAINING

This type of exercise forms the foundation of progressive exercise in cardiac rehabilitation because of its benefits on cardiovascular function and risk factors. It involves sustained activity of low to moderate intensity that increases the muscles' demand for oxygen. This results in a need for greater cardiac output. The primary conditioning effect of aerobic (endurance) training is an increase in muscle capacity to extract oxygen from blood. Thus, there is less need for cardiac output at any given workload. In addition, because of a decrease in the heart rate (HR) and a modest increase in stroke volume, the same amount of blood can be pumped more efficiently. Aerobic (endurance) training also decreases blood pressure (BP) at rest and during exercise. Functional benefits include being able to perform increasingly intense activities of daily living (ADLs) at the same cardiac workload.

RESISTANCE TRAINING

This is an important supplement to aerobic (endurance) training in cardiac rehabilitation. It utilizes an opposing force to induce overload and trigger the conditioning effect. The conditioning effects of supervised prescribed resistance training (RT) include improved BP, endurance, and strength (7,8). Functional benefits include increased independence, functional capacity, disability, quality of life, and adherence, as it adds variety to the exercise prescription (9). Common examples include conventional (strength) and circuit (endurance) RT.

CONVENTIONAL (STRENGTH) RT

This utilizes higher resistance (i.e., heavy weights), fewer repetitions, and longer rest periods to create a predominantly anaerobic overload to trigger adaptations that primarily increase muscular strength. Other conditioning effects include increases in lean body mass, basal metabolic rate, and quicker creation of adenosine triphosphate (ATP). This becomes increasingly important as exercise intensity increases, overwhelming the aerobic system's ability to create ATP fast enough to meet the demands of a task (10). Conventional (strength) RT may also improve the efficiency of muscle contraction by increasing the number, size, and synchronicity of motor unit recruitment. Functional benefits include being able to perform increasingly heavy ADLs at the same cardiac workload, as they require a smaller proportion of the total available motor units. Angina may still be triggered at the same level of cardiac work; however, this threshold may not be reached until a higher level of activity by the peripheral muscles. Important additional considerations include the fact that strength is inversely associated with all-cause mortality (11) and metabolic syndrome (12,13). Common examples of conventional (strength) RT include moderate-intensity weight lifting.

CIRCUIT (ENDURANCE) RT

This utilizes lower resistance (ie, lighter weights), more repetitions, and shorter rest periods to create a predominantly aerobic overload to trigger adaptations that primarily increase muscular endurance as well as aerobic capacity. Other conditioning effects include modification of cardiovascular disease (CVD) risk factors, similar to aerobic (endurance) training and more effectively than conventional (strength) RT. Functional benefits include features of both aerobic (endurance) training and conventional (strength) RT.

EXERCISE PRESCRIPTION

Specific instructions from a health care provider may be more effective than a general instruction to "get more exercise." A physician's endorsement of the effectiveness of cardiac rehabilitation is the main predictor of referral (4). Patient participation is more likely when they are referred, educated, and married, have high self-efficacy and easily accessible programs (4). Physiologic testing and monitoring should be used to determine appropriate exercise intensity levels. A balanced exercise prescription should include a combination of aerobic, resistance, and flexibility training.

PHYSIOLOGIC TESTING AND MONITORING

An exercise stress test (EST) can be used to determine safe levels of metabolic activity. Exercise intensity levels can also be subjectively gauged by the patient using the Rate of Perceived Exertion (RPE: see Table 16.1).

METABOLIC EQUIVALENTS OF TASK

The amount of energy required to perform an activity is measured in metabolic equivalents of task (METs). One MET is the energy requirement at rest. Increasingly strenuous activities require larger amounts of energy and higher MET levels, which correspond with increasing workload for the heart (Table 16.2). Guidelines for exercise and progressive return to activity are often quantified in terms of METs.

TABLE 16.1 ■ Borg Rate of Perceived Exertion Scale.

6	
7	Very very light
8	
9	Very light
10	
11	Fairly light
12	
13	Somewhat hard
14	
15	Hard
16	
17	Very hard
18	
19	Very, very hard
20	

Adapted from Ref. (18), with permission.

TABLE 16.2 ■ Energy requirements for daily activities.

Metabolic Equivalents of Task	Conditioning	Occupation	Recreation	Self-care/ Home Activity
<3	Walk <2 mph/ level ground	Vacuum/ light effort	Vacation with walk and ride	Feed animal, sit as sport spectator
3–5	Water aerobics	Take out trash/ moderate effort	Golf and carry clubs	Mow lawn, carry small child
5–7	Walk 3–4 mph/ run, play with animals	Brush, groom, shear farm animals	Tennis doubles	Carry object 30–60 lbs
7–9	Walk 5 mph	Dig ditch	Bicycling, general	Carry object 60–90 lbs
>9	Step aerobics (10–12"), run 7 mph	Heavy labor	Track and field hurdles	Carry object >90 lbs

Abbreviation: mph, miles per hour.
Modified with permission from Refs. (14,15).

EXERCISE STRESS TEST

Prognosis, risk stratification, and activity prescription are preferably guided by an EST (16). An initial EST should be conducted 6 to 8 weeks after hospital discharge. Patients who can perform *at least* 5 METs without ST depression or exercise-induced angina do not usually require further diagnostic testing (17). Treadmill testing is most common, though testing can also be done using a bicycle ergometer. The upper extremity ergometer can provide a viable alternative to treadmill testing for those unable to use the lower extremities, but HR will rise earlier at a lower workload.

RATE OF PERCEIVED EXERTION

The Borg RPE scale is a commonly used guide to exercise prescription, based on the subjective measure how hard the patient feels they are working. It is safe, effective, correlates well with MET levels, and is a practical means of prescribing and monitoring exercise intensity. The RPE scale is particularly useful for patients taking medications such as beta-blockers that attenuate the normal HR response to exercise. Most patients on cardiac rehabilitation should exercise "somewhat hard" to "hard" (level 13 or 14) on the RPE scale (Table 16.1).

AEROBIC (ENDURANCE) PRESCRIPTION

Generally, patients beginning cardiac rehabilitation 7 to 10 days after discharge from hospital exercise at 70% to 85% of the HR level they achieved without signs or symptoms of myocardial ischemia during an EST (performed before cardiac rehabilitation). A typical aerobic workout plan is 45 to 60 minutes on 3 (preferably nonconsecutive) days per week. A 5- to 10-minute warm-up including stretching and range of motion (ROM) calisthenics helps prevent injuries and allows for gradual acceleration of the cardiovascular system. Next, a stimulus phase of 20 to 30 minutes at 70% (for beginners) or 85% (experienced patients) stresses the body to stimulate physiologic adaptation (conditioning effect). Lastly, a 5- to 10-minute cool-down (again including stretching and ROM calisthenics) limits the risk of postexercise hypotension caused by pooling of blood in muscles (Figures 16.1 and 16.2).

To determine a patient's target pulse rate range, identify the highest rate safely achieved during the most recent exercise test on the top line (maximum pulse line) and then locate the corresponding 10-second counts on the 85% and 70% lines directly below. These 2 values represent the limits of target rate range for exercise conditioning (19).

CONVENTIONAL (STRENGTH) RT PRESCRIPTION

Conventional guidelines recommend a weight limit of 1 to 5 pounds for RT in the first 3 to 12 weeks after cardiac event or intervention (9). Subsequent initial RT prescription in cardiac patients should consist of 1 set of 12 to 15 repetitions using 8 to 10 exercises to cover the major muscle groups 2 to 3 d/wk, using weights at 30% to 40% of the 1-repetition

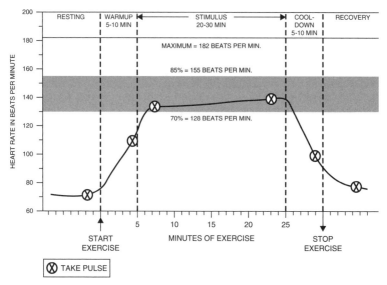

Adapted from Ref. (14), with permission.

FIGURE 16.1 ■ Pattern for an aerobic workout.

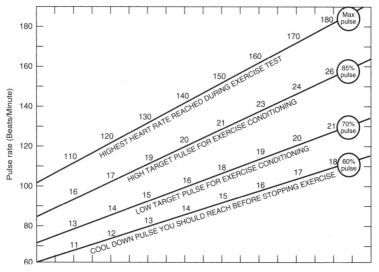

Adapted from Ref. (19), with permission.

FIGURE 16.2 ■ Target pulse rates for 10-second counts that should be measured the first 10 seconds after exercise.

maximum (1-RM) for upper body and 50% to 60% of the 1-RM for the lower body (9). To estimate the 1-RM, use Table 16.3. Single set programs in the initial training period allow nearly the same relative increases in strength as multiple set programs (20) and encourage adherence (9). The initial RT prescription should use moderate weights, emphasize good technique, and allow recovery time to allow the full repetition range without straining, breath-holding, or Valsalva. This should facilitate musculoskeletal adaptation and minimize injury and muscle soreness (Table 16.4). Performing RT after the aerobic exercise will allow adequate warm-up. By 3 weeks after MI, many patients can safely perform moderate-intensity RT (21). After the patient can comfortably perform 12 to 15 repetitions, the weight may then be increased approximately 5% (9). Similar to aerobic exercise, the RPE, HR, and BP should be monitored during RT (9) because

TABLE 16.3 ■ Load-repetition relationship for resistance training.

% 1-RM	Repetitions Possible
60	17
70	12
80	8
90	5
100	1

Adapted from Ref. (25), with permission.

TABLE 16.4 ■ Recommendations for the initial prescription of resistance training.

Resistance training should be performed:

1. in a rhythmical manner at a moderate to slow controlled speed
2. through a full range of motion, avoiding breath-holding and straining (Valsalva maneuver) by exhaling during the contraction or exertion phase of the lift and inhaling during the relaxation phase
3. alternating between upper and lower body work to allow for adequate rest between exercises
4. at an initial resistance or weight load that allows for and limits to 12–15 repetitions at a low level of resistance (eg, <40% of 1-RM) for cardiac patients
5. in a single set performed 2 d/wk
6. by the major muscle groups of the upper and lower extremities, eg, chest press, shoulder press, triceps extension, biceps curl, pull-down (upper back), lower-back extension, abdominal crunch/curl-up, quadriceps extension or leg press, leg curls (hamstrings), and calf raise

Modified from Ref. (9), with permission.

the BP measured between sets may underestimate the pressor response during the actual lift (22). The RPE should be 11 to 14, i.e., "fairly light" to "somewhat hard" (23).

CIRCUIT (*ENDURANCE*) RT PRESCRIPTION

Typical programs use a variety of lightweight machines continuously to create an aerobic workout. They alternate between 30 seconds of weight lifting at 40% to 50% of 1-RM and 30 seconds of rest in between sets (14). Weight machines may reduce the chances of injury by aiding in balance and acting as a spotter. Alternative exercises can use calisthenics, an elastic cord, pulley, dumb bell, or dowel (9). During these exercises, the grip on the equipment should be secure but not overly tight so as to avoid excessive BP elevation (24).

FLEXIBILITY TRAINING PRESCRIPTION

Stretching of major muscle and tendon groups should be conducted 2 to 3 times per week (9).

■ PHASES OF CARDIAC REHABILITATION
PHASE I

This period consists of the acute inpatient hospitalization. It is subdivided into acute and subacute subsections. During the subacute period, particularly complicated patients may warrant admission to a comprehensive integrated inpatient rehabilitation program (CIIRP).

ACUTE PERIOD

During the first 3 days in the critical care unit, the workload may generally include exercise at 1 to 2 METs. This can include passive ROM, protective chair posture, bedside commode on day 1 (instead of a bedpan, which requires a higher MET level) and walking at ≤1 mile per hour (mph). It is necessary to avoid Valsalva, isometric exercises, and raising legs above the heart during this period as these activities may unduly stress the heart. Progressive activities may include initiation of ambulation and ADLs on days 2 to 4 (1).

SUBACUTE PERIOD

After discharge from the critical care unit, the workload may generally be advanced to 3 to 4 METS. This can include walking at 2 mph, light resistance exercise, and propelling a wheelchair (26).

COMPREHENSIVE INTEGRATED INPATIENT REHABILITATION PROGRAM

During the subacute period of cardiac rehabilitation, patients with a complex cardiac event or significant comorbidities such as neuropathy, amputation, considerable arthritis, or a prior stroke may require admission to a CIIRP (1). CIIRP, formerly known as Acute Comprehensive

Inpatient Rehabilitation, consists of an in-hospital rehabilitation unit in which patients reside 24 hours daily for an average of 13 days to benefit from coordinated, integrated interdisciplinary medical and rehabilitation services. To qualify for CIIRP under CMS guidelines, patients must have one of the eligible cardiac diagnoses listed above, in addition to the demonstrated need for and ability to safely benefit from a skilled multidisciplinary environment, which incorporates daily medical management by a physician, skilled rehabilitation nursing, and >3 hours of therapy daily (consisting of physical therapy, occupational therapy, speech language pathology or prosthetics and orthotics). Other services such as those that address nutrition and psychology are often beneficial, but do not count toward the 3-hour requirement. For non-CMS payers, the required admission diagnoses, therapy needs, and reimbursement requirements may vary.

HOSPITAL DISCHARGE PLANNING
Before hospital discharge, patient education and family conferences should include information about cardiac symptoms such as angina, medications including sublingual nitroglycerin, coronary disease, modification of risk factors such as smoking and diet, and resumption of activities including work and sex. Written information such as *After a Heart Attack* (a free resource available from the American Heart Association [AHA]) should be provided.

FOLLOW-UP
Appointments should be scheduled with cardiology, primary care, or cardiac rehabilitation providers. These should include an opportunity to assess understanding of educational material after discharge. Where available, patient support groups lead by a cardiac rehabilitation professional in the first or second month (for instance, *http://www.mendedhearts.org/*) may be quite informative and supportive for the patient. Supervised physical conditioning or patient-run heart clubs are often available in local communities. For a directory of comprehensive outpatient cardiac rehabilitation (secondary prevention) programs and education materials, see *http://www.aacvpr.org* or the AHA at *http://www.americanheart.org* (14).

PHASE II
This period consists of supervised electrocardiogram (EKG)-monitored outpatient therapy, usually lasting 2 to 3 sessions weekly for up to 12 weeks. It should ideally include participation in a comprehensive outpatient cardiac rehabilitation (secondary prevention) program and return to community ADLs. To improve accessibility, low-risk patients (ie, minimal risk of activity-induced angina or arrhythmia) may participate in home-based programs during phase II with equal safety and efficacy (27).

COMPREHENSIVE OUTPATIENT CARDIAC REHABILITATION
(SECONDARY PREVENTION) PROGRAM

These programs take place during phase II cardiac rehabilitation and should include a medical evaluation, prescribed exercise, a program to modify cardiac risk factors (i.e., smoking, hyperlipidemia, hypertension, nutrition, obesity, and diabetes) and education and counseling on vocation, physical activity psychosocial factors, and proper use of prescribed medications. For most patients, important components of care after a myocardial event are easily remembered with the mnemonic ABCDE:

A. aspirin

B. beta-blocker

C. cholesterol-lowering medication (statin)

D. diet (for weight control, glycemic control, and improving the lipid profile)

E. exercise training

Comprehensive outpatient cardiac rehabilitation (secondary prevention) program facilities, under the supervision of a physician medical director, should be staffed by appropriately trained health care professionals (typically exercise physiologists, nurses, and physical therapists) and have continuous EKG, appropriate exercise, and resuscitative equipment. These providers should be trained in cardiopulmonary resuscitation and have readily accessible emergency care. Cardiac rehabilitation programs generally accept patients 1 to 2 weeks after hospital discharge (5,6).

RETURN TO COMMUNITY ADLS

Consider the activities listed in Table 16.2 and similar references in combination with the results of an EST, clinical signs, and symptomatology to gauge readiness to engage in progressive activities. Angina, arrhythmia, or congestive heart failure warrants a cardiology consult and reconsideration of readiness to advance activity levels.

SEX

Gradual return to sex can be recommended. If asymptomatic during ADLs, a patient may resume intercourse 4 to 6 weeks after MI. Foreplay and climax require 3 and 5 METS, respectively (28), approximately the same energy requirements as walking around the block briskly or climbing a flight of stairs (14). Positions with sustained weight on the arms should be avoided as this may increase BP. It is advised that the patient wait 2 to 3 hours after a large meal before engaging in sexual activity. Sublingual nitroglycerin can be considered in otherwise stable patients with sex-induced angina. Caution should be exercised, however, in those taking sildenafil, tadalafil, and vardenafil (approved for erectile dysfunction) and especially in hypotension or aortic stenosis. Resources such as the AHA brochure *Sex and Heart Disease* are available (*http:// www.americanheart.org/presenter.jhtml?identifier=9239*) (14).

WORK
Most MI patients can return to work as most jobs require <6 METs. Initially, consider a trial of progressive part-time work.

PHASE III
This period consists of supervised but non-EKG-monitored outpatient maintenance therapy. Seven to 8 METs of functional capacity and clinical stability are generally accepted criteria for transition to phase III. Repeat EST at the end of a few months of exercise training can help determine new target exercise levels.

■ **SAFETY CONSIDERATIONS**
Mild-to-moderate-intensity RT is considered safe as it generally causes a lower rate pressure product (RPP = HR × systolic BP [SBP]) than maximal treadmill aerobic exercise (29) and does not exceed hemodynamic levels attained by patients with heart failure during standard exercise testing (30). Most cardiac patients can perform combined aerobic and resistance (circuit) weight training (6,31,32) without orthopedic or cardiac complications (33). Cardiovascular risks are likely related to age, underlying CVD, fitness level, and intensity of RT. Low-risk cardiac patients without evidence of myocardial ischemia with exercise or at rest, complex ventricular dysrhythmias, or severe left ventricular dysfunction have reported no major adverse cardiovascular events (9). Supervised cardiac rehabilitation RT is considered safe in clinically stable women (34) and men (35) with CHD as it has been demonstrated to not induce angina, ischemic ST depression, complex ventricular arrhythmias, unusual hemodynamics, or cardiovascular complications in this population.

CONTRAINDICATIONS
CONTRAINDICATIONS TO CARDIAC REHABILITATION
The following conditions disqualify the patient from participation in cardiac rehabilitation. Generally, participation may proceed when the condition has resolved:

1. resting SBP >160 or diastolic BP >110 mmHg

2. poorly controlled angina

3. atrial fibrillation with rapid ventricular response

4. heart block (second or third degree)

5. complex arrhythmias

6. significant congenital or valvular heart disease

7. recent acute mental or physical illness

8. severe dyspnea at low workloads

9. significant pulmonary, neurologic, or orthopedic limitations

10. acute endocarditis or pericarditis

11. severe aortic stenosis

12. unstable congestive heart failure or severe left ventricular dysfunction

13. serious noncardiac comorbidity

CONTRAINDICATIONS TO RT
A list of absolute and relative contraindications to RT are listed in Table 16.5.

PRECAUTIONS
Cardiac rehabilitation is considered very safe and beneficial in most patients given the above exercise prescription parameters, proper patient

TABLE 16.5 ■ Absolute and relative contraindications to resistance training.

ABSOLUTE
Unstable CHD
Decompensated heart failure
Uncontrolled arrhythmias
Severe pulmonary hypertension (mean pulmonary arterial pressure >55 mm Hg)
Severe and symptomatic aortic stenosis
Acute myocarditis, endocarditis, or pericarditis
Uncontrolled hypertension (>180/110 mm Hg)
Aortic dissection
Marfan syndrome
Uncontrolled diabetes
High-intensity RT (80%–100% of 1-RM) in patients with active proliferative retinopathy or moderate or worse nonproliferative diabetic retinopathy

RELATIVE (SHOULD CONSULT A CARDIOLOGIST BEFORE PARTICIPATION)
Major risk factors for CHD
Uncontrolled hypertension (>160/100 mm Hg)
Low functional capacity (4 METs)
Musculoskeletal limitations
Individuals who have implanted pacemakers or defibrillators

selection, monitoring, precautions, and supervision (14). However, the provider must remain vigilant in considering the following factors.

CARDIOVASCULAR SEQUELAE

The provider should monitor for common medical complications following a cardiovascular event including angina, arrhythmias, symptomatic congestive heart failure, Dressler syndrome (pericarditis), and arterial embolization.

ENVIRONMENT

Conservative activity guidelines recommend avoidance of activities, which impose additional strain on the heart, especially during the first 3 months after MI. Thus, the patient should avoid working or exercising during very humid, hot, cold, or windy weather, taking very cold or hot baths or showers, exercising or walking on an inclined surface or hill, or engaging in any activity that creates worry or emotional stress (14).

MEDICATION EFFECTS

Cardiovascular medications should be considered during EST interpretation and exercise prescription formulation. For instance, beta-blockers decrease peak HR, making RPE, symptoms, and EKG more useful parameters for EST and exercise prescription. Common antihypertensive medication effects on peak HR are as follows:

1. Decrease: beta-blockers, clonidine, methyldopa, verapamil

2. No discernible effect: angiotensin-converting enzyme (ACE) inhibitors, angiotensin II receptor blockers, digitalis (in patients with CHF)

3. Increase: calcium channel blockers, hydralazine, minoxidil, nifedipine, nitrates, prazosin (36)

MONITORING

EKG monitoring is recommended in patients at high risk for ischemia (left ventricular ejection fraction [LVEF] <35%, New York Heart Association Grade III or IV congestive heart failure, systolic BP decrease of >10 mm Hg during exercise, postoperative angina, ischemia during EST, or poor cognition leading to inability to reliably self-monitor and report symptoms of ischemia) or arrhythmia (LVEF <30%, history of atrial fibrillation/rapid ventricular rate, ventricular tachycardia, ventricular fibrillation, pacemaker, automatic implantable cardioverter defibrillator or ST elevation MI within 6 weeks). Excessive elevations of BP are generally not a concern with the recommended low- to moderate-intensity RT without Valsalva (37). BP during RT in cardiac patients was reported in a clinically acceptable range when lifting 40% to 60% of the 1-RM (38).

PSYCHOLOGICAL COMPLICATIONS

Patients should be monitored for common psychological sequelae of cardiac disease including anxiety, depression, inappropriate fear of physical activity, denial of illness persisting beyond the first few days in hospital, and persistent or major depression. Depression and anhedonia occur in more than 25% of patients after MI (1). This correlates with mortality and recurrent coronary events (39). Selective serotonin reuptake inhibitors can be used safely in ischemic heart disease (40–43) and are preferred over tricyclic antidepressants (44).

SCREENING

Low-risk patients warrant a graded approach to cardiac rehabilitation, but probably do not require an extensive cardiovascular screening before participation in RT (9). Moderate- to high-risk patients can safely participate in RT with appropriate preparation, surveillance, and guidance (9). Medical screening is not required for RT initiated at a low level (9). Patients with stable CVD are recommended for low- to moderate-intensity RT without further medical diagnostic testing if they have a functional capacity ≥4 METs (9). This can be estimated by a questionnaire such as the Duke Activity Status Inventory (see Appendix).

TECHNIQUE

Avoid extended breath-holding while exercising, straining or lifting, working in a bent or stooped position or with arms held above head, doing work that requires continuous muscle tensing.

TIMING WITH MEALS AND ALCOHOL

Avoid exercising or working during the first hour after a meal, after consuming alcohol, or consuming excessive amounts of alcohol (14).

WHEN TO STOP EXERCISE

If a patient's health status changes or they experience chest discomfort or undue shortness of breath during RT, they should stop RT and undergo further medical consultation (9). Exercise should be ceased immediately if any adverse signs or symptoms arise such as chest pain, excessive shortness of breath, dizziness, or arrhythmias (22,23).

UNIQUE PATIENT POPULATIONS

ARRHYTHMIAS

Most patients with a history of ventricular tachycardia will experience ventricular tachycardia or ectopy during cardiac rehabilitation. Intense exercise and exercising in a supine position should be avoided as they increase the likelihood of arrhythmias (1).

CONGESTIVE HEART FAILURE

Isometric exercise should be avoided because of risk of arrhythmia. Exercise is beneficial because it can improve cardiac output and reduce plasma renin activity and sympathetic tone.

CORONARY ARTERY BYPASS GRAFT

Cognitive deficits exist in 22.5% of patients 2 months after coronary artery bypass graft (CABG) (45). These may dissipate by 1 to 3 years postoperatively when compared with nonsurgical controls with CAD (46).

ELDERLY

Frailty may warrant a low-intensity exercise regimen. Elderly individuals who exercise can decrease by 25% the usual age-associated decrements in cardiac output, LVEF, and maximum HR and increase in end diastolic volume (1).

HEART TRANSPLANT

ATHEROSCLEROSIS

Patients are at risk for accelerated atherosclerosis and cardiac disability. For instance, coronary artery disease can develop 5 to 10 years after transplant (1).

DENERVATION

Without vagus nerve input, HR changes are based on circulating catecholamines, which are much slower than vagus nerve control. Therefore, HR increases with exercise and decrease to baseline after exercise will be delayed. The heart has increased resting HR (100 beats per minute [BPM] is normal) and decreased maximum effort (peak HR is 20% to 25% lower than age-matched controls, and many parameters are lower including work capacity, cardiac output, VO_2, and systolic BP). Ischemia and arrhythmia must be identified by EKG because sensations including angina are no longer reliable. (Fortunately, these occur less frequently than in other cardiac patients.) Therefore, exercise intensity should be based on RPE 11 to 14 or a percentage of VO_2 or maximum workload (not HR or angina since denervated) (26).

MEDICATION SIDE EFFECTS

Posttransplant medication regimens may complicate medical management. For instance, immunosuppression may predispose to infection. Stroke risk is increased because of mycotic or embolic sources or sirolimus-induced vasculitis. Peripheral neuropathy or myopathy can arise from nerve impingement, critical illness, or posttransplantation medications including steroids and statins. Transplant medications may also cause tremor. Steroids can predispose to osteoporosis, especially given limited weight-bearing activity.

PROGNOSIS

Most patients increase exercise tolerance, work output, and return to community safely.

LIMITED RESOURCES

If a cardiac rehabilitation program is not available, it is appropriate to follow guidelines such as those listed in Table 16.6 in combination

TABLE 16.6 ■ Activity schedule and symptom recognition for patients recovering from a cardiac event.

I. Conservative activity schedule
Pace of these activities may be titrated according to early post-MI stress test when available.

Month	Metabolic Equivalents of Task
1	1–3
2	3–5

II. Recognizing heart symptoms
Recommend contacting a health care provider before resumption of exercise if the heart gives any warning signs or symptoms:

Pulse
1. increase ≥20 BPM after exercise

2. ≥120 per minute

3. irregular, fluttering, or jumping in chest or throat, very slow, or with sudden rapid bursts

4. early stress test or medications may modify values

Chest Pain
1. may include pressure in the chest, arm, or throat precipitated or following exercise (take any prescribed nitroglycerin and rest if there is chest pain)

2. atypical pain in abdomen or back, nausea, fatigue, or dizziness more common in women

Dizziness
1. may include light-headedness, or feeling faint during exercise

Breathing difficulty
1. may include shortness of breath during or after new exercise or awakening from sleep

Modified from Ref. (20), with permission.

with Table 16.2 or a more complete list of MET demands for common activities (14,18). The pace of these activities may be scaled up or down by results of early post-MI stress test when available. If no supervised program is available, patients' 2 months status after uncomplicated MI can use an EST to determine RPE and target HR.

NEUROPATHY
This warrants special caution because of risks of orthostasis and injuries related to poor proprioception and pain perception (9).

PACEMAKERS
Individuals with pacers should be carefully evaluated before RT, as pacer leads are prone to dislodgement or fracture during repetitive motion (47).

RETINOPATHY

Vigorous exercise is contraindicated with retinopathy because of risk of retinal detachment and vitreous hemorrhage (48).

STERNAL PRECAUTIONS

Sternal precautions are generally in place for 6 weeks postoperatively. Patients generally may not lift >10 lbs, reach overhead, or use arms to push up during transfers from sit to stand. Some studies have suggested that for the first 8 to 12 weeks after CABG, patients should avoid upper-body RT with >50% of maximum voluntary contraction to allow healing of the sternum (49). Restrictions should be specified on the discharge summary from the surgical team. During rehabilitation, pain at the surgical site must be considered during exercise prescription. The comprehensive outpatient cardiac rehabilitation (secondary prevention) program is generally delayed until sternal precautions are lifted.

STROKE AND AMPUTEE

Patients commonly have comorbid cardiac disease. Hemiplegic ambulation has a much higher energy cost, as does gait with an amputation (see Appendix). Lower limb impairments may necessitate upper limb ergometry.

VALVE SURGERY

Bio-prosthetic valves generally warrant aspirin, whereas artificial valves necessitate warfarin.

WOMEN

CVD is the most common cause of death in women worldwide, yet it is frequently unrecognized. Women most commonly present with typical signs and symptoms of myocardial ischemia, but frequently present with atypical symptoms including abdominal pains, nausea, or fatigue (50). They usually present with cardiac disease later in life and are half as likely as men to be referred to cardiac rehabilitation (51).

Admission to Phase II Outpatient Cardiac Rehabilitation

Erik Stanton Brand and Kerry J. Stewart

Diagnosis: acute myocardial infarction within the preceding 12 months, stable angina pectoris, coronary artery bypass surgery, heart valve repair/replacement, percutaneous transluminal coronary angioplasty or stenting, heart (or heart–lung) transplant, stable heart failure, claudication

Admit to: cardiac rehabilitation unit (phase II)

Condition: stable

Allergies: list known drug or other allergies

Precautions: sternal, fall, cardiac

Vital signs: before and after exercise regimen

Weight bearing status: full weight bearing (besides above precautions)

Activity: as tolerated without contraindications such chest pain, shortness of breath, new onset or uncontrolled peripheral edema, hypotension, uncontrolled or symptomatic hypertension, confusion

Cardiology: EKG STAT at clinician discretion or changes on cardiac monitor prn change in rate, rhythm, or interval

Therapies:
> **Cardiac rehabilitation staff:** perform the following procedures: exercise prescription, outline progression of patient through cardiac rehabilitation, instruct on phase II cardiac rehabilitation class outline, review screen of criteria and contraindications for patient to enter cardiac rehabilitation, risk stratification, behavior pretest, review risk factors with patient, instruct patient on use of Framingham 10-year risk calculator online
> **Physical therapy:** not needed normally but consider evaluation if appropriate to participate in cardiovascular conditioning
> **Occupational therapy:** not needed normally but consider evaluation if appropriate
> **Nutrition:** diet education
> **Prosthetics:** not needed normally but consider evaluation if appropriate, i.e., to reduce cardiac demands
> **Speech:** not needed normally but consider evaluation if appropriate
> **Psychology:** evaluation variable dependent on surrounding issues
> **Vocational rehabilitation:** may be appropriate
> **Social work:** family organization and communication

Modalities: not needed normally but consider evaluation if appropriate

Prophylaxis:
> **Cardiac:** ACE inhibitor, beta-blocker, acetylsalicylic acid 81 mg po (unless otherwise indicated or stent in place necessitating 325 mg po), statin

(or other lipid-lowering medication), smoking cessation counseling, antihypertensive medications as dictated by cardiology team

Stent: acetylsalicylic acid enteric coated 325 mg po 4 times a day, clopidogrel 75 mg po 4 times a day

Skin: sternal, inguinal, or saphenous vein graft harvest site wound care as appropriate

Pain: Cease exercise if angina occurs. Musculoskeletal pain from incisions may require small doses of opioid analgesics, nonsteroidal anti-inflammatory drugs (with caution if gastrointestinal bleed, hypertension or nephropathy) or acetaminophen.

> **Chest pain protocol:** Notify House Officer/physician for all episodes of chest pain. EKG STAT, vital signs before and with each dose of morphine or nitroglycerin, O_2 2 L/min by nasal canula (titrate to ≥95% up to 5 L/min), nitroglycerin 0.4 mg sublingual q5min prn up to 3 doses (call House Officer if chest pain persists), morphine 2 mg inject q5min prn chest pain not relieved by nitroglycerin (contraindicated if respiratory rate <10/min or unstable vital signs; do not exceed 10 mg/hr).

DVT: not needed normally but consider evaluation if appropriate

GI: gastritis: H2 blocker, proton pump inhibitor; indigestion: aluminum/magnesium hydroxide oral suspension 30 mL po bid prn

Constipation: especially if on opioids: docusate 100 mg po q12h with bisacodyl 5 mg tabs 1 to 2 po qd prn no bowel movement or suppository PR prn constipation, senna 1 to 2 tablets po qd prn constipation, magnesium hydroxide oral susp 30 mL po bid prn

Medications:

Home medications: per individual

Pain: Control pain to facilitate therapy participation and minimize risk of chronic pain. Consider administration before therapy to ensure participation.

> **Neuropathic:** gabapentin 100 or 300-mg tabs titrate q2 days (4 times a day to twice a day) until up to 1800 mg/d,
> amitriptyline 25- to 75-mg po qhs, duloxetine 30- to 60-mg po q12 h or pregabalin 50- to 75-mg po q12 h

> **Musculoskeletal:**
> > **Short acting:** oxycodone 5- or 10-mg tabs po q6-8h prn breakthrough pain, acetaminophen/oxycodone 5/325 to 10/325 mg 1 to 2 po q6-8h prn breakthrough pain, hydrocodone/acetaminophen 5/500 or
> > 7.5/650 mg 1 to 2 po q8h prn breakthrough pain
> > or acetaminophen 325 mg tabs po q4h prn pain or temp >101 F max dose 4000 mg/d

> > **Long acting** use with caution if pain is uncontrolled and using short acting: morphine sulfate controlled release 15 mg po qd to q12h, methadone 2.5 to 5 mg po q12h, oxycodone controlled release 10 mg po q12h or fentanyl 12 mcg/h or 25 mcg patch q72 hours

> **Incisional:** light massage to scar and incision once healed or healing to prevent long-term pain, monitor for skin breakdown, erythema,

drainage, warmth, swelling, lidocaine patch 5% apply peri-incisional q12h, lidocaine 1% to 2% cream apply twice a day to 4 times a day prn, marcaine 0.5% to 0.75% cream apply twice a day to 4 times a day prn, compound lidocaine 1% to 2% or marcaine 0.5% to 0.75% (longer duration) with or without gabapentin and anti-inflammatory twice a day to 4 times a day prn

Anxiety: oxazepam 15 to 30 mg po 4 times a day prn

Labs: lipid profile

EKG: baseline on file for comparison

Imaging: baseline chest x-ray on file for comparison

Length of stay: 4 to 11 weeks usually

Goals: Use cardio-pulmonary conditioning to increase aerobic fitness and muscle strength. Verbalize and maintain sternal, cardiac, fall, or other precautions. Provide incision care and pain control.

■ ACKNOWLEDGMENT

Special thanks to Robert Samuel Mayer, MD.

■ REFERENCES

1. Mayer RS. MOC|3 Cardiac and Cancer Rehabilitation Online Review Course. American Academy of Physical Medicine & Rehabilitation. http://me.e-aapmr.org/shared/courseDescription.aspx?courseID=12813&clientID=587&URL=http://me.e-aapmr.org.

2. Taylor RS, Unal B, Critchley JA, Capewell S. Mortality reductions in patients receiving exercise-based cardiac rehabilitation: how much can be attributed to cardiovascular risk factor improvements? *Eur J Cardiovasc Prev Rehabil.* 2006;13(3):369–374.

3. Wenger NK, Froelicher ES, Smith LK, et al. Cardiac Rehabilitation as Secondary Prevention. Clinical Practice Guideline. Quick Reference Guide for Clinicians, No. 17. Rockville, MD: U.S. Department of Health and Human Services, Public Health Service, Agency for Health Care Policy and Research and National Heart, Lung, and Blood Institute. AHCPR publication 96-0673. October 1995.

4. Jackson L, Leclerc J, Erskine Y, Linden W. Getting the most out of cardiac rehabilitation: a review of referral and adherence predictors. *Heart.* 2005;91(1):10–14.

5. Centers for Medicare & Medicaid Services. NCD for Cardiac Rehabilitation Programs (20.10) *http://www.cms.hhs.gov/Transmittals/Downloads/R52NCD.pdf.* Accessed May 21, 2010

6. Leon AS, Franklin BA, Costa F, et al. Cardiac rehabilitation and secondary prevention of coronary heart disease: an American Heart Association scientific statement from the Council on Clinical Cardiology (Subcommittee on Exercise, Cardiac Rehabilitation, and Prevention) and the Council on Nutrition, Physical Activity, and Metabolism (Subcommittee on Physical Activity), in collaboration

with the American Association of Cardiovascular and Pulmonary Rehabilitation. *Circulation*. 2005;111(3):369–376. [Erratum in: Circulation. 2005 Apr 5;111(13):1717.]

7. Cornelissen VA, Fagard RH. Effect of resistance training on resting blood pressure: a meta-analysis of randomized controlled trials. *J Hypertens*. 2005;23:251–259.

8. Kelley GA, Kelley KS. Progressive resistance exercise and resting blood pressure: a meta-analysis of randomized controlled trials. *Hypertension*. 2000;35:838–843.

9. Williams MA, Haskell WL, Ades PA, et al. Resistance Exercise in Individuals with and without cardiovascular disease: 2007 update. a scientific statement from the American Heart Association Council on Clinical Cardiology and Council on Nutrition, Physical Activity, and Metabolism. *Circulation*. 2007;116:572–584.

10. Pratley R, Nicklas B, Rubin M, et al. Strength training increases resting metabolic rate and norepinephrine levels in healthy 50 to 65-yr-old men. *J Appl Physiol*. 1994;76:133–137.

11. Fitzgerald SJ, Barlow CE, Kampert JB, Morrow JR, Jackson AW, Blair SN. Muscular fitness and all-cause mortality: prospective observations. *J Physical Activity Health*. 2004;1:7–18.

12. Jurca R, Lamonte MJ, Barlow CE, Kampert JB, Church TS, Blair SN. Association of muscular strength with incidence of metabolic syndrome in men. *Med Sci Sports Exerc*. 2005; 37:1849–1855.

13. Jurca R, Lamonte JM, Church TS, et al. Associations of muscle strength and fitness with metabolic syndrome in men. *Med Sci Sports Exerc*. 2004;36:1301–1307.

14. Stewart KJ, Ziegelstein RC. Postmyocardial Infarction Care and Cardiac Rehabilitation. In Fiebach NH, Kern DE, Thomas PA, Zeigelstein RC, eds. *Principles of Ambulatory Medicine*. Philadelphia, PA: Lippincott Williams and Wilkens, 2007:971–992.

15. Ainsworth BE, Haskell WL, Whitt MC, et al. Compendium of physical activities: an update of activity codes and MET intensities. *Med Sci Sports Exerc*. 2000;32(9) (suppl): S498–S504.

16. Gibbons RJ, Balady GJ, Bricker JT, et al. American College of Cardiology/American Heart Association Task Force on Practice Guidelines (Committee to Update the 1997 Exercise Testing Guidelines). ACC/AHA 2002 guideline update for exercise testing: summary article: a report of the American College of Cardiology/American Heart Association Task Force on Practice Guidelines (Committee to Update the 1997 Exercise Testing Guidelines). *Circulation*. 2002;106:1883.

17. American College of Physicians. Evaluation of patients after recent acute myocardial infarction (position paper). *Ann Intern Med*. 1989;110:485.

18. Borg G. Subjective effort in relation to physical performance and working capacity. In: Pick HL, ed. *Psychology: From Research to Practice*. New York: Plenum; 1978:333.

19. Haskell WL. Design and implementation of cardiac conditioning programs. In: Wenger NK, Hellerstein HK, eds. *Rehabilitation of the Coronary Patient*. New York: Wiley; 1978:209.

20. Feigenbaum MS, Pollock ML. Strength training: rationale for current guidelines for adult fitness programs. *Physician Sports Med*. 1997;25:44–64.

21. Wilke NA, Sheldahl LM, Tristani FE, Hughes CV, Kalbfleisch JH. The safety of static-dynamic effort soon after myocardial infarction. *Am Heart J.* 1985;110:542–545.
22. MacDougall JD, Tuxen D, Sale DG, Moroz JR, Sutton JR. Arterial blood pressure response to heavy resistance exercise. *J Appl Physiol.* 1985;58:785–790.
23. American Association of Cardiovascular and Pulmonary Rehabilitation. *Guidelines for Cardiac Rehabilitation and Secondary Prevention Programs.* 4th ed. Champaign, IL: Human Kinetics; 2004.
24. American College of Sports Medicine. *ACSM's Guidelines for Exercise Testing and Prescription.* 7th ed. Philadelphia, PA: Lippincott Williams and Wilkins; 2006.
25. Dingwall H, Ferrier K, Semple J. Exercise prescription in cardiac rehabilitation. In: Thow M, ed. *Exercise Leadership in Cardiac Rehabilitation.* West Sussex, England: Whurr Publishers Ltd; 2006:97–131.
26. Jafri, I. Cardiac rehabilitation. In: Cuccurullo SJ, ed. *Physical Medicine and Rehabilitation Board Review.* New York: Demos, 2004:610–628.
27. Dalal HM, Zawada A, Jolly K, Moxham T, Taylor RS. Home based versus centre based cardiac rehabilitation: cochrane systematic review and meta-analysis. *BMJ.* 2010 19;340:b5631. doi: 10.1136/bmj.b5631.
28. Hellerstein HK, Friedman EH. Sexual activity in the post-coronary patient. *Arch Intern Med.* 1970;125:987.
29. Featherstone JF, Holly RG, Amsterdam EA. Physiologic responses to weight lifting in coronary artery disease. *Am J Cardiol.* 1993;71:287–292.
30. McKelvie RS, McCartney N, Tomlinson C, Bauer R, MacDougall JD. Comparison of hemodynamic responses to cycling and resistance exercise in congestive heart failure secondary to ischemic cardiomyopathy. *Am J Cardiol.* 1995;76:977–979.
31. Pollock ML, Franklin BA, Balady GJ, et al. Resistance exercise in individuals with and without cardiovascular disease: benefits, rationale, safety, and prescription: an advisory from the Committee on Exercise, Rehabilitation, and Prevention, Council on Clinical Cardiology, American Heart Association: position paper endorsed by the American College of Sports Medicine. *Circulation.* 2000;101:828–833.
32. Kelemen MH, Stewart KJ, Gillilan RE, et al. Circuit weight training in cardiac patients. *J Am Coll Cardiol.* 1986;7:38.
33. Stewart KJ, Mason M, Kelemen MH. Three year participation in circuit weight training improves muscular strength and self-efficacy in cardiac patients. *J Cardiopulm Rehab.* 1988;8:292.
34. Izawa K, Hirano Y, Yamada S, Oka K, Omiya K, Iijima S. Improvements in physiological outcomes and health-related quality of life following cardiac rehabilitation in patients with acute myocardial infarction. *Circ J.* 2004;68:315–320.
35. Wenger NK Froelicher ES, Smith LK, for the Cardiac Rehabilitation Guideline Panel. Cardiac Rehabilitation as Secondary Prevention: Clinical Practice Guideline No. 17. Rockville, MD: US Department of Health and Human Services, Public Health Service, Agency for Health Care Policy and Research and the National Heart, Lung, and Blood Institute; October 1995. AHCPR publication 96–0672.
36. Powles AC. The effect of drugs on the cardiovascular response to exercise. *Med Sci Sports Exerc.* 1981;13(4):252–258.

37. McCartney N. Acute responses to resistance training and safety. *Med Sci Sports Exerc.* 1999;31–37.

38. Haslam DR, McCartney SN, McKelvie RS, MacDougall JD. Direct measurements of arterial blood pressure during formal weightlifting in cardiac patients. *J Cardiopulm Rehabil.* 1988;8:213–225.

39. Davidson KW, Burg MM, Kronish IM, et al. Association of anhedonia with recurrent major adverse cardiac events and mortality 1 year after acute coronary syndrome. *Arch Gen Psychiatry.* 2010;67(5):480–488.

40. Shapiro PA, Lesperance F, Frasure-Smith N, et al. An open-label preliminary trial of sertraline for treatment of major depression after acute myocardial infarction (the SADHAT Trial). Sertraline Anti-Depressant Heart Attack Trial. *Am Heart J.* 1999;137:1100.

41. Roose SP, Laghrissi-Thode F, Kennedy JS, et al. Comparison of paroxetine and nortriptyline in depressed patients with ischemic heart disease. *JAMA.* 1998;279:287.

42. Strik JJ, Honig A, Lousberg R, et al. Efficacy and safety of fluoxetine in the treatment of patients with major depression after first myocardial infarction: findings from a double-blind, placebo-controlled trial. *Psychosom Med.* 2000;62:783.

43. Glassman AH, O'Connor CM, Califf RM, et al. Sertraline antidepressant heart attack randomized trial (SADHEART) group. Sertraline treatment of major depression in patients with acute MI or unstable angina. *JAMA.* 2002;288:701.

44. Roose SP, Glassman AH. Cardiovascular effects of tricyclic antidepressants in depressed patients with and without heart disease. *J Clin Psychiatry.* 1989;50(suppl):1.

45. van Dijk D, Keizer AM, Diephuis JC, Durand C, Vos LJ, Hijman R. Neurocognitive dysfunction after coronary artery bypass surgery: a systematic review. *J Thorac Cardiovasc Surg.* 2000;120(4):632–639.

46. Selnes OA, Grega MA, Borowicz LM Jr, et al. Cognitive outcomes three years after coronary artery bypass surgery: a comparison of on-pump coronary artery bypass graft surgery and nonsurgical controls. *Ann Thorac Surg.* 2005;79(4):1201–1209.

47. Lampert R, Cannom D, Olshansky B. Safety of sports participation in patients with implantable cardioverter defibrillators: a survey of Heart Rhythm Society members. *J Cardiovasc Electrophysiol.* 2006;17:11–15.

48. Aiello LP, Wong J, Cavallerano J, Bursell SE, Aiello LM. Retinopathy. In: Ruderman N, Devlin JT, Schneider SH, Kriska AM, eds. *Handbook of Exercise in Diabetes.* 2nd ed. Alexandria, VA: American Diabetes Association; 2002:401–413.

49. Vincent KR, Vincent HK. Resistance training for individuals with cardiovascular disease. *J Cardiopulm Rehabil.* 2006;26:207–216.

50. World Heart Federation web site. Available at *http://www.world-heart-federation.org/what-we-do/go-red-for-women/get-the-facts/.* Accessed May 21, 2010.

51. Jackson L, Leclerc J, Erskine Y, Linden W. Getting the most out of cardiac rehabilitation: a review of referral and adherence predictors. *Heart.* 2005;91:10–14.

For further references and resources related to this chapter, visit *www.hopkinsbayview.org/PAMreferences* Chapter 63.

Geriatric Rehabilitation

Lauren T. Shapiro

■ SPECIAL CONSIDERATIONS WHEN CARING FOR GERIATRIC PATIENTS
PHYSIOLOGIC CHANGES

Significant physiologic changes occur as people age, which may impact a patient's functional abilities and increase one's susceptibility to illness and injury. Loss of muscle mass and strength occurs with aging. Cardiovascular changes include a decline in maximal heart rate and maximum oxygen consumption, rise in blood pressure, and decreased baroreceptor sensitivity; the latter predisposes older patients to orthostatic hypotension. Creatinine clearance (Cr Cl), vital capacity, glucose tolerance, and peristalsis through the gastrointestinal tract also decrease with age. Older adults are also more susceptible to infections and may be less likely to mount a fever or leukocytosis in response to infection.

ILLNESSES AND IMPAIRMENTS

Older adults are more likely to have potentially disabling chronic illnesses, including osteoarthritis, osteoporosis, cerebrovascular disease, and Parkinson's disease. They may also have multiple medical comorbidities, cognitive impairment, visual and/or hearing impairments.

HOSPITALIZATION, BED REST, AND DECONDITIONING

Elderly patients often demonstrate impaired abilities to ambulate and to perform activities of daily living (ADLs) following an acute illness, making it essential to assess their mobility and independence with ADLs prior to discharge. Bed rest orders are often unnecessary and may have deleterious effects for older adults, including significant declines in lower extremity strength, power, and aerobic capacity. The use of mechanical restraints should be avoided as there is no evidence that they reduce the risk of falls in hospitalized patients, and they may be associated with an increased risk of injuries and agitation. Patients remain at risk for falls, pressure sores, delirium, and adverse drug reactions while hospitalized, which are further discussed below.

■ FALLS AND COMMON INJURIES

A number of factors increase the risk of falls among older adults, including lower limb weakness, impaired vision, cognitive impairment, orthostatic hypotension, and medications. Injuries commonly seen in older adults following falls are discussed in the following sections, but it should be noted that these injuries can also occur with minimal or no trauma.

HIP FRACTURES

Hip fractures often result from falls among the elderly and should be suspected in patients reporting groin pain and in those who are unable to rise or bear weight on their injured leg following a fall. External rotation and a shortened appearance of the leg suggest a displaced femur fracture. Radiographs including an anteroposterior view of the pelvis and a lateral view of the proximal femur should be obtained as soon as possible. The presence of a fracture should prompt consultation with an orthopedic surgeon and preparation for surgery. Should radiographs fail to demonstrate a fracture but strong clinical suspicion for a fracture remains, additional imaging may be necessary. An older adult who sustains a hip fracture likely has osteoporosis, and as such, necessary precautions are required during physical activity to prevent further fractures.

PELVIC FRACTURES

Pelvic fractures may result from forward or backward falls. Patients may initially complain of groin pain and subsequently of sacral pain. Radiographs may fail to reveal the fracture, necessitating bone scan or MRI for diagnosis. These fractures usually heal well, and bed rest should be avoided.

VERTEBRAL COMPRESSION FRACTURES

Vertebral compression fractures may result from falls as well. Patients may report the sudden onset of back pain, typically worse with standing or walking and may have tenderness to palpation over the fracture. Plain radiographs should be the initial imaging study performed and may demonstrate the classic wedge-shaped deformity. Compression fractures are usually stable fractures and can be treated conservatively with a short period of relative rest and pain medication.

SUBDURAL HEMATOMAS

Subdural hematomas may occur in older adults who fall, especially those receiving anticoagulation. Symptoms may take time to emerge and may include headache, dizziness, and altered mental status. Head CT scan should be performed when a hematoma is suspected.

■ PRESSURE SORES

The elderly are predisposed to developing pressure sores, especially during periods of acute illness and immobility. Daily skin assessments should be performed while hospitalized. Patients should be repositioned every

2 hours, and the use of pressure-reducing devices should be considered to prevent sores. Nutritional consultation is beneficial in patients who develop pressure sores to determine if nutritional deficiencies are affecting healing.

■ DELIRIUM AND AGITATION

Delirium is an acute cognitive impairment with associated change in consciousness. It may have a fluctuating course with periods of lucidity. It is a clinical diagnosis, the differential for which is quite broad. The underlying cause(s) should be identified to allow for proper treatment and return to the patient's baseline mental status.

THE EVALUATION OF DELIRIUM

HISTORY

History taking should begin with obtaining information regarding the onset of symptoms, which is of the utmost importance given the difficulty discerning between delirium and dementia in older adults. All medications, and particularly any newly added medications, should be carefully reviewed.

PHYSICAL EXAMINATION

Vital signs including pulse oximetry should be obtained. A comprehensive examination should be performed, including a thorough neurological assessment and examination for signs of infection and other medical conditions.

LABS

A bedside glucose reading should be taken. A complete blood count, comprehensive metabolic panel, and blood and urine cultures should be obtained. Coagulation studies should be obtained in patients receiving anticoagulants and in those with suspected liver dysfunction. Other lab work, such as blood alcohol levels or medication levels, may be clinically warranted. Lumbar puncture should be performed and cerebrospinal fluid sent for analysis when suspicion exists for meningitis or encephalitis.

IMAGING

A chest radiograph will help exclude pneumonia or congestive heart failure as the precipitating cause. A head CT should be performed in patients presenting with a significant change in mental status and in those with focal neurologic deficits.

SUNDOWNING

Sundowning refers to behavioral disturbances that occur in the late afternoon or evening among some older adults with dementia. Interventions may include structuring activities during usual times of agitation, redirection, reassurance, and meeting patients' physical needs, such as for pain control or toileting. Antipsychotic medications are most commonly used to treat the associated agitation, but must be used with caution as there is increased risk of mortality with these agents when used in individuals with dementia. When medication is required to manage the agitation, the lowest effective dose should be given.

■ MEDICATIONS AND ADVERSE DRUG REACTIONS

Adverse drug reactions (ADRs) are a significant cause of morbidity and mortality in the elderly.

FACTORS CONTRIBUTING TO INCREASED RISK OF ADRs AMONG THE ELDERLY

NONCOMPLIANCE WITH DRUG THERAPY

Reasons may include the cost of medication, inability to read instructions, and cognitive impairment. Compliance may be improved by patient education, use of a pill box or medication calendar, large type prescription labels, the use of less expensive generic medications, and the use of once-daily medications.

POLYPHARMACY

The use of some combinations of medications may put a patient at higher risk for an ADR; for example, there is an increased risk of gastrointestinal bleeding with concomitant use of nonsteroidal anti-inflammatory drug and anticoagulants. One drug may also inhibit or increase the metabolism of another. Fluoxetine and paroxetine, for example, can inhibit the metabolism of other medications via the cytochrome P450 system, thereby prolonging their half-life. Thus, the use of alternative selective serotonin reuptake inhibitors is preferable in elderly adults with depression.

BODY WEIGHT AND COMPOSITION CHANGES

Fat-soluble drugs, including benzodiazepines, tend to accumulate more in the fatty tissue of elderly patients, prolonging their half-life. Use of lorazepam is preferred over diazepam in older adults because of its more rapid pharmacokinetics.

DECREASED PLASMA PROTEIN BINDING CAPACITY

This can lead to higher free drug plasma concentrations and may increase the risk of drug interactions. Consider checking free levels of medications that are highly protein-bound, including phenytoin.

ALTERED HEPATIC CLEARANCE

Hepatic clearance of medications may be impaired in the elderly, though liver function tests may remain normal. The content of cytochrome P450 enzymes within the liver diminishes with age, affecting the phase I metabolism of some medications.

Decreased Renal Excretion

Creatinine clearance (Cr Cl) declines significantly with age and cannot be determined solely on the basis of the serum creatinine. Dose adjustment of some medications, including gabapentin and allopurinol, is required when a patient's Cr Cl is less than 60 ml/min. Cr Cl calculators are available online and for personal digital assistant (PDA). Cr Cl can also be estimated using the Cockroft–Gault formula below:

$$\text{Cr Cl} = [(140 - \text{age}) \times \text{weight in kg}]/[72 \times \text{serum creatinine} (\times 0.85 \text{ for women})]$$

Increased Sensitivity of the Central Nervous System

A number of changes occur in the central nervous system (CNS) pathways of the aging brain that predispose elderly patients to neurologic side effects of medications. Older adults with neurologic diseases, including Alzheimer's disease and Parkinson's disease, may especially be at high risk for ADRs. Anticholinergic medications, which include tricyclic antidepressants, tolterodine, oxybutynin, scopolamine, and trihexyphenidyl, may precipitate delirium. First generation antihistamines, including diphenhydramine, have anticholinergic properties and may cause confusion as well. Opioid medications and drugs used to treat Parkinson's disease, including levodopa, may also contribute to delirium.

POTENTIALLY INAPPROPRIATE MEDICATIONS IN THE ELDERLY

The Beers criteria, established by expert consensus, have identified medications that are potentially inappropriate for use in adults aged 65 and older. Medications included in the criteria that are commonly prescribed by physiatrists can be found in Table 17.1.

TABLE 17.1 ▪ Medications prescribed by physiatrists that may be inappropriate for older adults.

Amitriptyline (Elavil)	Ketorolac (Toradol)
Barbiturates (all)	Lorazepam (Ativan)
Bisacodyl (Dulcolax)– long-term use	Meperidine (Demerol)
Carisoprodol (Soma)	Metaxalone (Skelaxin)
Chlordiazepoxide (Librium)	Methocarbamol (Robaxin)
Cyclobenzaprine (Flexeril)	Naproxen (Naprosyn, Aleve)
Diazepam (Valium)	Nitrofurantoin (Macrodantin)
Diphenhydramine (Benadryl)	Oxybutynin (Ditropan)
Doxepin (Sinequan)	Propoxyphene (Darvon)
Fluoxetine (Prozac)	Promethazine (Phenergan)
Hydroxyzine (Atarax and Vistaril)	Temazepam (Restoril)
Indomethacin (Indocin)	Triazolam (Halcion)

STRATEGIES TO PREVENT ADRs IN THE ELDERLY

■ Patient education

■ Consultation with pharmacist regarding proper drug dosages and potential interactions

■ Use of nonpharmacologic treatments whenever possible

■ Having patients bring with them all of their medications, including herbal supplements, to physician visits to allow for proper accounting of what they are taking

■ Using the lowest efficacious dose of a medication available and increasing it gradually

■ Avoidance of high risk medications.

■ EXERCISE AND THE ELDERLY
RECOMMENDATIONS FOR OLDER ADULTS BEGINNING AN EXERCISE PROGRAM

There are many demonstrated benefits of regular exercise in older adults, but it remains important for patients to discuss their plans with their physician prior to beginning an exercise regimen. Elderly patients should first undergo a history and physical examination to identify physical limitations and cardiac risk factors. Exercise stress testing can be useful to determine the patient's fitness level and appropriate level of exercise intensity, as well as to identify patients who are at risk for a cardiac event during periods of increased metabolic demand. Older patients should be advised to gradually increase the intensity of their exercise and should not exceed the intensity at which they can no longer comfortably carry on a conversation.

EXERCISE PRECAUTIONS IN OSTEOPOROTIC PATIENTS

People with osteoporosis should avoid some forms of exercise, including high impact exercises such as jumping or running, and contact sports. They should also refrain from any exercise that vigorously or repeatedly flexes or rotates the spine, including sit-ups, toe touches, and the use of gym equipment with reciprocal arm movements. Such exercises may increase the risk of vertebral fractures.

■ PHYSICAL MODALITIES, TRACTION, AND MANIPULATION

Caution is required with the use of these treatments in older adults, as is summarized in the following sections.

HEAT AND COLD THERAPY

Heat and cold therapy are contraindicated in those with arterial insufficiency, impaired sensation, and in those who are unable to communicate or respond to pain. Older adults may have atrophic skin, increasing their risk of thermal damage with such therapies. Inquire about the presence of metal implants, including pacemakers and deep brain stimulators, prior to ordering deep heat modalities.

MANUAL TRACTION
Caution is advised with use of manual traction in the elderly and is absolutely contraindicated in patients with osteoporosis.

SPINAL MANIPULATION
Spinal manipulation is also absolutely contraindicated in people with osteoporosis. Relative contraindications include severe spondylosis, osteopenia, and anticoagulation.

■ BIBLIOGRAPHY

1. Bachman D, Rabins P. "Sundowning" and other temporally associated agitation states in dementia patients. *Annu Rev Med.* 2006;57:499–511.
2. Brault JS, Kappler RE, Grogg BE. Manipulation, traction, and massage. In: Braddom RL, ed. *Physical Medicine and Rehabilitation*, 3rd ed. Philadelphia, PA: Saunders Elsevier; 2007;437–457.
3. Clark GS, Siebens HC. Geriatric Rehabilitation. In: DeLisa JA, Gans BM, Walsh NE, eds. *Physical Medicine and Rehabilitation: Principles and Practice*. 4th ed. Philadelphia, PA: Lippincott Williams & Wilkins; 2005;1531–1560.
4. Cornell CN, Sculco TP. Orthopedic disorders. In: Duthie EH Jr, Katz PR, Malone ML, eds. *Duthie: Practice of Geriatrics.* 4th ed. Philadelphia, PA: Saunders Elsevier; 2007:511–527.
5. Fick DM, Cooper JW, Wade WE, et al. Updating the beers criteria for potentially inappropriate medication use in older adults. *Arch Int Med.* 2003;163:2716–2724.
6. Ginsberg G, Hattis D, Russ A, Sonawane B. Pharmacokinetic and pharmacodynamic factors that can affect sensitivity to neurotoxic sequelae in elderly individuals. *Environ Health Perspect.* 2005;113(9):1243–1249.
7. Gay RE, Bauer BA, Yang RK. Integrative medicine in rehabilitation. In: Braddom RL. *Physical Medicine and Rehabilitation.* 3rd ed. Philadelphia: Saunders Elsevier; 2007;511–513.
8. Graf C. Functional decline in hospitalized older adults. *Am J Nurs.* 2006;106(1):58–67.
9. Keefe KP, Sanson TG. Elderly patients with altered mental status. *Emerg Med Clin North Am.* 1998;16(4):701–715.
10. Kortebein P, Symons TB, Ferrando A, et al. Functional impact of 10 days of bed rest in healthy older adults. *J Gerontol: Med Sci.* 2008;63A(10):1076–1081.
11. Lyder CH, Preston J, Grady JN, et al. Quality of care for hospitalized medicare patients at risk for pressure ulcers. *Arch Int Med.* 2001;161:1549–1554.
12. National Osteoporosis Foundation. Rehabilitation of patients with osteoporosis-related fractures. *Osteoporos: Clin Updates.* 2003;1–10.
13. Nied RJ, Franklin B. Promoting and prescribing exercise for the elderly. *Am Fam Physician.* 2002;65(3):419–426.

14. Pham CB, Dickman RL. Minimizing adverse drug events in older patients. *Am Fam Physician*. 2007;76(12):1837–1844.
15. Routledge PA, O'Mahony MS, Woodhouse KW. Adverse drug reactions in elderly patients. *Br J Clin Pharmacol*. 2003;57(2):121–126.
16. Weber DC, Hoppe KM. Physical agent modalities. In: Braddom RL. *Physical Medicine and Rehabilitation*. 3rd ed. Philadelphia, PA: Saunders Elsevier; 2007;459–477.
17. Williams CM. Using medications appropriately in older adults. *Am Fam Physician*. 2002;66(10):1917–1924.

18

Orthopedic Rehabilitation

Lisa S. Barrett

■ INTRODUCTION

Admission to inpatient orthopedic rehabilitation depends on the patient's degree of disability, their medical complexity, and social factors that would affect their functional independence in post hospital discharge such as availability of support and the accessibility of their home. According to the Centers for Medicaid and Medicare Services, recognized impairment categories include major multiple trauma, lower extremity fracture, lower extremity joint replacement, extremity amputation, and debilitating arthritides.

A multidisciplinary team consisting of physicians, nurses, and therapists create a structured rehabilitation program based on comprehensive medical and functional evaluations and the patient's goals. Goals of therapy focus on improving mobility, balance, strength, range of motion, gait, and activities of daily living (ADLs). Therapy goals should carryover to the outpatient setting. Due to the risk of developing complications in the acute postoperative period, physician monitoring and medical management in an inpatient setting are often a necessary first step to facilitate the patient's successful functional recovery.

■ PELVIC FRACTURES

The pelvic ring or girdle is formed by the ilium, ischium, pubis, sacrum, and coccyx. It supports the spine and joins the trunk to the lower extremities. Any or all of these bones can be broken. In the United States, 3% of skeletal fractures involve the pelvis (Mechem).

Pelvic fractures can result from low- to high-energy blunt trauma (eg, motor vehicle collisions 50%–60%, motorcycle collisions 10%–20%, motor vehicle vs pedestrian collision 10%–20%, and falls 8%–10%). In elderly women with osteoporosis, a fractured pelvis can result from a fall.

Determination of the stability of the fracture is paramount as it affects treatment and prognosis. The pelvic ring (alignment) is preserved and hence stable in a nondisplaced fracture. A displaced fracture is unstable as the pelvic alignment is compromised and is often associated with internal organ injury. The stability of the fracture is best determined by imaging.

Two classification systems for pelvic fractures are often used.

The Tile classification system is based on the integrity of the posterior sacroiliac complex.

■ In type A injuries, the sacroiliac complex is intact. The pelvic ring has a stable fracture that can be managed nonoperatively.

■ Type B injuries result in partial disruption of the posterior sacroiliac complex. These are often rotationally unstable.

■ Type C injuries are characterized by complete disruption of the posterior sacroiliac complex and are rotationally and vertically unstable.

The Young classification system is based on mechanism of injury: lateral compression (LC), anteroposterior compression (APC), vertical shear, or a combination of forces. LC fractures involve transverse fractures of the pubic rami, either ipsilateral or contralateral to a posterior injury.

■ Grade I—Associated sacral compression on side of impact

■ Grade II—Associated posterior iliac ("crescent") fracture on side of impact

■ Grade III—Associated contralateral sacroiliac joint injury

APC fractures involve symphyseal diastasis or longitudinal rami fractures.

In conjunction with the patient's mechanism of injury and symptoms, physical exam findings can be suggestive of pelvic fracture and associated internal organ trauma.

■ Tenderness, laxity, or instability on palpation of the bony pelvis suggests fracture.

■ Hematuria, vaginal, or rectal bleeding; a hematoma over the ipsilateral thigh, inguinal ligament, or in the perineum; neurovascular deficits in the lower extremities; and hemodynamic instability.

■ Instability on hip adduction and pain on hip motion suggests an acetabular fracture, with or without an associated hip fracture.

■ Signs of urethral injury in males include a high-riding or boggy prostate on rectal examination, scrotal hematoma, or blood at the urethral meatus.

Anteroposterior pelvic radiographs with inlet and outlet views are commonly used to detect pelvic fracture. CT scan and/or ultrasound of the pelvis and abdomen are important to survey for internal organ laceration and fluid collection.

If blood is found in the urine, urology consultation should be considered. Urethrography and cystography may be used to evaluate associated injuries to the urethra and bladder, respectively.

Arteriography might be necessary to evaluate vascular integrity and identify the source of intraabdominal blood loss if identified in previous studies.

Open reduction and internal fixation (ORIF) is preferred for definitive management of unstable fractures in hemodynamically stable patients with the goal of bone healing and prevention nonunion and malunion.

Potential complications include the following:

- Infection
- Hemodynamic instability
- Deep vein thrombosis
- Pulmonary embolism
- Acute pain
- Sexual dysfunction
- Gait dysfunction
- Pelvic misalignment can result in chronic back pain.
- Fractures of the acetabulum include posttraumatic arthritis, femoral head osteonecrosis, neurovascular injury, and sciatic nerve palsy.

REHABILITATION

Weight-bearing restrictions depend on the degree of fracture instability and are determined by the managing surgeon. Three months of non-weight bearing is usually recommended for vertically unstable fractures.

Physical therapy goals include protected weight-bearing with crutches or a walker in minimally displaced pelvic fractures until radiographic evidence of fracture healing is present. Once the fracture is stable (6–12 weeks), trunk and lower extremity strengthening and range of motion exercises may be introduced. Occupational therapy goals include upper extremity strengthening, transfer training, and instruction in use of adaptive equipment.

Full recovery from a pelvic fracture and resumption of normal activities may take 6 to 12 months.

■ HIP FRACTURES

Hip fractures involve any aspect of the proximal femur from the femoral head to approximately 4 to 5 cm distal to the subtrochanteric area. Patients may complain of localized pain in their hip, groin, and/or knee that is aggravated by walking or an inability to walk.

A fracture of the hip can result from a low-velocity injury (ie, fall and running) or high-velocity injury (ie, motor vehicle collision). In the elderly, hip fracture risk factors include decreased bone mineralization (eg, osteoporosis), visual impairment, cognitive impairment, decreased depth perception, and decreased mobility. The disability resulting from a hip fracture in this population is associated with significant morbidity and mortality. Approximately 15% to 20% die within 1 year.

Hip fractures are classified as follows.

- Femoral neck (intrascapular): (45% of fractures)—proximal to greater and lesser trochanter.

- Intertrochanteric (extracapsular): (45% of fractures)—between the greater and lesser trochanters

■ Subtrochanteric: (10% of fractures)—distal to lesser trochanter.

Physical examination findings include the following:

■ Limb shortening and external rotation

■ Limited passive range of motion

■ Antalgic gait

■ Inability to stand

■ Tenderness in groin or proximal thigh

■ Ecchymosis

The following complications may occur after hip fracture:

■ Avascular necrosis of the femoral head (femoral neck fractures)

■ Hip osteoarthritis

■ Deep vein thrombosis

■ Pulmonary embolism

■ Fat embolism

■ Blood vessel injury

■ Compartment syndrome

■ Internal bleeding

■ Peripheral nerve injury

■ Osteomyelitis

■ Reflex sympathetic dystrophy

Femoral neck fractures compromise the tenuous blood supply to the proximal femur. The femoral head is at risk of avascular necrosis if the lateral and medial circumflex femoral arteries and the foveal artery are disrupted.

Diagnostic imaging should include radiographs of hip (AP/lateral) with 15° to 20° internal rotation. MRI should be considered if plain radiographs are negative and index of suspicion is high. Bone scan is more sensitive than plain radiographs and less specific than MRI.

MANAGEMENT

Nonsurgical management includes casting and traction. Most of these fractures are treated surgically.

External fixation is indicated in cases involving severe soft tissue injuries or contamination. A frame around the leg is attached to the bone with pins. Early mobilization of the limb is an advantage of external fixation, but pin insertion sites are a nidus for infection requiring daily inspection and care. Pins may also interrupt arterial blood flow prolonging healing process.

Arthroplasty is indicated for treatment of femoral neck fractures. Advantages of arthroplasty include early mobilization, mechanical stability, and decreased pain. Range of motion restrictions is necessary for 12 weeks after surgery: no hip flexion greater than 90°, no internal rotation past neutral, and no adduction past neutral.

Open Reduction and Internal Fixation (ORIF) is the preferred treatment option for intertrochanteric fractures. Patients can be mobilized early after the procedure and there is no range of motion restrictions. Disadvantages of the procedure include infection and pain.

Intramedullary fixation is an alternative treatment method for intertrochanteric fractures. An intramedullary nail is inserted into the femur, spanning the fracture site. The nail is removed after the fracture heals. This procedure provides great fracture stability, but insertion of the nail can interrupt arterial blood flow prolonging healing process, femoral shaft fractures.

REHABILITATION

Weight-bearing restrictions, determined by the surgeon, depend on the degree of fracture instability and method of surgical stabilization. The rehabilitation program can be introduced at the bedside level and advanced as appropriate.

If no weight-bearing restrictions are in place, rehabilitation can proceed as follows.

Postoperative day 1: bed or chair level exercises consisting of active range of motion of the quadriceps, and ankle dorsiflexors and plantar flexors. Instruction in peforming activities of daily living safely to reduce pain and further injury and the proper use of adaptive equipment is introduced.

Postoperative day 2 to 5: bed to chair mobility and transfer training, gait training with assistive devices, and wheelchair mobility training.

Postoperative day 6 to 10: advanced transfer training (eg, car) and mobility training (eg, stairs).

Outpatient rehabilitation is recommended for progressive strengthening and endurance training 8 to 12 weeks postdischarge.

■ KNEE ARTHROPLASTY

Knee arthroplasty is indicated for treatment of advanced degenerative joint disease (osteoarthritis, rheumatoid arthritis, and traumatic arthritis) that is unresponsive to conservative management.

Symptoms and signs include the following:

- Intractable pain
- Functional mobility impairment
- Knee instability
- Valgus, varus, and knee flexion deformities

Common complications after knee arthroplasty include the following:

- Deep vein thrombosis
- Infection
- Patellofemoral instability, patellar fracture
- Arthrofibrosis
- Aseptic loosening
- Peroneal nerve palsy

Diagnostic imaging anteroposterior view, a lateral view, a 45° posteroanterior view of the knee, and a skyline view (or sunrise view) of the patella. Loss of joint space, cysts, subchondral sclerosis, and osteophytes confirm the diagnosis of osteoarthritis.

Rehabilitation after knee arthroplasty usually progresses as follows.

Postoperative day 1:

Bed or chair level exercises consisting of active range of motion of the quadriceps, gluteals, and ankle dorsiflexors and plantar flexors.

Postoperative day 2:

Knee flexibility exercises introduced measuring the degree of active knee flexion, active assisted knee flexion, and terminal knee extension to reduce the risk of contracture and gait abnormality.

Strengthening exercises—ankle dorsiflexors and plantar flexors, quadriceps and gluteal sets, straight leg raises, and isometric hip adduction.

Gait training with an assistive device and functional transfer training (eg, sit-to-stand, toilet transfers, and bed mobility).

Postoperative days 3 to 5:

Progression of ADL training, range of motion, strengthening exercises, and ambulation on level surface and stairs with assistive device.

Orthopedic Sample Order Set

Scott J. Lepre

Specific Challenges

Orthopedic procedures are one of the most common reasons for referral to inpatient rehabilitation units. And while these patients may seem straightforward, they present unique challenges that must be addressed and properly managed.

It must always be remembered that each patient is unique, and the physiatrist cannot expect each patient to have the exact same rehabilitation process even when the same procedure has been performed. There are many different variables that will need to be considered for each patient, including the following:

■ Premorbid medical issues (especially previous surgical interventions)

■ Postoperative medical complications (ie, wound infection, post operative anemia, etc)

■ Previous exposure to pain medications (if patient has taken narcotics in the past, they might need higher doses to manage their pain; if the patient has never taken narcotics before, they might be more sensitive to them)

■ Different surgical techniques (ie, use of a cemented vs uncemented prosthesis)

■ Different life circumstances/functional responsibilities

■ Different emotional/coping mechanisms

■ Premorbid functional status

This sample order set will serve as a guideline to address the most common and critical issues encountered during the inpatient rehabilitation of the orthopedic patient. Not all items will apply to every patient, and the patient's unique circumstances must always be considered.

Diagnosis: Describe the specific orthopedic procedure performed and be sure to specify the side (ie, Open Reduction Internal Fixation of Left Femur Fracture, Right Total Hip Arthroplasty)

Admit To: Acute rehabilitation unit (CIIRP—Comprehensive Integrated Inpatient Rehabilitation Program)

Condition: Stable, guarded, and so on. (All patients should be medically stable upon admission to inpatient rehabilitation, but each patient must be assessed in this regard.)

Nursing:

■ Vital sign frequency (ie, q shift, q8 hours)

■ Wound care/surgical dressing orders (ie, wet to dry, leave open to air, etc— should be specified in the transfer orders; if not, check with the surgeon)

■ Bladder scan orders if needed (if patient has recently had a foley catheter removed, check post void residual (PVR) and write parameters for clean intermittent catheterization (CIC); usually performed if PVR is >300 mL)

■ IV access (depends on the policy of the specific rehabilitation unit if IV access is needed for all patients or just when indicated)

■ Line care orders (write for PICC line care if patient has a PICC)

■ Trach care orders (if patient has a trach)

■ PEG care orders (if patient has a PEG)

■ Parameters for when to notify M.D. (ie, notify M.D. for systolic blood pressure >180 (parameters may vary based on patient and national guidelines) or fever >38.5, blood sugar <60 or >400 etc)

■ Patient education/teaching (ie, diabetes teaching, nutritional counseling, and self injection teaching for lovenox)

■ Oxygen requirements (ie, put patient on nasal canula oxygen to keep O2 sats >90%)

■ Brace use (if the patient has a brace, specific usage instructions should be provided with the transfer orders, ie, wear knee immobilizer at all times)

■ continuous passive movement or CPM for Total Knee Arthoplasty (use of these devices is controversial).

Precautions: Fall precautions, hip precautions (for hip replacement)

Activity: As tolerated, ambulate with assistance, weight-bearing limitations (be sure to specify exactly what the weight-bearing limitations are, for example non-weight-bearing, partial weight-bearing, toe touch weight-bearing, etc)

Allergies: List if any present (be sure to confirm with the patient and to ask the type of reaction) or NKDA if none

Medications:

Bowel Regimen (important since most patients will be on opioids for pain):
■ Colace 100 mg PO BID

■ Senna 2 tabs PO Daily

■ Bisacodyl suppository prn constipation

Pain Control: The first step is to determine the exact etiology of the pain (surgical pain vs DVT if pain is in the calf; muscle soreness vs neuropathic pain, especially if patient has concomitant risk factors such as DM). It is critical in these patients to achieve and maintain adequate pain control, in order to enable the patient to participate fully in therapies and achieve their goals. There are many options for pain control, from nonnarcotics, to narcotics, and to other agents. The choice of which medication to use should be based on the patient's current medical status, prior use of pain medications, age, and specific nature of the pain. The specific agents used and doses may vary depending on surgical or patient factors. The agents and dosages below are examples of common starting doses unless otherwise specified.

Short-Acting Narcotics:

■ Oxycodone 5 to 10 mg PO q4 to q6 hours prn breakthrough pain

■ Morphine Sulfate Immediate Release (MSIR) 15 mg PO q4 hours prn breakthrough pain

■ Oxycodone/Acetaminophen (Percocet®) 5/325mg 1 to 2 tabs PO 4 to 6 hours prn breakthrough pain

Long-Acting Narcotics:
■ Oxycodone extended release (Oxycontin®) 10 mg PO q12 hours

■ MSSR 15 mg PO BID

■ Fentanyl Transdermal Patch 12.5 or 25 mcg q72 hours

Other:

■ Lidocaine Transdermal Patch 5% (Lidoderm®) q12 hours (on for 12 hours, then off for 12 hours; patch should not be placed directly on the incision but can be cut and placed on either side of the incision)

■ Acetaminophen 650 mg PO q4 to q6 hours prn breakthrough pain (can have a synergistic effect when used with narcotics; use with caution in patients with liver disease, maximum daily dose — 4000 mg)

■ Nonsteroidal antiinflammatories (ie, Ibuprofen 400 mg PO q6 hours prn breakthrough pain—use with caution in patients with kidney disease)

Diet: Per patient's PMH and current dietary needs (regular vs carb control for diabetics vs cardiac diet for patients with cardiac history). It is important to ensure that the patient is getting adequate PO nutrients in order to provide the body with the materials it needs to allow proper wound healing.

Therapies/Consults

Physical Therapy: Specific therapies will depend on the nature of the operation, the joint/bone involved, patient's premorbid level of functioning, and expected goals for discharge. The majority of orthopedic patients will need significant attention to ROM (especially joint replacements), strengthening of affected limbs, endurance (due to increased energy requirement of mobility), gait, balance, transfers, and stairs.

Occupational Therapy: ADLs, strength, use of adaptive equipment, and fine motor coordination (UE injuries).

Speech and Language Pathology: Not needed normally. Consider evaluation if other conditions exist and appropriate.

Orthotics: Depending on the nature of the injury/surgery, certain orthotics may be needed (ie, knee immobilizer)

Psychology: Evaluation variable depending on surrounding issues.

Vocational Rehab: May be appropriate depending on the nature/severity of the injury/surgery and nature of the patient's work.

Social Work: Discharge planning, family training.

Modalities: Use of heat or ice can be helpful for treating swelling and pain.

Prophylaxis
Skin: Monitor surgical site for signs of wound infection (erythema, drainage, and warmth). It is normal for there to be some redness directly surrounding individual surgical staples (staple erythema), but further investigation is warranted if the erythema extends further. Monitor for signs of skin breakdown over common areas of pressure sores (heels, sacrum). Educate on pressure relief and use multipodus boots as needed.

Edema: Postoperative edema of the affected limb is common; however, unilateral edema must always be investigated for DVT as a potential etiology. Calf tenderness, chest pain (PE), and tachycardia (PE) are warning signs of a more serious problem. Venous Doppler of the affected limb or spiral CT/VQ scan of the chest should be ordered, and therapy held until results are obtained.

DVT: The specific agents and dosages used generally depend on the surgeon's discharge instructions.

■ Lovenox

■ Heparin

■ Coumadin

Gastrointestine:

■ H2 blocker

■ Proton pump inhibitors

Labs: Routine labs should be ordered on admission to establish baseline (CBC, BMP). INR should be checked daily if patient is on Coumadin until therapeutic. Albumin and prealbumin should be checked if patient is at nutritional risk.

Estimated Length of Stay: Should be patient and situation dependent. Simple unilateral joint replacements may require as little as 3 days. More complex orthopedic procedures, multiple traumas, and procedures resulting in limitations in weight-bearing can prolong the rehabilitation stay. In general, the majority of orthopedic patients should be able to achieve their rehabilitation goals within 5 to 10 days.

Rehabilitation Goals: Will depend on the patient and their unique life circumstances. If the patient lives alone and will not have any assistance, they will need to be independent in ambulation, transfers, and self-care. If they will not be alone, then these goals may vary from independence to some level of assistance.

1. Ambulation/Mobility

2. Transfers

3. Self-care/ADLs

4. Pain control

5. Strengthening/ROM

6. Endurance

Equipment: Braces, limb immobilizers, and other equipment should be detailed. Other equipment needs are to be determined during rehab stay.

■ **BIBLIOGRAPHY**

1. Cifu D, Burnett, McGowan J. Rehabilitation after hip fracture. In: Grabois M, ed. *Physical Medicine & Rehabilitation*. Cambridge, MA: Blackwell Science, Inc.; 1997.

2. Dechert TA, Duane TM, Frykberg BP, Aboutanos MB, Malhotra AK, Ivatury RR. Elderly patients with pelvic fracture: interventions and outcomes. *Am Surg.* 2009;75(4):291–295.

3. Egan M, Jaglal S, Byrne K, Wells J, Stolee P. Factors associated with a second hip fracture: a systematic review. *Clin Rehabil.* 2008;22(3):272–282.
4. Flanagan SR, Ragnarsson KT, Ross MK, Wong DK. Rehabilitation of the geriatric orthopaedic patient. *Clin Orthop Relat Res.* 1995;316:80–92.
5. Lyons AR. Clinical outcomes and treatment of hip fractures. *Am J Med.* 1997;103(2A):51S–64S.
6. Schneider M, Kawahara I, Ballantyne G, et al. Predictive factors influencing fast track rehabilitation following primary total hip and knee arthroplasty. *Arch Orthop Trauma Surg.* 2009;129(12):1585–1591.

Osteopathic Medicine in Musculoskeletal Conditions

Nathan J. Neufeld and John M. Jones

■ INTRODUCTION

Osteopathic manipulative medicine (OMM) is a diagnostic and thera-peutic tool used in many types of illness and disease. Hands-on treat-ment of musculoskeletal structures is used to reduce pain and normalize performance by reestablishing normal function of the body. This prag-matic approach to the neuromusculoskeletal system is ideally suited to address many complaints in physical medicine and rehabilitation. Osteopathic medicine has the goal of removing obstructions to the body's normal movement and fluid flow (vascular and lymphatic) to optimize function, given the patient's circumstances.

In this chapter, we will give examples of simple OMM (also known as osteopathic manipulative treatment, or OMT) for common bother-some syndromes seen by physiatrists. OMM has minimal side effects, and with an appropriate selection of techniques, it is safe to be used on the vast majority of patients. The suggested treatment schemes of this chap-ter are for both those trained in OMM and those without formal OMM training who are interested in understanding some very straightforward approaches to patient care. These options of treatment are not meant to be exhaustive, but rather a quick reference of initial treatment ideas for common syndromes. For further inquiry and or study, please see listed references. The American Academy of Osteopathy, an osteopathic medi-cal specialty college, offers courses which are open to interested allo-paths. Those who identify specific value of OMM for a patient but are not interested in doing this type of treatment may refer to a physician who practices OMM (visit www.osteopathic.org to find a physician).

■ TYPES OF OMM

The sample treatments are based on 4 commonly taught OMM tech-niques: muscle energy (ME), counterstrain, myofascial release, and Still technique. Each of these is a system of diagnosis and treatment. OMM is based on analysis and treatment of the whole body, as biomechani-cal issues in one region affect all regions. The treatments presented, however, will often improve the patient's condition when used in isolation. If they do not, a more holistic analysis is warranted.

■ EPICONDYLITIS

Common findings:

Radial head somatic dysfunction

Restricted forearm pronation

Restricted forearm supination

Tenderness of epicondyle to palpation

Pain:

Elbow pain

Wrist pain

Treatment:

- Patient seated

- Physician facing patient

- Have the patient flex the forearm

- Support the proximal forearm with one hand, placing your index finger laterally and posteriorly behind the radial head

- Restricted supination:

  - With your other hand, grasp the distal forearm and introduce supination to the initial point of restriction

  - Have the patient attempt and maintain pronation against physician resistance for 3 to 5 seconds

  - After contraction, wait 2 seconds in the same position, then gently reengage forearm supination restriction

  - Repeat the procedure 3 to 5 times, slightly increasing the range of supination each time

- Restricted pronation:

  - Start as above. With your other hand, grasp the distal forearm and introduce pronation to the initial point of restriction

  - Have the patient attempt and maintain supination against physician resistance for 3 to 5 seconds

  - After contraction, wait 2 seconds in the same position, then gently reengage forearm pronation restriction

  - Repeat the procedure 3 to 5 times, slightly increasing the range of pronation each time

■ CARPAL TUNNEL SYNDROME (MEDIAN NEUROPATHY AT THE WRIST)

Common findings:

Tight transverse retinaculum

Tinel test

Weakness of affected hand

Pronator teres syndrome (proximal median nerve impingement)

Pain:

Tingling and numbness in digits on affected side

Radiating pain into hand

Radiating pain proximally in forearm

Treatment: Direct myofascial release

■ Patient in seated position

■ Physician facing the patient

■ Grasp the patient's affected wrist with both hands

■ Position thumbs over the transverse retinaculum

■ Apply deep and lateral pressure for 1 to 2 minutes to patient tolerance, stretching the soft tissue by slowly moving your thumbs outward as the tissue relaxes

■ Repeat on several visits as needed for symptoms to resolve

■ Can be done prophylactically on unaffected side

SELF-TREATMENT

Teach the patient to stretch the transverse retinaculum by pulling the tendons deeper into the carpal tunnel.

■ Have the patient place the affected hand palm down, with the middle and distal phalanges of the long and ring fingers against a flat surface

■ Place downward pressure on the long and ring fingers, while using the other hand to pull the thumb posteriorly for about 30 seconds

■ This can be done several times a day

■ LOW BACK PAIN
Possible diagnoses

Idiopathic low back pain (LBP)

Musculoskeletal LBP

Non-radiating LBP

Low back strain

Iliolumbar ligament syndrome

Psoas syndrome

Lumbar somatic dysfunction

Common findings

Tenderness to palpation of lumbar paravertebral musculature

Accentuated or diminished normal spinal curves

Compensatory postural or gait patterns

Functional leg length discrepancy

Pain

Lumbar myofascial pain

Abdominal pain

Groin pain

Treatment: Modified Still technique
   First, rule out ruptured disk, bony, neurologic, or soft tissue pathology. Once more, serious diagnoses are ruled out and a functional musculoskeletal condition remains, treat the musculoskeletal dysfunction.
   The treatment given is for the very common L5 somatic dysfunction; however, the same principle can be applied at superior lumbar segments after treating L5. LBP can come from many different causes and somatic dysfunctions, and the scope of this publication does not permit a full analysis. The sample below is for articulatory dysfunction at L5/S1 and multifidus/myofascial soft tissue texture abnormalities.

■ Position patient supine on the exam table with space for the examiner to move freely

■ Place the fingers of your most cephalad hand under the patient at L5 to monitor the segment; check for tenderness lateral to the spinous process (if treating at superior levels, at the transverse processes)

■ Flex hip and knee toward the abdomen with most caudal hand on the patient's knee of side nearest the examiner

■ Continue to slowly flex hip to point where you feel motion at your finger behind the vertebra

■ Adduct the thigh slightly, noting whether abnormal tissue texture decreases at your palpating finger (if so, this is a flexion somatic dysfunction of L5)

   ■ The patient should feel some degree of pain or tension resolution

   ■ If no resolution is noticed, slowly abduct the hip to about 60° while retaining flexion to L5 This should be accompanied by a palpable release of tissue tension (if so, this is an extension somatic dysfunction of L5)*

- ■ Ideally, complete resolution of the tenderness is noticed when the area is re-palpated; however, significant improvement without complete resolution may yield success

■ Once the position of greatest resolution is found:

- ■ Apply a slight compressive force through the knee toward the lumbar spine

- ■ While maintaining this compression, slowly move the knee laterally (for a flexion dysfunction, medially across the midline for an extension dysfunction), then extend it and the hip in a smooth arc, ending up with the leg fully extended on the table.

ADDITIONAL LBP OMM TREATMENTS

Virtually, any form of OMM can be selected and used to treat LBP, depending on the training of the physician, the condition of the patient, and the application of good clinical judgment.

Lumbar spine, pelvis, or sacral somatic dysfunctions are often treated with the following:

ME

Counterstrain

Myofascial release

High velocity low amplitude

Still technique

Craniosacral

■ PSOAS SYNDROME

Possible diagnoses:

Lumbar sprain/strain

LBP

Acute iliopsoas strain

Hypertonic Iliopsoas

Common findings:

Patient is unable to straighten up, and is leaning toward affected side

Tenderness in the iliac fossa

+Thomas test (functional)

---

*If neither flexion nor extension positions decrease the L5 tissue texture abnormalities and eliminate the majority of tenderness, the somatic dysfunction is probably Type I. Refer to the reference for this treatment position.

Pain:

Deep LBP

Leg, groin or pelvic pain

Sacroiliac joint pain

TREATMENT

Counterstrain technique:

- Patient in the supine position
- Physician on the side of the dysfunction
- Find the tender point about 5 cm medial to the anterior superior iliac spine (ASIS) and deep in the iliac fossa
- Maintain a monitoring finger on the tender point
- Have the patient flex the hips and knees to about 90°, placing your thigh under the distal legs
- Have the patient spread the knees apart, so that the thighs are abducted and in external rotation
  - Fine tune the position by passively flexing the patient's hips farther, or inducing further external rotation on the affected side by moving the affected thigh into further abduction
- Hold for 90 seconds in this position
- Slowly and passively return the patient's hips, thighs, and legs to neutral position
- Retest the tender point

Goal: Achievement of at least 70% reduction of tenderness after the patient is returned to neutral position

■ FUNCTIONAL LEG LENGTH DISCREPANCY

Possible diagnoses:

Short leg syndrome

Runner's short leg syndrome

Pelvic somatic dysfunction

Common findings:

Limp

Functional scoliosis

Foot arch asymmetry

Pelvic asymmetry

Pain:

LBP—secondary to compensatory scoliosis

Sacroiliac pain

Pelvic pain

Knee pain

Foot arch pain

TREATMENT: ME TECHNIQUE
Pelvic asymmetry

Short leg treatment—posterior rotation of ipsilateral pelvis

- Patient in prone position
- Physician on side opposite to the dysfunction
- With your caudad hand, grasp the flexed knee of affected side
- Place your cephalad hand over the posterior superior iliac spine (PSIS) on the side of dysfunction
- Passively extend the hip until you feel motion at the PSIS
- Have the patient pull the knee down toward the table
- Have the patient maintain this muscle contraction for 3 to 5 seconds
- Have the patient relax, then wait 2 seconds in same position; gently reengage the hip extension barrier
- Repeat patient contraction 3 to 5 times, resetting to the barrier after each contraction

Long leg treatment—anterior rotation of contralateral pelvis

- Patient in supine position
- Physician on the side of the dysfunction
- With your caudad hand, grasp the thigh under the ipsilateral flexed knee
- Place your cephalad hand on the ASIS on the side of the dysfunction
- Passively flex the hip until motion is sensed at the ASIS
- Have the patient push the thigh against your hand, and maintain the contraction for 3 to 5 seconds
- Have the patient relax, then wait 2 seconds in the same position; gently reengage the hip flexion barrier
- Repeat patient contraction 3 to 5 times, resetting to the barrier after each contraction

■ PIRIFORMIS SYNDROME

Common findings:

History of fall on buttocks

Postpartum

Pelvic asymmetry

Pain:

Buttock pain

Hip pain/greater trochanteric pain

LBP

Pelvic pain

Tender point location:

■ Find while patient is in the prone position

■ The tender point is located half to two-thirds of the way on a line between the inferior lateral angle (ILA) of the sacrum and the greater trochanter (muscle body/musculotendinous junction of the piriformis)

Treatment: Counterstrain technique

■ Patient in supine position*

■ Physician on the affected side

■ Find the tender point and monitor it with one finger

■ Flex the hip (90° or more) and knee on the affected side

■ Shorten the muscle further by adding hip abduction and external rotation until tenderness is decreased by 70% or more

■ Hold for 90 seconds in this position of least tension

■ Slowly and passively return the lower extremity to neutral

■ Reassess the tender point by palpating it with your monitoring finger

Goal: Achievement of at least 70% reduction of tenderness after the patient is returned to neutral position

■ PROXIMAL TIBIOFIBULAR JOINT PAIN

Common findings:

Decreased range of ankle motion

Tenderness of fibular head to palpation

Pain with running or walking

---

*This technique can also be done in the prone position with affected leg over side of table, accompanied by hip flexion, external rotation, and abduction.

Pain:

Fibular head glide restriction with malalignment

Impingement of deep peroneal nerve

Treatment: Modified Still technique

- Patient in seated position
- Find ankle direction of least movement
    - Decreased ankle plantar flexion—fibular head has restricted posterior glide
    - Decreased ankle dorsiflexion—fibular head has restricted anterior glide
- Place the affected knee into about 15° of flexion; place the ankle in the direction opposite to its restriction
- Have the patient relax the leg
- Apply a small axial force through the ankle with one hand while resisting force with the other hand at the fibular head
- With hand at the knee, apply translational force to the fibular head
    - Decreased ankle plantar flexion—apply an anterior to posterior force on the fibular head
    - Decreased ankle dorsiflexion—apply a posterior to anterior force on the fibular head
- While continuing to apply axial force and translational force on fibular head, start with the ankle in the most relaxed position and place it through the range of motion toward the direction of the restriction
- Retest the proximal fibular head glide

■ INVERSION ANKLE SPRAIN

Possible diagnoses:

Lateral ankle sprain

Recurrent ankle sprain

Chronic ankle pain

First- and second-degree acute ankle sprains

Common findings:

Weak tibialis anterior

Weak fibularis (peroneal) musculature

Restricted dorsiflexion

Ankle instability

Pain:

Lateral ankle pain

Knee pain

Low back pain

Proximal tibiofibular pain

Treatment: Counterstrain technique

■ Patient in lateral recumbent position with affected side down on table

■ Have the patient flex the knee, placing the affected foot and lateral malleolus over the edge of the table

■ Place a rolled towel under the distal fibula to provide padding for comfort

■ With monitoring hand, grasp the affected ankle proximal to the malleolus

■ Find the diagnostic tender point in a depression about 3 cm anterior to and inferior to the posterior portion of the lateral malleolus

■ With operating hand, grasp the planter aspect of the mid-foot

■ Place the foot in eversion

■ Apply up to 15 kg of pressure (promoting eversion) through the thenar eminence of the operating hand, focused at a point approximately 3 cm distal to the medial malleolus

■ Adjust the position and patient comfort with external rotation and plantar flexion, until tenderness is reduced by at least 70%

■ Hold in this position for 90 seconds

■ Slowly and without patient assistance, return ankle to neutral

■ Retest tender point

Goal: Achievement of at least 70% reduction of tenderness after the patient is returned to neutral position

■ **PLANTAR FASCIITIS**

Common findings:

Tenderness to palpation of plantar fascia

Tight gastrocnemius and Achilles tendon

Flat arches

High arches

Pain:

Plantar fascia

- Inflammation
- Muscle hypertonicity

Heel pain

Calf pain

Treatment: Counterstrain technique

- Patient in prone position
- Physician on the affected side
- Find the tender point on the plantar surface at the most distal aspect of the calcaneus where the plantar fascia attaches
- Flex the knee on the affected side to about 70°
- Place your foot on the table, and the dorsal surface of the patient's foot on your thigh
- With your cephalad hand, push the calcaneus toward your thigh, shortening the plantar fascia
- At the same time, use your other hand to push the distal foot toward the tender point, shortening the plantar fascia from the distal end until the tenderness is decreased by at least 70%
- Hold for 90 seconds in this position of least tension
- Slowly and without patient assistance return ankle back to neutral
- Reassess the tender point by palpating it with your monitoring finger

Goal: Achievement of at least 70% reduction of tenderness after the patient is returned to neutral position

■ ACKNOWLEDGMENTS
We would like to acknowledge the contributions and suggestions of Christopher C. Smith, DO, Florida Hospital East Orlando, Department of Osteopathic Family Medicine, to the writing of this chapter.

■ FURTHER READING
1. Jones LH, Kusunose R, Goering E. Jones Strain-Counterstrain. American Academy of Osteopathy; Indianapolis, 1995. ISBN: 0964513544. *www.jonesinstitute.com.*
2. Rennie PR, Glover JC, Carvalho C, Key LS. Counterstrain & Exercise: An Integrated Approach. 2nd ed. American Academy of Osteopathy; Indianapolis, 2001. ISBN: 0971275815. *www.renniematrix.com.*

3. Van Buskirk RL. The Still Technique Manual: Applications of a Rediscovered Technique of Andrew Taylor Still, MD. 2nd ed. American Academy of Osteopathy; Indianapolis, 2006, 1995. ISBN: 0940668114.

4. Ward RC, Hurby RJ, Jerome JA, Jones JM, Kappler RE. Foundations for Osteopathic Medicine. 2nd ed. Lippincott Williams & Wilkins; Philadelphia, 2003. ISBN: 0781734975.

20

Pain Management

Jarrod David Friedman

Pain is a more terrible lord of mankind than even death itself.
—Albert Schweitzer

■ EPIDEMIOLOGY

According to the National Center for Health Statistics, 76.2 million people a had pain issue or were treated for pain during 2006 at an estimated cost of approximately 100 billion dollars, in health care expenses, lost income, and lost productivity. In the same report it was noted that 37% of Americans aged 20 years or more and almost 60% of those aged 65 years or more reported pain (1,2). For comparison, there are 23.6 million people with diabetes or 23.3 million people with coronary artery diseases in the United States according to the American Diabetes Association and American Heart Association, respectively.

Of the 40 millio5n visits for new pain to primary care physicians (PCPs), 41% was for musculoskeletal pain issues (3). Acute pain issues made up 15% to 20% of those complaints, subacute pain 50% to 60%, and chronic pain 25% to 30%. Of all complaints, low back pain was the most common diagnosis and cause for missed workdays with an annual incidence of 15% to 20% of the adult population and a lifetime incidence of 60% to 85% of the population (4). Approximately 14% of U.S. adults have serious chronic back conditions.

■ PAIN EVALUATION

"See things as they truly are and not as you wish them to be!"
—Jack Walsh

Pain is a subjective experience. Currently, there is no system that definitively provides independent data to determine a patients' degree of pain. There are tools that help determine how a patient's pain is affecting or impairing their function, but these are for the most part subjective. They rely on patients being sincere and honest in their answers, but they have good reliability. A list of some common questionnaires is noted below (Table 20.1). Refer to Table 20.2 for the Functional Pain Scale.

TABLE 20.1 ■ Scales used for evaluating pain.

Questionnaire	Description
McGill Pain Questionnaire	Developed in 1971 by Melzack and Torgerson, these 20 questions group various descriptive words together and patients are to pick 1–2 words that describe their pain.
Pain Disability Index	Developed 1987 by Tait et al, it is designed to measure the impact of chronic pain on various daily activities.
Cancer Total Quality Pain Management Patient Assessment Tool (TQPM)	Developed by Paice et al, in 1998, it measures pain management outcomes, expectations, barriers, and satisfaction of inpatients as well as outpatients.
Profile Fitness Mapping (PFM)	This was developed between 1992 and 1994 at the Alfta Rehabilitation Center in Sweden as a clinical-based back-specific questionnaire that incorporates both functional limitation and a symptom scale along with subclassification of severity and temporal aspects of symptomatology (5).
Becks Depression Inventory-II	Originally developed in 1961 and revised and republished in 1996 by Dr. Aaron T. Beck, it includes 21 multiple-choice questions. The score (0–63) is reliable for measuring the severity of depression. No depression (0–9); mild to moderate (10–18); moderate to severe (19–29); and severe (30–63) (6) 1996.
Functional Pain Scale (FPS)	This scale was developed specifically to incorporate both subjective and objective components and reliably assess pain in older adults (7).

TABLE 20.2 ■ Functional pain scale (Adult).

Functional Pain Scale	Simple	Description
0	No pain	No functional impairment
1	Tolerable	Does not interfere with activities
2	Tolerable	Interferes with some activities
3	Intolerable	Able to use phone, TV, or read
4	Intolerable	Unable to use phone, TV, or read, ambulate
5	Intolerable	Unable to verbally communicate

Treating pain like most other areas of medicine requires skills in the evaluation, observation, and interpretation of diagnostic, radiologic, and interventional techniques to determine the cause of a patient's pain as well as to evaluate their response to medications and other treatments.

PAIN MANAGEMENT GUIDELINES
There are several basic approaches to the treatment of pain, and clinical guidelines also vary depending on the group's point of view. There are 4 societies whose mission is primarily pain management that have very different perspectives on treatment and different algorithms for the treatment of pain (Table 20.3).

As an example, many health care payers and some physicians question the validity of discography (for discogenic pain) based on a single randomized controlled trial (8) in 2000 concluding that discography was affected by somatization. Other studies challenge this conclusion. A study by Manchikanti et al. in 2001 (9) reported that when properly performed, discography is not affected by somatization disorder at all (10). Other studies by Derby et al (11,12) and Bogduk (13,14) showed that when properly performed by a trained interventional pain physician, the technique was approximately 80% specific. This is one example of how conflicting evidence can affect clinical practice and the development of practice guidelines. Because of this, we recommended that all practitioners involved in pain management be familiar with guidelines from the groups mentioned in Table 20.3 and that in areas of conflicting evidence, practitioners review the primary literature to draw conclusions.

PHYSICAL EXAMINATION
The physical examination is a very important component of any evaluation. Pain patterns are suggestive but not always consistent with the origin of a pain. The goal of the physical examination is to help narrow the differential diagnosis, as it pertains to the potential causes of a patient's pain.

The spine is the most common source of pain. The intricacy of spinal anatomy complicates diagnosis because any of the multiple parts of the

TABLE 20.3 ■ Source and focus of available pain management guidelines.

Society	Focus
American Pain Society	Noninvasive focus—medications and Physical Therapy
American Society of Interventional Pain Physicians	Combination of medications and interventional therapy
North American Spine Society	Surgical focus
International Spine Interventional Society	Interventional focus

spine can refer pain to the same area or cause pain focally. Nerve compression, nerve root irritation, and facet joints can all cause pain both in the spinal area and pain referred to the extremities. It is important to understand that facet joints and nerve root irritation can result in pain in the extremities. Intervertebral disc issues can cause both axial back pain and pain in the extremity by causing nerve root irritation.

The spine is commonly divided into 3 columns to describe stability and the need for surgical intervention.

The 3-column principle can be used for localizing common spinal pathologies or causes of spinal pain, which is again the most prevalent source of back pain. The 3-column primary reference point is the spinal canal, thus, dividing the spine into anterior canal, intraspinal canal, and posterior spinal canal areas (Table 20.4). Thinking about the spine in this context provides a framework to systematically evaluate spinal sources of pain and to determine appropriate treatment. Figure 20.1 illustrates how to apply this approach in the case of lumbar pain.

The usual general physical evaluation of the patient with a painful complaint should include inspection, palpation, range of motion (ROM), sensation, and strength. Below are some physical signs or symptoms that are useful when evaluating these patients.

GENERAL APPEARANCE

Overall appearance can give some insights as to the presence and severity of pain. These nonspecific signs cannot be correlated to pain severity objectively (Table 20.5).

PROVOCATIVE MANEUVERS

Physical examination maneuvers can help the diagnostician to narrow down the possible areas of pathology (Table 20.6).

A study has shown that a positive response to interventional facet joint therapy or diagnostic medial branch block (which if confirmed twice will respond to radiofrequency ablation of the medial branch

TABLE 20.4 ■ The 3-column division of the spine.

Anterior Spinal Column or Anterior Spine	Middle Spinal Column or Intraspinal Canal	Posterior Column or Posterior Spine
Posterior longitudinal ligament	Spinal cord	Lamina
Vertebral body	Nerve roots	Facet joints
Intravertebral disc	Pedicles	Intraspinal ligament
Anterior longitudinal ligament	Epidural space	Spinous process
	Contents of spinal canal	Paraspinal muscles

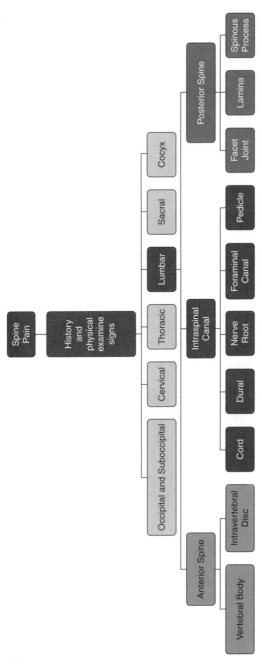

FIGURE 20.1 ■ Example of using the 3-column approach for lumbar spinal pain. Using this approach, all the potential sources of pain are evaluated systematically.

TABLE 20.5 ■ General appearance of signs of distress in patients with pain.

General Signs	Female Specific	Male Specific
Facial grimacing	Makeup absent	Unshaven
Crying	No jewelry	Hair not brushed
Decreased general movement	Unkempt hair/ not done	No shower
Strained or pressured voice	Unkempt clothes	Unkempt clothes
Decreased concentration		
Constant movement or no movement		

TABLE 20.6 ■ Provocative maneuvers and physical examination signs to determine site of spinal pathology.

Location	Methods of Evaluation	Description and Findings
Facet joints	Facet loading	Rotation and extension focal at suspected level of pathology results in pain being produced at the involved level.
	Extension/ hyperextension	Pain will be noted during the extension phase as the problematic level of the facets is activated.
	Rising from a flexed position	From a seated position the patient arises. Patient reports pain focally in the back at the levels involved.
	Focal palpation	In patients where soft tissue allows, palpation occurs lateral to the spinous process over the region of the facets. Pressure to the facet capsule will result in pain. In some cases, muscle spasms will prevent this palpation.
	Decreased or impaired range of motion in suspected spinal segment not otherwise expected	Instructions: Palpate over each spinal segment as the individual segment is activated in the movement of extension, flexion, or rotation. Alteration in normal movement, a halt to the movement process, or pain noted by the patient as an individual segment is activated will suggest that the segment is involved in the pain process.

(Continued)

TABLE 20.6 ■ (*Continued*)

Location	Methods of Evaluation	Description and Findings
	Blot maneuver	Posterior to anterior load performed by placing the palm across the area of the 1–2 individual spinous levels while the patients is lying flat on his/her stomach and then applying a light to moderate light load briefly. This should produce pain at the involved segment.
Vertebral body or disc	Spinal loading	Produces pain
	Prolonged sitting	Produces pain
	Blot maneuver	Palm over only 1 segment with moderate load will result in pain.
	Prolonged standing	Produces pain
Vertebral body or disc	Movement avoidance	Patient may prefer to stay still with no rotation, extension, or flexion
	Flexion or extension	Pain on flexion is suggestive
	Blot maneuver	Produces pain (as described above but with moderate to heavy pressure)

TABLE 20.7 ■ Pain duration descriptors.

Pain Type	Duration/Time
Acute pain	0–4 weeks
Subacute pain	1–6 months
Chronic pain	6 months or more

nerve) is likely if 5 or more of the facet joint maneuvers detailed in Table 20.6 are positive (92% positive predictive value) (15).

PAIN TIMELINE

Pain duration should be described in every case. Commonly accepted terminology is described in Table 20.7.

SPECIFIC PAIN CONDITIONS

ACUTE PAIN

Acute pain makes up 15% to 20% of all pain issues or 40 million visits a year to PCPs. The approach for treating acute pain differs between different health care professionals. For a physiatrist, the primary goal is to determine and treat risk factors, biomechanical imbalances, and pathologies that result in acute pain. Once the aforementioned problems are determined, a treatment program will be developed to educate, adapt, or fix biomechanical imbalances and treat the primary pathology causing the patients pain (Figure 20.2).

ACUTE PAIN SAMPLE CASE

The patient is a 34-year-old male with acute new onset back pain.

History of present illness: A 34-year-old male reports with a 2-week history of back pain after lifting a box at home. Pain was immediate. Pain worsened with bending and sitting at work for long periods. He was seen by his PCP who ordered a magnetic resonance imaging (MRI), which was negative. Currently, he only reports back pain without leg pain. He has no pain when coughing. No previous episodes of pain were reported.

Patient's goal: To regain full ROM and return to all his normal activity.

Medical history: Negative, healthy otherwise.

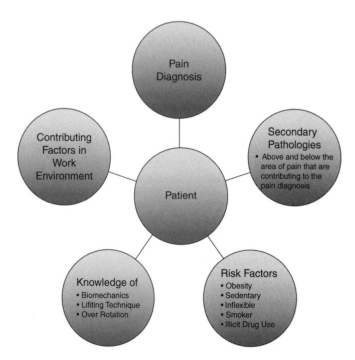

FIGURE 20.2 ■ Areas to consider in the evaluation of the patient with acute pain.

Family history: History of low back pain (mother, father, and 2 brothers, with multiple associated surgeries) and prostate cancer (father and brother).

Functional history: Completely independent before onset.

Social history: He has been smoking 1 pack per day for the past 20 years. He consumes approximately 6 beers a day and does not exercise regularly. He works full-time as a computer technician.

Medications: None

Review of systems: No bowel or bladder issues, no weakness.

Radiography: X-rays: normal alignment. MRI: no abnormalities.

Physical examination

General: Obese male, unkempt, poor sitting posture noted, pain score FPS 3 (intolerable but able to use phone, watch TV, and read paper).

Cervical spine

ROM: Decreased extension, flexion, rotation, and side bending.

Palpation: Tightness in muscles, facets negative free movement.

Specialty tests: Spurling's negative, facet loading negative.

Upper extremities: Within normal limits, shoulder examination negative.

Thoracic spine: Within normal limits, except for decreased ROM on rotation and side bending. Tightness on palpation of paraspinal muscles.

Abdominal: Obese, unable to go supine-sit without using secondary muscles.

Lumbar

ROM: Flexion to mid-thigh, extension normal, side bending decreased, rotation 10% to 20% of expected.

Palpation: bilateral paraspinal tenderness, no spinous process or intraspinous tenderness.

Strength: unable to perform extension secondary to pain.

Specialty test: Facet loading negative (no increase in pain), straight leg raise—no pain, cross straight leg raise—no pain, blot maneuver—negative for pain.

Pelvis: Bilateral hip ROM decreased on extension, flexion, and internal and external rotation. Ober's test positive. Faber's negative. No pain on sacroiliac joint palpation, pelvic rock negative, sacral blot negative.

Lower extremity: Within normal limits, strength 5/5 but tightness in all muscle groups.

Neurologic: No changes in sensation.

Assessment: A 34-year-old male with a 2-week history of low back pain with strong family history of lumbar disease with no neurologic signs.

Pain diagnosis: *Acute Lumbar Strain*

Secondary diagnoses:
1. Deconditioning
2. Obesity
3. Nicotine addiction
4. Core muscles weakness
5. Tightness of spinal musculature
6. Tightness of pelvic, bilateral hips, and lower extremities musculature
7. Poor posture and mechanics
with no history of training or education

Plan:

Diagnostic testing: None

Medication options

Antiinflammatories: Ibuprofen 600 to 800 mg orally three times a day for 2 to 4 weeks or Aleve 400 to 800 mg orally twice a day for 2 to 4 weeks.

If pain worsening or increased impairment: Consider oral steroids

Pain Medications

Tylenol 500 to 1000 mg orally 3 to 4 times a day as needed (no alcohol while taking), or

Tramadol 50 to 100 mg orally 2to 3 times a day as needed (maximum 300 mg/d)

Muscle relaxants: Cyclobenzaprine, Tizanidine, or Metaxalone

THERAPIES
Physical therapy: 2 to 3 per week for 4 to 6 weeks. Focus initially (first 2 weeks) on ROM and stretching of the lumbar spine, lower extremities, and hips then transition to strengthening and posture training. Upon discharge, patient should be instructed on a home exercise program for maintaining strength and ROM and proper lifting, sitting, and posture. Modalities: Heat and/or ice, transcutaneous electrical nerve stimulator as needed.

Education

1. Back school and education (physical therapy, seminars, and group classes that teach proper back mechanics and posture and safety techniques for lifting, pulling, pushing, etc.)

2. Referral to nutrition and dietary care

3. Weight loss program

4. Smoking cessation program

5. Alcohol consumption or alcohol-use cessation education

Complementary or alternative medicine:

1. Massage therapy 2 to 3 times per week for 4 to 6 weeks

2. Acupressure/acupuncture referral

Work recommendations: Consider workstation ergonomic evaluation.
Reevaluation: 2 to 4 weeks.

SUBACUTE PAIN

Subacute pain is the most prevalent type of pain that requires evaluation
and treatment according to initial visit to both the emergency room and
PCPs (16). In this setting, most patients have had the pain for a minimum
of 4 weeks and as long as 6 months. In these cases, an initial diagnosis
may have already been given.

*The primary components of a subacute pain evaluation are the
following:*

1. Ensure that all the underlying pathologies or disease processes
have been halted if possible.

2. Ensure all related pathologies and diagnoses have been determined
and treated.

3. Ensure that the pain is not referred from other areas or undiag-
nosed biomechanical dysfunction.

4. Ensure appropriate adherence to initial medical recommendations
or other recommendations.

SUBACUTE PAIN SAMPLE CASE

The patient is a 65-year-old female former factory worker with a known
diagnosis of cervical radicular pain and a C5 disc herniation with continued pain despite 6 weeks of physical therapy. She reported 60% pain
relief with the initial treatment plan and has undergone 2 epidural steroid injections.

Repeat epidural steroid injection or surgical referral for possible cervical discectomy and fusion are considerations; however, it would be
reasonable to reevaluate this patient and ensure that there is no residual
pain secondary to other spinal pathology such as facet-mediated pain
or shoulder pathology. For example, a previous otherwise stable partial rotator cuff tear could be aggravated by altered mechanics because
of severe radicular pain. These concomitant painful pathology overlaps
can be missed. Ensuring early pain control and adherence to treatment
are also necessary to prevent the development of a chronic pain syndrome. Educating the patient regarding all factors that contribute to their

pain is crucial. These include comorbid diseases, social behaviors (smoking, inactivity, or others), poor body mechanics, and work environment. Important factors to consider for the patient with subacute pain are summarized in Figure 20.3. Creating a treatment program that focuses on the multiple factors that may be contributing to continued pain is extremely important and can help minimize the conversion of a patient from subacute to chronic pain issues.

DIAGNOSTIC TESTING

As time goes by and painful complaints remain unresolved, the decision on further diagnostic testing should be based on the initial impression while considering other contributing factors as described above.

An important consideration is the patient's age. With increased age, the number of intraspinal or general pathologies that can be present on imaging evaluation increase without necessarily contributing to their pain issues. The multitude of spinal pathologies in the older population complicates evaluation and make more difficult to determine which is the primary pain generator. In those cases, diagnostic injections become increasingly

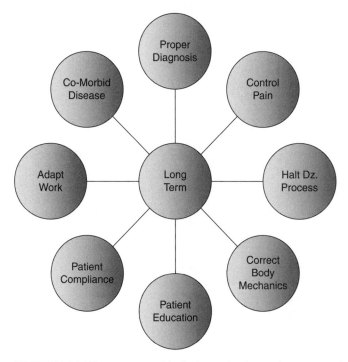

FIGURE 20.3 ■ Factors to consider in the evaluation and treatment of patients with subacute pain.

important to aid in making an accurate diagnosis. The diagnostic tests in a particular case should be based on the most likely pain generator (ie, bone, joint, muscle, nerve, spine, or soft tissues). The decision-making process is described in Figure 20.4. In the case of joint pain, the decision process for ordering diagnostic testing is described in Figure 20.5.

OPIOID PAIN MEDICATIONS
Opioids can be useful in managing pain in selected cases. The most common delivery routes are oral, intravenous, intramuscular, and transdermal. Opioids can have both short and long duration of effect from 15 to 20 minutes to 72 hours and are metabolized by either the liver or kidney or both.

The choice to start a patient on opioids varies depending on the physician's background, education, and experience level with opioid medication. The comfort level and experience a physician has prescribing opioids can affect their choices and use of these drugs.

Physicians should consider the following factors when deciding whether opioid pain medications are appropriate for a patient:

1. Pain is a subjective experience not fully understood. The ability of a particular patient to tolerate pain varies.

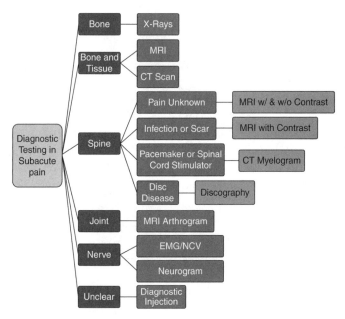

FIGURE 20.4 ■ Determination of appropriate diagnostic testing based on the primary pain generating system.

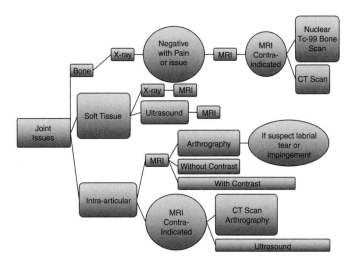

FIGURE 20.5 ■ Decision-making algorithm in cases of joint pain. Adapted from Ref. 19.

2. Patients respond to opioids differently. Some studies suggest that there might be genetic polymorphism for human opioid sensitivity (17). Patients with decreased opioid sensitivity may require higher doses of medication for appropriate pain relief and demonstrate drug-seeking or addictive behaviors that resolve when the pain is appropriately treated (also known as pseudoaddiction).

3. The purpose of any medication is to improve the quality of life, improve function, and when reasonable to return to normal function without resulting in additional damage to the injured region or another region.

There are some basic steps and factors to consider when deciding to start a patient on an opioid for pain management:

1. Opioids are medications and the disease they treat is pain.

2. Balancing risks, benefits, and side effects is crucial.

3. Patient should be

    a. consistent and dependable with follow-up visits and following instructions and

    b. able to understand the risk and the potential adverse-events associated with their medication

4. Contraindications or relative contraindications include the following:

    a. Nonorganic pain

    b. Patients providing inconsistent history and not making previous medical records available

    c. History of addiction to opioid medications

    d. Untreated psychiatric disease

    e. History of substance abuse (alcohol, cocaine, marijuana, etc.)

    f. Refusal or failure to follow physician recommendations

The choice between short- or long-acting opioids should be based on the individual patient and their pain generator, duration, and intensity. Short-acting opioids are better suited for pain that last for brief periods of time, occurring in association with specific activities, or occurring at specific times of the day. Long-acting opioids are designed for constant pain or for pain occurring during the majority of the day impairing function, quality of life, and participation in society. Long-acting opioids do not automatically increase a patient's risk for addiction, but dependence can develop and cessation of use can cause withdrawal symptoms (at higher doses). Short-acting pain medications such as oxycodone, hydrocodone, and morphine sulfate (immediate release) can be used to treat brief periods of break-through pain in patients using long-acting opioids to treat spikes of pain during the day (usually associated with increased levels of activity).

Most physicians will start with short-acting opioids and later convert the medication to a long-acting dosage when it becomes evident that 24-hour pain relief is necessary. The total daily dose of a short-acting opioid can be added and converted to a long-acting opioid medication used once or twice a day. Conversion from one opioid to another can be done using an equianalgesic opioid dose conversion table.

Physicians who treat their patients with regular opioid prescriptions should consider the following safeguards:

1. The practice should have clear guidelines and rules for opioid prescription.

2. Request the use of a single pharmacy for filling the prescriptions (the address and contact information should be provided to the clinic).

3. Request regular follow-up with a PCP.

4. Establish policies and procedures for performing drug screening, collecting urine sample, and performing pill count protocols.

5. One must understand and know the individual state and DEA guidelines and laws for prescribing Narcotic medications.

Diagnostic injections are helpful to determine the pain generators. The determination of what and where to inject is based on the clinical presentation and radiologic findings, but is also the art of interventional pain management. Diagnostic injections are not intended to permanently alleviate pain, though in some cases these injections can break the pain cycle and alleviate pain for some period of time. Please refer to the appendix for details on how to determine what interventional procedures can be used to diagnose the cause of a patient's pain.

CHRONIC PAIN

The factors noted in Figures 20.2 and 20.3 are involved and contribute in the process of acute and subacute pain progressing into chronic long-term pain. When comorbidities and precipitating factors are not treated and pain is not controlled, early pain worsens. Multimodal approaches as noted in Figure 20.6 can help minimize or halt pain progression.

Common issues that can preclude improvement if unnoticed include:

1. Obesity

2. Lack of flexibility of hips and legs, increasing stress across the spine, or general lack of flexibility

3. Depression

4. Sleep dysfunction

5. Obstructive sleep apnea

6. Poor posture

7. Poor body mechanics

8. Poor core and proximal strength

9. Smoking or illicit drug use

10. Psychological issues or psychiatric disease

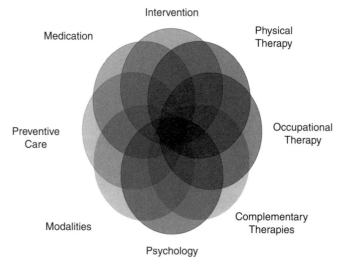

FIGURE 20.6 ■ Multimodal approach for pain management.

11. Poor understanding and knowledge of condition

12. Poor nutrition

13. Work ergonomics

14. Home ergonomics

15. Social stressors

Proper management of the patient as a whole addressing physical, emotional, and social stressors can help prevent pain from becoming chronic.

FACTS ABOUT INJECTIONS AND INJECTION AGENTS
Most injections will use a combination of an anesthetic and a corticosteroid.

ANESTHETICS
The faster the onset, the shorter the medication half-life. Fast agents should be considered when immediate local anesthesia is desired. Slow-acting anesthetics should be considered when a longer duration of analgesia is needed.

Fastest Onset		**Slowest Onset**	
Procaine	Lidocaine	Ropivacaine	Bupivicaine

The 2 most common anesthetics used are Lidocaine and Bupivicaine.

A. Lidocaine is supplied in concentrations of 1% to 5%. It has one of the fastest onsets (depending on the tissue onset, it is usually between 30 and 120 seconds). Duration of effect is approximately 1 to 2 hours.

B. Bupivicaine is supplied in concentrations of 0.25%, 0.50%, and 0.75% and has a slower onset but the duration can be between 2 and 6 hours.

STEROIDS
Common steroids used and their relative potency are listed below.

Generic	**Trade**	**Potency**
Cortisone		1
Hydrocortisone	Same	1.25
Triamcinolone	Kenalog	6
Prednisone		5
Methylprednisolone	Depo-Medrol	6
Dexamethasone	Decadron	33
Betamethasone	Celestone	41

For more information, visit the following Web sites:

Society	Web Site
American Academy of Pain Medicine	painmed.org
American Board of Pain Medicine	abpm.org
American Pain Society	AMPAIN.org
American Society of Interventional Pain Physicians	ASIPP.org
American Society of Regional Anesthesia and Pain Medicine	ASRA.com
International Association for the Study of Pain	iasp-pain.org
International Neuromodulation Society	neuromodulation.com
International Spine Interventional Society	Spinalinjection.org
North American Neuromodulation Society	neuromodulation.org
World institute of Pain	worldinstituteofpain .org/site/home.php
American Chronic Pain Association	theacpa.org (patient-based association)

Additional algorithms can be found in the appendix section.

■ REFERENCES

1. National Centers for Health Statistics, *Chartbook on Trends in the Health of Americans 2006, Special Feature: Pain.* http://www.cdc.gov/nchs/data/hus/hus06.pdf.
2. National Centers for Health Statistics, *Chartbook on Trends in the Health of Americans 2006, Special Feature: Pain;* Page 6.
3. National Centers for Health Statistics, Chartbook on Trends in the Health of Americans 2006, Special Feature: Pain.
4. National Centers for Health Statistics, Chartbook on Trends in the Health of Americans 2006, Special Feature: Pain.
5. Bjorklund M, Hamberg J, Heiden M, Barnekow-Bergkvist M. The assessment of symptoms and functional limitations in low back pain patients: validity and reliability of a new questionnaire. *Eur Spine* J. 2007;16(11):1799–1811
6. Beck AT, Steer RA, Ball R, Ranieri W. Comparison of beck depression inventories IA and II in psychiatric outpatients. J Pers Assess. 67(3):588–597.
7. Gloth FM III, Scheve AA, Stober CV, Chow S, Prosser J. The Functional Pain Scale: reliability, validity, and responsiveness in an elderly population. *J Am Med Dir Assoc.* 2001;2(3):110–114.
8. Carragee EJ, Chen Y, Tanner CM, Truong T, Lau E, Brito JL. Provocative discography in patients after limited lumbar discectomy: a controlled, randomized study of pain response in symptomatic and asymptomatic subjects. *Spine* (Phila Pa 1976). 2000;25(23):3065–3071.

9. Manchikanti L, Singh V, Pampati V, et al. Provocative discography in low back pain patients with or without somatization disorder: a randomized prospective evaluation. *Pain Physician*. 2001;4:227–239.

10. Manchikanti L, Singh V, eds. *Interventional Techniques in Chronic Spinal Pain*. Paducah, KY: ASIPP publishing; 2007.

11. Derby R., Howard M, Grant JM, Lettice JJ, Van Peteghem PK, Ryan DP. The ability of pressure controlled discography to predict surgical and non-surgical outcomes. *Spine*. 1999;24:364–371.

12. Derby R, Kim BJ, Lee SH, Chen Y, Seo KS, Aprill C. Comparison of discographic findings in asymptomatic subject discs and the negative disc and chronic LBP patients: can discography distinguish asymptomatic discs among morphologically abnormal discs? *Spine J*. 2005;5:389–394.

13. International Interventional Spine Society, Discography Review Course, 2007.

14. Bogduk N. Lumbar disc stimulation (provocation discography) in: practice Guidelines for Spinal Diagnostic and Treatment Procedures. ISIS 2004, pp 20–46.

15. Schwarzer AC, Aprill CN, Derby R, et al. Clinical features of patients with pain stemming from the lumbar zygapophyseal joints. Is the lumbar facet syndrome a clinical entity. *Spine*. 1994;19:1132–1137.

16. Manchikanti L, Singh V, eds. *Interventional Techniques in Chronic Spinal Pain*. Paducah, KY: ASIPP publishing; 2007.

17. Rathmell JP. *Atlas of image-guided interventional in Regional Anesthesia and Pain Medicine*. Philadelphia, PA: Lippincott; 2006:26–27.

Prosthetics, Orthotics, and Amputee Care*

Mark S. Hopkins and Katherine E. Binder

■ ORTHOTISTS AND PROSTHETISTS AND THE MULTIDISCIPLINARY REHABILITATION TEAM

The complete multidisciplinary rehabilitation team should include the prosthetist, orthotist, and Pedorthist. These health care professionals are uniquely trained to provide orthoses, prostheses, and pedorthic services. Prosthetists, orthotists, or prosthetist/orthotists (CP, CO, CPO) are health care professionals with the education and clinical training to evaluate, design, fit, and fabricate prostheses and/or orthoses. Pedorthics is the design, manufacture, and modification of pedorthic devices to prevent or alleviate foot problems caused by disease, congenital defect, overuse, or injury. A certified pedorthist is an individual who has studied foot anatomy and pathology, biomechanics, shoe construction and modification, foot orthosis fabrication and materials, footwear fitting, and patient/practice management. A limited number of states currently provide licensure for orthotists, prosthetists, and pedorthists professionals. Private credentialing organizations provide oversight and accreditation of educational programs, clinical residency, board certification examinations, professional conduct, and continuing education; The American Board for Certification in Orthotics, Prosthetics, and Pedorthics and The Board for Orthotist and Prosthetist Certification are 2 such organizations.

MATERIALS AND FABRICATION CONSIDERATIONS

Three primary issues are to be considered in the fabrication of an orthotic or prosthetic device: (1) the detailed selection of components and materials, (2) the level of customization, and (3) the process of evaluation and provision of the device. There are a wide array of fabrication materials available including plastics, leather, metals and elastomeric gels. All have properties that make them suitable for use as a part of an external appliance. Customization generally involves the selection of either a custom fabricated or a prefabricated device. The decision for custom fabricated or prefabricated involves questions about pathology, clinical outcomes, the need for a total contact fit vs a limited contact fit, body type, acute vs chronic use, cost, practitioner preference, patient prior use, and market availability.

*Illustrations by Katherine E. Binder.

■ **PROSTHESES**
External limb prostheses i.e. replacement limbs.

LOWER LIMB PROSTHESES
Evaluating a patient for and prescribing a prosthesis begins with a functional assessment. Specifically, assessing the **potential** of the client to use a prosthesis and thereby determine the appropriate prosthesis design necessary to achieve the goal of maximizing pain-free functional independence. Functional prosthesis use includes safe basic mobility as well as a normalized gait pattern for those clients with the ability to achieve it. Prosthesis design and prescription are based on (1) the durability of the residual limb; length, strength, skin integrity, sensation, proximal joint health, and so on; (2) the assessed functional ambulatory potential of the client; (3) prior prosthesis use; and (4) the patient's goals and lifestyle. Preparatory prostheses are valuable in making these assessments as they allow the user time to integrate the prosthesis into their daily routine. The individual's medical history, physical presentation, and **current** function are used to establish their functional potential. There are many standardized tests available to assist with this assessment. The most widely utilized system in the United States has been provided by The Centers for Medicare and Medicaid Services (CMS) to assist with lower limb prosthesis knee and foot/ankle selection (1). Functional categories labeled 0 through 4 describe progressively increasing potential ambulatory function with a prosthesis (Figure 21.1). The Amputee

MFCL Level	Foot/Ankle Assembly	Knee Units
0 No functional potential with prosthesis	Not eligible for a prosthesis	Not eligible for a prosthesis
1 Transfers and limited household distances	SACH or single axis only	No fluid control allowed
2 Household and limited community distances	Flexible keel or multi-axis allowed	No fluid control allowed
3 Community distances; variable cadence; traverse environmental barriers	Any foot/ankle assembly; including energy storage and multi-axial dynamic response	Most knee units; includes fluid, micro-processor fluid control; No High Activity Knee Frames
4 High activity, impact and stress; active adult, athlete or child.	Any foot/ankle assembly	Any knee unit

FIGURE 21.1 ■ CMS components and functional levels chart.

Mobility Predictor (AMP) by Robert Gailey is another particularly useful performance assessment tool (2).

Prosthesis design in general reflects the level of limb loss (Figure 21.2) and the intended functional use of the prosthesis. General types of prostheses are (1) immediate and early postoperative prostheses (IPOP/EPOP), (2) preparatory prostheses, (3) definitive prostheses, and (4) specialty or activity-specific prostheses. Immediate and early postoperative prostheses are provided shortly after amputation, often in the operating room, with the goals of (1) preventing edema, (2) protecting the incision line and limb to relieve pain and promote healing, and (3) facilitating early functional independence. Preparatory prostheses are provided as soon as the limb can tolerate the forces of the removable socket and are intended for the achievement of 3 primary goals: (1) limb maturation (volume reduction, shaping, strengthening, and desensitization), (2) maximizing early functional independence, and (3) assessing for the definitive prosthesis. The definitive prosthesis is provided when the aforementioned goals are achieved and is intended to be used for a longer period of time with the option of a more cosmetic restoration. The definitive prosthesis is modified or replaced when there are (1) significant changes in limb size or volume, (2) significant changes in function, and/or (3) due to wear and tear.

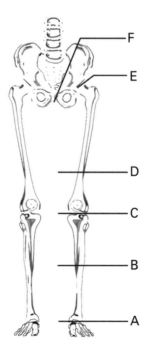

FIGURE 21.2 ■ Lower limb amputation levels.

Specialty or activity-specific prostheses may be provided for vocational or avocational activities wherein the primary prosthesis is not appropriate such as aquatics, sprinting, or use in extreme environments.

The basic components of lower limb prostheses are the (1) user and machine interface (socket + suspension), (2) construction, (3) replacement functional units (foot/ankle, knee, hip), and (4) socks, liners, and accoutrements.

The prosthesis interface includes concepts of the socket (stance or weight-bearing control) and suspension (swing or non-weight-bearing control) as a system. The specifics of the interface vary based on level/type of residual limb and the details of the potential user.

Construction considerations that apply for all lower limb prostheses include materials, connectors and the alignment of the various functional segments. The general construction techniques used in lower limb prostheses are (1) Exoskeletal; composed of a rigid external shell as the supporting structure and (2) Endoskeletal; composed of a rigid internal, modular (pylon and connectors) supporting structure. Exoskeletal construction remains an option primarily for prior users and has been replaced by endoskeletal systems in most cases. Modular endoskeletal components and fabrication have become the predominant construction technique primarily due to the reduction in weight and the relative ease of adjustments and repairs when compared to exoskeletal construction. Dynamic endoskeletal pylons are available that allow for shock and torque attenuation through spring loaded pistoning and rotation action or as flexible pylons that absorb force via bending. These functions would be in addition to the function of the selected foot/ankle. The alignment of the prosthesis refers to the spatial relationship of the major functional segments of the prosthesis in all 3 planes so that the interface, and thereby the user, is located over the functional segments (foot/ankle, knee, hip) to create a balance of stability and mobility. An even roll over shape and control of torque in the frontal plane (varus/valgus), sagittal plane (flexion/extension), and transverse plane (internal/external rotational) during stance phase allows for comfortable and efficient gait. Mal-alignment of the prosthesis can lead to (1) safety issues such as knee buckling, (2) limb pain and skin problems from uncontrolled shear and pressure, (3) gait deviations and inefficiencies, and (4) premature wearing of mechanical components.

Prosthetic foot/ankle systems remain largely passive devices using dynamic materials to accommodate but not actively adapt to the ground surface. They can be categorized into 2 main groups with a few subgroupings (Figure 21.3). The solid ankle cushion heel (SACH) nonarticulated foot uses a compressible foam heel to simulate plantarflexion and a rigid shortened anterior keel to allow for stance phase roll over or third rocker. The anterior support of the SACH foot is often insufficient for active users creating a drop-off effect at the end of stance. The flexible keel foot allows for a longer and more accommodating toe lever

Foot Category	Foot Sub-Category	Foot Function	CMS level
Non-Articulated	SACH	Soft compressible heel, short rigid keel simulates PF and DF	1
	Flexible Keel	Soft compressible heel, longer flexible keel simulates limited tri-planar motion	2
	Energy Storing	Long elastic keel to maximize simulated push off effect	3
Articulated	Single Axis	Sagittal plane motion only; PF at heel strike and DF stop at heel off	1
	Multi-Axis	Tri-planar motion with rigid keel	2
	MultipAxis, Dynamic Response	Tri-planar motion with long elastic keel to maximize simulated push off effect	3

FIGURE 21.3 ■ Prosthesis foot chart.

which improves control on uneven terrain and with variable cadence. The energy storing foot is designed with a long and dynamic anterior lever arm which allows for greater simulated push off and control at the end of stance due to the leaf spring effect of the keel. The energy storing foot is appropriate for users with the functional potential to walk at variable speeds and manage environmental obstacles such as stairs, ramps, and uneven terrain. Articulated feet with either a single axis or multiple axes allow for greater accommodation to the ground surface. The multiaxis, dynamic response foot provides this ground accommodation with the additional feature of an energy storing anterior lever arm or keel for users with the ability to vary their cadence. Stand alone modular ankle units are available and are designed to allow multiaxial motion or patient adjustable heel height. Microprocessor-controlled ankles are available. They provide a greater degree of adaptation to the ground surface instead of simple accommodation and are a new design focus.

Prosthetic knee mechanisms can be categorized based on the function of the knee during the stance and swing phases of gait and by the number of mechanical axes, single axis or polycentric (Figure 21.4). Polycentric knee joints allow for shortening of the shank section during flexion and are therefore often provided for users with long residual limbs. The polyentric knee joint configuration is also designed for stability and maximizes

	Common Terminology	Prescription Notes
Stance Control (Stance or Weight bearing control)	Knee Joint Alignment	Ground reaction force at knee axis is biased towards extension under a weight bearing load
	Weight Activated Stance Control	Mechanical breaking mechanism supports user within a small range of flexion (0-25) under a weight bearing load
	Fluid Control	Hydraulic stance control for flexion damping
	Fluid Control with Micro-processor	Hydraulic stance control for flexion damping wider and automated resistance range adjustment; hydraulic only
Swing Control (Swing or Non-weight bearing control)	Friction	Constant rabe, not cadence responsive
	Extension Assist	Promotes knee extension at end of swing
	Fluid Control	Variable cadence responsive; pneumatic and/or hydraulic
	Fluid Control with micro-processor	Variable cadence responsive with wider and automated resistance range adjustment; pneumatic and/or hydraulic
Single Axis Construction	One axis of rotation	Most common design for stance fluid control with or without micro-processor
Multi-Axis/ Poly-Centric Construction	Multiple axes allows for shortening of shank during swing phase and sitting flexion.	Inherently stable by design; limited stance fluid control options

FIGURE 21.4 ■ Prosthesis knee chart.

the use of the ground reaction force as an extension bias during stance. Alignment of the major components of the prosthesis and the management of the ground reaction force are commonly used to create an extension torque bias at the knee for weight-bearing stability and to reduce the risk of buckling. In addition to this alignment technique, many prosthetic knee joints have flexion resistance mechanisms such as weight-activated brakes or hydraulic damping units to further stabilize the knee against inadvertent knee flexion or buckling and the risk of a fall. Manual locking knees are often provided to prosthesis users who are unable to control the knee. They provide the maximum resistance to buckling as they are locked in extension during standing and walking. Fluid controlled knees provide a flexion damping under load during stance phase and also assist with the control of the knee during swing under variable speed conditions. Knee mechanisms without this fluid control allow for only single speed swing phase movement. This single speed knee swing creates gait deviations such as terminal impact or excessive heel rise if the user changes their pace. Microprocessor- and fluid-controlled prosthetic knee units provide automated control of the hydraulic damping mechanism through a broad range of force and speed. They rely on sensors built into the knee and/or pylon to determine position and torque. The potential for variable cadence (swing control) and need for advanced stability (stance control) for both stumble recovery and flexion damping (down ramps, stairs, and curbs) are indications for swing and stance phase hydraulics. Knee and foot/ankle components should be considered one integrated system to maximize the balance of stability and mobility. Knee units with powered extension force are limited at this time, but are a new design focus.

PARTIAL FOOT PROSTHESES

General considerations in the design of partial foot prostheses are based on the level of amputation and function of the remaining foot (Figure 21.5). Common amputations levels are (1) Toe; the hallux being the most disruptive of function, (2) ray resection, (3) Lisfranc, (4) Chopart, and (5) Boyd and Pirogoff. The biomechanical goals of the partial foot prostheses are to (1) support the residual foot structure, (2) control the distribution of forces, (3) replace the lost anterior lever arm, and (4) allow for shoe fit. The prosthesis structure and lever arm control are determined by the height of the device and the materials selected therefore; typically the shorter the residual limb the higher the device. Three general designs based on the height of the prosthesis are (1) Submalleolar, (2) Supramalleolar, and (3) Tibial tubercle height. The residual limb length, available ankle and foot ROM, strength, sensation, and weight-bearing stability all help to determine the required prosthetic leverage to achieve a normalized gait pattern. Drop off at the end of stance phase, and subsequent compensations, due to an insufficient anterior lever are common gait deviations. Selection of the

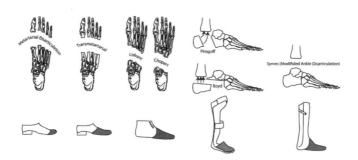

FIGURE 21.5 ■ Partial foot amputation.

height of the prosthesis, the materials, socks, or other interface additions, as well as, the appropriate footwear make up the basic prescription.

SYME ANKLE DISARTICULATION PROSTHESES

The basic components of the Syme's prosthesis are (1) the interface (socket + suspension), (2) the construction, (3) the foot/ankle, and (4) socks, liners, and accoutrements (Figure 21.6).

Syme ankle disarticulation prostheses are designed to maximize the advantages of this amputation level. These advantages are (1) distal weight bearing allowing for reduced proximal loading, (2) a bulbous distal shape allowing for reduced proximal suspension, and (3) a long lever arm and surface area for distribution of force and greater control of the prosthesis. The disadvantages of the Syme ankle disarticulation prosthesis are the limited space distal to the socket for prosthetic foot and ankle mechanisms and the difficulty achieving satisfactory cosmetic restoration for many clients. With the Syme ankle disarticulation prosthesis, the interface is commonly designed for full distal weight bearing and for self-suspension. Due to limits on space distal to the end of the limb, the socket is generally mounted directly onto the foot with a short modular connector. The socket either has a window or door (medially or posteriorly) to allow donning or is created in a cylindrical shape with a soft foam insert. Socks or gel liners are used as additional interface materials. Foot selection is limited due to the available space (approximately 2–3 inches for adults) and requires the use of a lower profile ankle/foot design. Despite this limited space, energy storage feet remain an option.

TRANSTIBIAL PROSTHESES

The basic components of the transtibial prosthesis are (1) the interface (socket + suspension), (2) the construction, (3) the foot/ankle, and (4) socks, liners, and accoutrements (Figure 21.7).

The design of the transtibial prosthesis reflects the anatomy of the residual limb creating an interface that optimizes weight-bearing and swing-phase forces over a relatively small surface area. By definition the transtibial region extends from the distal Syme's ankle disarticulation to the proximal knee disarticulation level; however, there are surgical considerations which determine optimal length. Leverage and surface area increase with longer limbs, but at the distal levels of the shank, soft tissue coverage may be limited and may predispose the limb to skin problems. Proximally the extensor mechanism must be maintained to allow for knee control, and the short leverage and surface area would generally indicate socket designs that extend above the knee joint such as supracondylar/suprapatellar or joints and corset resulting in a more cumbersome fitting. Mid-shank lengths approximating the musculoskeletal junction of the gastrocnemius/soleus muscle group are considered the ideal length region providing for reasonable distal soft tissue coverage and leverage for control. Full distal end loading is not generally tolerated without

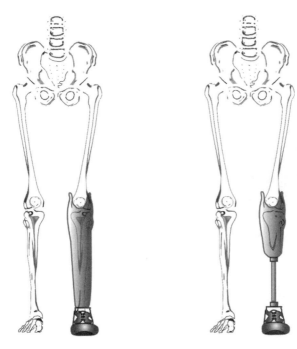

FIGURE 21.6 ■ Syme's prosthesis.   **FIGURE 21.7** ■ Transtibial prosthesis.

specialized osteoplastic procedures so that weight is borne over the entire limb with considerations for pressure sensitive areas. Many design options are available for the transtibial interface with the ultimate goal of comfort and control (Figure 21.8). The use of gel liners have become common practice. Gel liners are intended to provide for improved suspension; control for variances in sheer and pressure; and loading of the residual limb in a more uniform, reliable pattern. Gel liners can be used with mechanical locks or with sealing sleeves to create a suction or elevated vacuum fitting which significantly reduces pistoning thereby improving swing phase control. With more room for prosthetic components distal to the end of the residual limb, all foot/ankle designs are an option including the longer "J" shaped energy storage feet with leaf spring levers extending to the shank, multiaxial dynamic response feet, as well as integrated shock, and torque attenuation pylon systems.

KNEE DISARTICULATION PROSTHESES
The basic components of the knee disarticulation prosthesis are (1) the interface, which is the combination of the socket and suspension as a

	Common Terminology	Prescription Notes
Socket (Stance or weight bearing control)	Patella Tendon Bearing (PTB)	Specific weight beaning on pressure tolerant areas and relief of pressure sensitive areas
	Patella Tendon Bearing, Supra-condylar & Supre-patellar (PTBSCSP)I	Variance of PTB that encapsulates the knee for suspension or control
	Joints and Corset	Variance of PTB that encapsulates the knee for suspension or control Medial and lateral metal knee joints and thigh lacer for residual limb weight bearing reduction and knee support
	Total Surface Weight Bearing	Designed for use with gel liners to more evenly distribute forces and allows for improved suction and vacuum
Suspension (Swing or non-weight bearing control)	Supra-Condylar Cuff, Fork Strap and Waist Belt	Strap suspension above knee and extended to the waist; simple
	Supra-Condylar and Supra-patellar	Solf suspension over femoral condyles
	Suspension Sleeve	May be primary or secondary suspension; used for sealing suction or vacuum sockets
	Silicone Suction Socket	Use of gel liners with a pin and locking mechanism or without (with sleeve)
	Elevated Vacuum Socket	Mechanical or electro-mechanical pump and sealed socket with gel liner creates elevated vacuum 12-20 in Hg

FIGURE 21.8 ■ Transtibial interface chart.

system, (2) the construction and materials, (3) the prosthetic knee mechanism, (4) the foot/ankle mechanism, and (5) the required socks or liners.

Knee disarticulation prostheses are designed to maximize the advantages of this level of amputation. The advantages of the knee disarticulation or through knee amputation limb are (1) distal weight bearing allowing for reduced proximal loading, (2) full hip motor power available allowing for improved control and gait efficiency, (3) a bulbous distal shape allowing for reduced proximal suspension, and (4) long lever arm and surface area for control of prosthesis. The disadvantages of the knee disarticulation limb and prosthesis are the limited space distal to the socket for prosthetic knee mechanisms and the difficulty achieving satisfactory cosmetic restoration for many clients. Socket design for the knee disarticulation level prosthesis is often relatively simple when compared to the transfemoral prosthesis. In particular, the availability of distal limb weight bearing may eliminate or significantly reduce the need for pelvic (ischial tuberosity) weight bearing and the use of aggressive proximal socket brim designs for control. Self-suspension also reduces the need for proximal suspension systems such as belts (Figure 21.9). These advantages make the interface of the knee disarticulation prosthesis less cumbersome for the user and allow for improved comfort in both walking and sitting. As with transtibial prostheses, endoskeletal construction is common. Polycentric knee joint mechanisms are commonly prescribed as they allow for the shortest possible thigh length and sitting comfort. Foot and ankle selection is based on the functional potential of the user and is determined along with the function of the knee unit for an integrated foot/ankle and knee system.

	Common Terminology	Prescription Notes
Socket (Stance or weight bearing control)	Quadrilateral	Pelvic weight bearing on the ischial tuberosity which is outside of the socket
	Ischial Containment	Pelvic weight bearing on the ischial tuberosity which is captured in the socket for greater limb control
Suspension (Swing or non-weight bearing control)	Silesian Belt	Flexible belt that attaches to the lateral proximal socket and wraps over the contralateral illiac crest
	Hip joint, pelvic band and belt	Rigid metal hip joint and band creates improved frontal plane control
	Full Suction	Socket and limb in direct contact creating a suction effect; commonly used with a "pull in" stocking and an auto-expulsion air valve
	Silicone Suction Socket	Use of gel liners with a pin and locking mechanism or without (with sleeve)
	Elevated Vacuum Socket	Mechanical or electro-mechanical pump and sealed socket with gel liner creates elevated vacuum 12-20 in Hg

FIGURE 21.9 ■ Transfemoral/KD interface chart.

TRANSFEMORAL PROSTHESES

The basic components of the transfemoral prosthesis are (1) the interface (socket + suspension), (2) the construction and materials, (3) prosthetic knee mechanism, (4) the foot, ankle and pylon system, and (5) associated socks, liners, and accoutrements (Figure 21.10).

At the transfemoral level, residual length becomes a primary consideration. The shorter levels of amputation create significantly reduced surface area and leverage for controlling forces. This is of particular concern for prosthetic knee control. In the frontal plane, the balance between hip abductors and adductors and the desired adducted position of the femur in the prosthetic socket become difficult to maintain. The imbalance can lead to gait deviations such as Trendelenburg's gait or the gluteus medius lurch compensation which compromise gait efficiency and user comfort. Accommodations for short limbs must be made in the design of the prosthesis often leading to a more cumbersome fitting with aggressive socket brims and pelvic suspension straps for stance and swing phase control, respectively. Very short transfemoral limbs may be fit with a hip disarticulation style prosthesis. While long residual limbs are desirable for leverage and control, there may be limited room for some knee units with very long limbs approaching the femoral condyles.

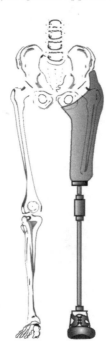

FIGURE 21.10 ■ Transfemoral prosthesis.

The primary transfemoral socket shapes are Quadrilateral and Ischial Containment (Figure 21.9). Both require pelvic weight bearing on the ischial tuberosity and thereby unload the distal end of the residual limb. The quadrilateral socket shape relies on a narrowed anterior–posterior socket dimension to maintain the ischial position, and the user sits on the posterior-medial aspect of the top of the socket when bearing weight on the prosthesis. The ischial containment socket relies on a narrowed medial–lateral dimension and an extended capture of the medial aspect of the tuberosity and descending ramus for weight bearing and frontal plane control. The ischial containment socket design is intended to provide greater control of the femur and thereby reduce socket instabilities leading to gait deviations such as lateral trunk lean. The primary goal for the transfemoral socket remains user comfort and control.

Knee selection is based on the functional potential of the user and the available residual limb leverage among other factors as mentioned previously (Figure 21.4). With loss of the knee and the foot/ankle complex, shock and torque attenuation become concerns. Dynamic pylons with shock and torque absorbing mechanisms may be provided. Foot/ankle selection should be considered with the knee as a system (Figure 21.3).

HIP DISARTICULATION AND TRANS-PELVIC PROSTHESES

The basic components of the hip disarticulation or trans-pelvic prosthesis are (1) interface (socket + suspension), (2) construction, (3) hip joint, (4) knee joint, (5) foot/ankle, and (6) socks, liners, and accoutrements (Figure 21.11).

General considerations in the design of the hip disarticulation and trans-pelvic prosthesis are based on the residual pelvic structure and, in particular, the availability of the ischial tuberosity for weight bearing and the iliac crest for suspension. Without these 2 boney anchors, socket control is reliant on soft tissue compression and may be less stable. The socket interface is most commonly fabricated as a single piece with a rigid attachment to the hip joint and a flexible closure wrapping around and encapsulating the entire residual pelvis for weight bearing, suspension, and rotational control. Pelvic motions (posterior pelvic tilt) are used to initiate swing phase. Weight-bearing stability is built into the alignment with extension biased at the knee and hip joints under load. Hip joints are largely single axis joints with extension assist mechanisms and are aligned with the axis placed on the distal anterior aspect of the socket for maximal extension bias and for sitting comfort. Without active control of the hip joint, knee and foot/ankle component selection is largely based on the need for stance stability and safety.

TRANS-LUMBAR PROSTHESES

General considerations are based primarily on the client's general health and on upright positioning potential. If the client is medically

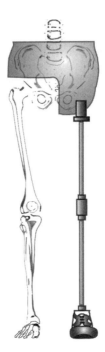

FIGURE 21.11 ■ Hip disarticulation prosthesis.

stable and can tolerate an upright position, a custom seating socket can be fabricated to allow for sitting and for wheelchair mobility. The custom socket is made from a casting of the residual body and extends to at least mid-thoracic level. Custom air chambers are commonly used to maintain support and even pressure distribution. Ambulation with prosthetic legs is not currently an option. Selection of materials and the connection of the custom seating socket with an appropriately prescribed wheelchair are essential for successful functional outcome. The details of this prescription are best left as a multidisciplinary task with input from all members of the team.

UPPER LIMB PROSTHESES
The population of upper limb prosthesis users is quite different than lower limb prosthesis users representing a very small minority of the limb loss population. This is primarily due to the limited number of upper limb amputations and to the much higher prosthesis rejection rate. Unilateral upper limb amputees will quickly become ADL proficient with the remaining limb. There is generally considered to be a 3 to 6 month critical period for upper limb amputees to be successfully fitted

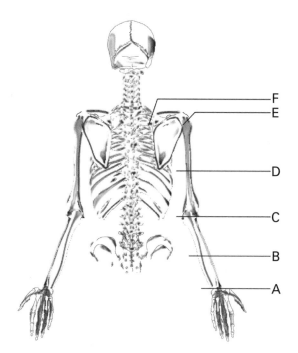

FIGURE 21.12 ■ Upper limb amputation levels.

with a prosthesis after which time they are much more likely to reject a prosthesis. Bilateral upper limb amputees can become independent in the majority of the essential ADLs with appropriate training. The description of upper limb prostheses mirrors the level of amputation (Figure 21.12). Long, medium, short and very short level descriptions as percentages of the intact limb are used as guidelines. There are 6 basic options for clients with upper limb loss: (1) no prosthesis, (2) passive or static terminal device, (3) body powered, (4) externally powered, (5) hybrid, or (6) specialty prostheses.

PARTIAL HAND PROSTHESES

General considerations are based on (1) the level of amputaion, (2) the function of the remaining hand with potential prehension abilities being critical, and (3) unilateral or bilateral involvement. Levels of amputation include (1) partial or complete digit(s) disarticulation, (2) ray resection, (3) trans-metacarpal, and (4) trans-carpal. Partial hand prostheses are more likely to be rejected than any other level of prosthesis due to their limited function and poor aesthetics. The device provided may be considered more an orthosis than a prosthesis depending on the functional intent. Occupational therapists are critical to successful prosthesis prescription and should be involved as early as possible. As the function of the hand is so complex and the function of most partial hand prostheses so inadequate, more than one device may be required to provide necessary functional restoration. Three design concepts should be considered: (1) aesthetic restoration, (2) protection, and (3) prehension; static or dynamic prehension designs are possible.

WRIST DISARTICULATION AND TRANSRADIAL PROSTHESES

The basic parts of the wrist disarticulation or transradial prosthesis are (1) interface (socket + suspension), (2) control system, (3) wrist unit, (4) terminal device, and (5) associated socks, liners and accoutrements (Figure 21.13). The design of the wrist disarticulation and transradial prosthesis are based on the length of the residual limb and the available forearm rotation (pronation and supination). With the wrist disarticulation level, full forearm length and an intact radius and ulna allow for improved control, distal pressure tolerance, and full pronation and supination. However, there is limited space at the end of the socket for a wrist and terminal device so that the prosthetic limb may be longer than the intact contralateral limb. At the transradial level, the length of the lever

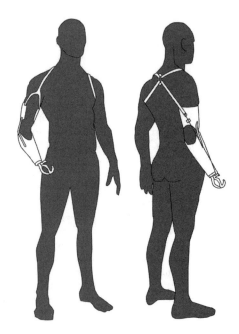

FIGURE 21.13 ■ Transradial prosthesis.

arm determines the control system, component, and interface (socket and suspension) selection. A short residual limb length requires a prosthetic interface that captures more of the limb and may extend above the elbow joint. The self-suspending supraepicondylar Muenster socket is a common design. The use of silicone liners and sleeves as used with lower limb prostheses has become more prevalent. Control system options are (1) passive, (2) body power, or (3) external power. The term passive refers solely to the terminal device which may not be activated to open or close however; the prosthesis is functional as an extension of the residual limb for bi-manual activities and for manipulating objects in space. Passive systems are often more cosmetically acceptable. Body powered systems are cable and harness operated and require the user to provide tension to the cable via biscapular abduction or gleno-humeral flexion or abduction. Externally powered systems at this level are largely myo-electrically controlled through electro-myographic (EMG) signals from the residual wrist/hand flexors and extensors. Terminal device options are (1) hook or (2) hand. Hook terminal devices can be body powered and are either voluntary opening or voluntary closing. They are available in a wide range of shapes and sizes. Externally powered hooks are available as well. The prescription of more than one hook and the combination of a hook and a hand is common to allow the user to interchange terminal devices based on desired function. The most common wrist unit is the friction wrist which allows passive rotational positioning of the terminal device. Mechanical flexion wrist units are available to assist with midline activities. Powered, myoelectric wrist rotators are also available.

ELBOW DISARTICULATION AND TRANSHUMERAL PROSTHESES
The basic components of the elbow disarticulation or transhumeral prosthesis are (1) interface (socket + suspension), (2) control system, (3) elbow unit, (4) wrist unit, (5) terminal device, and (6) associated socks, liners, and accoutrements (Figure 21.14). Residual limb length and control of the prosthesis are primary concerns in the design of the elbow disarticulation and transhumeral prosthesis. At the elbow disarticulation level, full humeral length, broad and tolerant distal humeral end, and full leverage allow for improved control of the prosthesis. However, there is limited room for a prosthetic elbow mechanism often requiring the use of external hinges or an elbow unit which is positioned much lower than the contralateral/nonamputated limb. At the transhumeral level, the length of the lever arm determines the control system, component, and interface (socket and suspension) selection. Longer limbs allow the socket trimlines to remain relatively low and end distal to the shoulder joint. At mid length levels, socket extensions onto the pectoralis area anteriorly and the scapular area posteriorly for rotational control are common. At higher levels with shorter lever arms, the socket may extend over the acromion process as a shoulder cap; and at very proximal levels, clients are fit with a shoulder disarticulation level

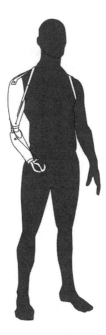

FIGURE 21.14 ■ Transhumeral prosthesis.

prosthesis as the residual humerus does not provide sufficient lever-age for control. The use of silicone liners and sleeves as used with lower limb prostheses has become more prevalent. Control system options are (1) passive, (2) body power, (3) external power, or (4) hybrid, a combination of body and external power. Body powered systems are cable and harness operated and require the user to provide tension to the cable via biscapular abduction or gleno-humeral flexion or abduction. For a fully body powered transhumeral prosthesis, a single cable controls both elbow movement and terminal device open/close. A separate cable locks and unlocks the prepositioned elbow. This requires a sequential control pattern: (1) preposition the elbow and terminal device in space, (2) lock the elbow in position, and (3) operate the terminal device. Externally powered systems at this level are largely myoelectrically controlled through EMG signals from the residual elbow flexors and extensors. Selection of the elbow unit is based on the control system selected. Terminal device and wrist unit selection is then made based on the control system and elbow unit selected. A common hybrid control system is a body powered elbow unit and an externally powered hand terminal device.

SHOULDER DISARTICULATION AND INTRA-SCAPULAR/ THORACIC PROSTHESES

The basic parts of the shoulder disarticulation or intra-scapular/thoracic prosthesis are (1) interface (socket + suspension), (2) control system, (3) shoulder unit, (4) elbow unit, (5) wrist unit, (6) terminal device, and (7) associated socks, liners, and accoutrements. General considerations in the design of prostheses at these proximal levels involve the availability of the shoulder girdle for control of both the interface (suspension and force control) and for potential myoelectric sites at the pectoralis, upper trapezius, and scapular muscles. Without the shoulder girdle, control is diminished, and, most clients choose to forgo prosthesis fitting and may be fit with a shoulder cap only which allows for proper fitting of clothing and protection of the body segment. Passive systems are common at this level and often have manual locking elbow units operated and prepositioned with the contralateral limb. Full body powered systems are possible at this level but often require the use of inguinal control straps and chin nudge switches which are cumbersome and make the prosthesis likely to be rejected. Hybrid systems with body power and external power combinations are more common. Full externally powered systems are the current design focus. Efforts at expanding myoelectric sites through surgical intervention such as targeted reinnervation as well as the use of powered shoulders, elbows, wrists, and hand for increased movement and sequential control are now possible and have demonstrated significant functional gains (3).

■ ORTHOSES

An orthosis is a device, applied to the exterior of the body, for the purpose of supporting, correcting, aligning, or improving the function of moveable parts of the body or reducing pain of the head, spine, or extremities. General terminology for orthoses may be organized into the following: (1) lower limb, (2) upper limb, and (3) spinal categories. Further subcategories are based on the joints affected by the orthosis. Standardized terminology includes the use of simple initialisms describing the joints affected and ending with "orthosis." For example, ankle foot orthosis (AFO), wrist hand orthosis (WHO), and thoracic lumbar sacral orthosis (TLSO) are standardized terms that allow for quick communication of the basic device. Further descriptors may be added to specify the desired function, materials, or design criteria. For example, articulated, dorsiflexion (DF) assist AFO; or wrist powered tenodesis WHO; or rigid, tri-planar control, custom molded TLSO. These standardized terms allow quick communication, although still commonly used terms such as splints, braces, and supports are nonstandard and nonspecific and should be avoided in favor of the aforementioned terminology.

Orthosis users are a heterogeneous group and not easily categorized by diagnosis alone. Therefore, in many cases the focus of orthotic prescription is on orthosis design and function, and less on the underlying etiology and diagnosis. Evaluation for orthoses involves a functional assessment and the establishment of reasonable functional goals, anticipated outcomes, and duration of use. Selecting materials for the construction of the orthosis includes the decision on custom fabricated or prefabricated. This decision involves questions about pathology, clinical outcomes, the need for a total contact fit vs a limited contact fit, body type, acute vs chronic use, cost, practitioner preference, patient prior use, and market availability.

LOWER LIMB ORTHOSES
The prescription and design of a lower limb orthosis begins with a clear diagnosis and physical exam including functional assessment and gait analysis and involves the selection of (1) the joint control (ankle/foot, knee, and/or hip), (2) construction and materials (custom fabricated vs prefabricated; metal, plastic, and hybrid), (3) straps and fitting modifications for control, and (4) recommendations for appropriate footwear.

Shoes
The shoe is considered part of the lower limb orthosis system and should be prescribed with the orthosis (Figure 21.15). In the case of traditional double upright metal orthosis systems, the orthosis is physically attached to the shoe. Shoes may be custom molded and are often modified to improve fit or create a specific biomechanical effect. Common shoe modifications are (1) heel lift to accommodate a plantar-flexion (PF) contracture, (2) heel and sole lift to accommodate a leg length

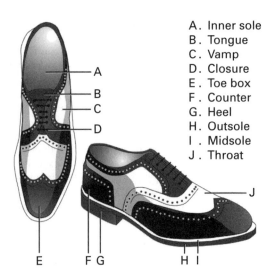

A. Inner sole
B. Tongue
C. Vamp
D. Closure
E. Toe box
F. Counter
G. Heel
H. Outsole
I. Midsole
J. Throat

FIGURE 21.15 ■ Shoe.

discrepancy, (3) rocker sole to simulate ankle PF and DF, (4) extended rigid shank to limit forefoot extension, (5) cushioned heel to simulate PF, (6) heel flares (medial and/or lateral) to control for frontal plane instability (varus or valgus), (7) Thomas and reverse Thomas heel to support the medial and lateral longitudinal arches, respectively, and (8) heel and sole wedge to accommodate inversion/varus or eversion/valgus deformity. These can be combined to address a wide variety of lower limb problems. Shoes to be used with plastic orthoses generally have removable innersoles and are often fit ½ size larger for extra depth, width, and length. Shoes to be used with metal systems must have a firm sole for attachment of the stirrup or caliper box.

FOOT ORTHOSES

Foot orthoses (FOs) are employed to directly support and align the foot to prevent or correct foot deformities and, thereby, improve the function of the foot and lower limb. FOs can (1) reduce stress on the foot, ankle, knee, hip, pelvis, and spine by correcting faulty alignments and properly controlling the motion within the foot, (2) support the longitudinal and transverse arches of the foot, (3) provide relief for painful areas, (4) provide an even distribution of the weight-bearing stresses over the entire plantar surface of the foot, and (5) equalize leg length discrepancy. FOs can be either prefabricated or custom and are made with a wide range of materials that span an almost unlimited spectrum of durometer. FOs can be generally described as either accommodative or corrective/functional with further classification into soft, semi-rigid, or rigid subcategories. The detailed design of the foot orthosis includes (1) posting or wedging under the rearfoot, forefoot, or both, (2) metatarsal arch support, (3) reliefs or cut outs for painful areas, and (4) forefoot extension modifications. The University of California Biomechanics Lab (UCBL) foot orthosis is a rigid orthosis with higher trim-lines thereby providing more transverse plane control of the flexible flatfoot. Matching FOs to appropriate shoes is critical.

ANKLE FOOT ORTHOSES

The general indications for an AFO are (1) motor control deficits of the lower limb and resultant functional deficits (safety, mobility limitations, and gait inefficiency), (2) foot, ankle or knee instability causing pain, deformity, or limited function, (3) immobilization required for pain control, fracture stabilization, burns, trauma, or wound management, and (4) foot/ankle joint contracture management. The orthosis includes the foot and ankle and therefore has lever arms extending proximal and distal to the ankle joint. The length of the lever arms, the ankle joint control, and the materials used to fabricate the AFO determine the control.

Traditional AFOs (Figure 21.16) are made of 2 metal side bars and joints connected proximally by a leather covered calf band and attached

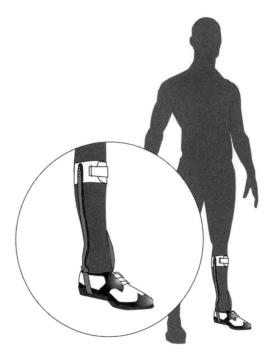

FIGURE 21.16 ■ AFO metal.

distally to the shoe. Molded plastic AFOs (Figure 21.17) are intended to be in contact with the limb for more control, are lighter weight, and allow for easier use with more than one shoe. The ankle joint control provided by an AFO can be considered to either limit or assist motion and can be constructed either with or without an ankle joint (Figure 21.18). Common nonarticulated versions are (1) solid ankle which significantly limits motion and (2) posterior leaf spring (PLS) which assists DF during swing phase and creates only limited restriction of stance phase motion. Common articulated designs include (1) free motion in the sagittal plane for frontal plane control only, (2) DF assist, and (3) limited motion. A very common limited motion adjustable ankle joint is the bichannel adjustable ankle locking (BiCAAL) joint, also known as the dual channel joint. The BiCAAL joint allows for control of both plantar flexion and DF with either springs for assist or rigid pins for stops. The addition of straps and padding to the orthosis allows for more aggressive control of instability either due to weakness or due to ROM limitations from spasticity or contracture.

Many variations on the concept of the AFO are available. The supramalleolar ankle foot orthosis with a short proximal lever arm

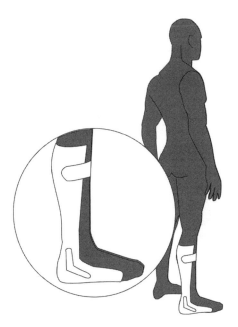

FIGURE 21.17 ■ AFO plastic.

Joint Type	Function	Construction
Free Motion	Free sagittal motion, limited frontal and transverse plane motion	Articulated; metal or plastic joints are available
Limited Motion	Plantar-flexion and/or dorsi-flexion stops	Articulated; metal or plastic joints are available Non-articulated, sold ankle creates both PF and DF stops
Dorsi-flexion Assist	Spring assisted dorsi-flexion during swing phase	Articulated; metal or plastic joints are available Non-articulated, posterior leaf spring construction creates this effect

FIGURE 21.18 ■ Orthotic ankle joints.

is used for frontal and transverse plane control of the subtalar, mid-tarsal, and forefoot. The patellar tendon bearing orthosis is commonly prescribed without an ankle joint for a rigid solid ankle restriction and a rigid attachment to an orthopedic shoe with extended rigid shank

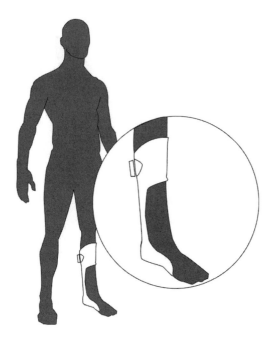

FIGURE 21.19 ■ AFO floor reaction.

for axial unloading and immobilization of the ankle joint following major trauma or reconstruction. The floor reaction AFO (Figure 21.19) uses a DF stop and a molded pretibial shell to create a knee extension stabilizing force for patients with knee buckling from quadriceps weakness or other pathology. The Charcot Reducing Orthosis Walker (CROW) is a removable custom molded walking boot and alternative to total contact casting. Myo-orthoses provide user friendly and reliable functional electrical stimulation (FES) foot drop correction and may be used as an AFO replacement for some cases of upper motor neuron related DF paralysis or weakness resulting in foot drop.

KNEE ORTHOSES
Knee orthoses (KOs) are prescribed for support of the tibiofemoral and/or patella-femoral joints. Common designs include neoprene sleeves with buttress pads to control for patellar tracking dysfunction and rigid frame style orthoses with medial and lateral joints for tri-planar control. A commonly prescribed KO the compartment unloader style. This KO creates a varus or valgus thrust to open either the lateral or medial compartment of the arthritic knee for pain relief. This type of KO is fabricated as a rigid frame with either 1 or 2 knee joints and an

adjustable alignment feature for frontal plane thrust control. Selecting prefabricated vs custom, articulated or nonarticulated including joint type, and the rigidity of the device are primary concerns.

KNEE ANKLE FOOT ORTHOSES

Knee ankle foot orthoses (KAFOs) provide support for the lower limb with indications which mirror that of the AFO but, with the direct knee control (Figure 21.20). Mechanical knee joints can either be built as double upright systems (medial and lateral) or as a single upright system with a single knee joint most commonly on the lateral side of the knee. The long mechanical lever arms of the KAFO extending as far as the hip joint proximally and including the foot and ankle distally allow for direct control of the knee joint for frontal plane (varus/valgus), sagittal plane (flexion/hyperextension), or transverse plane (rotation) limits. Foot and ankle control options remain the same as for the AFO (articulated or nonarticulated; free motion, DF assist, or limited motion). Knee joints can be organized as either single axis or polycentric and based on the mechanical resistance to stance phase flexion, that is, knee

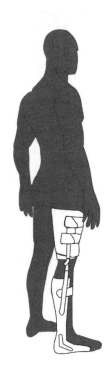

FIGURE 21.20 ■ KAFO.

Knee Joint	Function
Free motion	Free motion into flexion; 0 degree knee extension stop
Locked	Locked during weight bearing and released for flexion in sitting. Drop locks, lever locks or pawl /bail locks are common.
Posterior Offset	Similar to free motion joint with full flexion and 0 degree knee extension stop. The axis of rotation is offset posteriorly to enhance the knee extension torque when weight bearing.
Polycentric	Multiple axes of rotation, Allows for more intimate tracking and alignment of the orthotic and anatomic knee joints. Commonly used in knee orthoses for sports.
Stance Control	Selective locking in extension during stance and unlocking to allow flexion during swing. Mechanical and electro-mechanical versions available.

FIGURE 21.21 ■ Orthotic knee Joints.

buckling prevention (Figure 21.21). The majority of knee joints have a 0 or 180 degree stop built into the design to prevent hyperextension. Resistance to flexion is commonly either (1) static lock mechanism, (2) floor reaction effect often with posterior offset axes of rotation, or (3) stance control orthotic knee joints which allow selective lock and unlock during the stance and swing phases, respectively. Construction techniques include (1) traditional all metal and leather systems with shoe attachment, (2) molded plastic, and (3) hybrid combinations of metal and plastic construction. The majority of KAFOs are custom due to the complexity of crossing multiple joints and maintaining accurate orthosis and anatomic joint alignment. Additional designs include axial unloading with ischial weight-bearing proximal brims, femoral fracture orthoses, and contracture management designs with either static progressive or dynamic knee joints.

Ambulatory potential and issues of donning and doffing of the KAFO should be addressed prior to prescription particularly when upper limb function is compromised. As the KAFO is concerned with direct control of the knee, the first decision is the knee joint control mechanism (free flexion, posterior offset stability, locked static or locked dynamic stance control). The ankle joint and knee joint control should be considered as system for a balance of stability and mobility with the goal of providing the least restrictive device possible. Knee joint control, ankle joint control, construction, additional straps, and the appropriate footwear make the basic prescription.

Hip Knee Ankle Foot Orthoses and Hip Orthoses

Orthoses that cross the hip joint fall into 1 of 2 categories: those that extend to the foot and ankle (Hip Knee Ankle Foot Orthoses, HKAFOs) and those that do not (Hip Orthoses). A separate category of orthoses are the reciprocating gait orthoses (RGOs) (Figure 21.22). The general design of the HKAFO mirrors that of the KAFO but with the addition of a hip joint, pelvic band, and pelvic belt. This addition allows for direct control of hip instability either in the frontal plane to reduce lateral trunk lean (Trendelenburg's Gait or gluteus medius lurch compensation) or in the sagittal plane to limit posterior lean of the trunk. Transverse

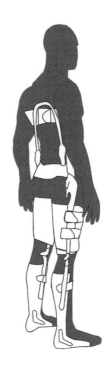

FIGURE 21.22 ■ RGO.

plane or rotational control is inherent in the design of the HKAFO with pelvic connection proximally and foot/ankle leverage distally. Unilateral HKAFOs are prescribed for significant paralysis and instability of the entire lower limb and require a high level of custom fitting and user training. Unilateral hip abduction orthoses may be prescribed to limit hip flexion, adduction, and internal rotation following total hip arthroplasty. The RGO is a bilateral HKAFO with a molded spinal extension and mechanical reciprocating leg assist system mounted posterior and proximal to the hip joints. This reciprocating system can be a cable or rocker bar configuration and creates a linked hip flexion force on one side with hip extension of the other. The user creates the reciprocal pattern by unloading one limb and extending the trunk with the assist of the arms pushing on an assistive device (walker or bilateral crutches). This pattern is an alternative to a swing to or swing through pattern for clients with paraplegia. RGO prescription requires a full evaluation and commitment to ambulation training from the client and rehabilitation team. Full ROM, intact skin, managed spasticity and upright posture need to be assessed in advance and complicating issues of orthostatic hypotension and osteoporosis must be ruled out.

UPPER LIMB ORTHOSES

Upper limb orthoses are provided based on issues including the duration of anticipated orthosis use, materials and fabrication techniques, integration of the orthosis into a therapeutic care plan, referral patterns, preferences, and professional availability. Role delineations and the specific function of the Orthotists and Therapists (Physical, Occupational, and Hand) within the rehabilitation team vary considerably. In general, Orthotists provide devices that are intended for long-term use and those that require more complex construction (eg, high temperature plastics and metals). Orthoses fabricated from low temperature thermoplastics, directly molded to the client's limb and fully integrated into a specific therapy treatment program are primarily the responsibility of the therapist.

HAND ORTHOSIS

Hand orthoses (HOs) have several functions. They are (1) to maintain the palmar arch, (2) to keep the thumb in opposition, (3) to maintain the web space, and (4) to act as a vehicle for the attachment of other orthotic systems and assistive devices. Features of the HO may include (1) an opponens bar, (2) a thumb adduction stop, (3) metacarpal–phalangeal extension stops, (4) interphalangeal joint extension assists, and (5) molded palmar arch support. HOs are often designed to immobilize a specific joint to assist with healing after trauma or over-use type injury. The orthosis may be prefabricated or custom fabricated and composed of a wide array of materials.

WRIST HAND ORTHOSIS

WHOs may have many of the features of the HO with an extension across the wrist for more control of the hand and direct control of the wrist. WHOs may be categorized as static or dynamic in basic design. Prefabricated wrist stabilization WHOs of the wrist gauntlet style are commonly prescribed for over-use injuries and soft tissue trauma. Static, palmar wrist cock-up WHOs (Figure 21.23) are a very common orthosis and are provided for the passive positioning of the hand and wrist in the functional position following trauma, neurological insult with paralysis or postsurgical reconstruction. Support of the hand and wrist with a WHO following peripheral nerve injury is common with the design and trimlines specific to the injury and paralysis.

An example of a dynamic orthosis is the Tenodesis style WHO (Figure 21.24) which assists prehension through a wrist driven flexor hinge parallelogram linkage system. Wrist extension provides an MP flexion force. The tenodesis WHO is indicated in cases of C6 or C7 quadriplegia primarily but could be used for C5 level cases with either

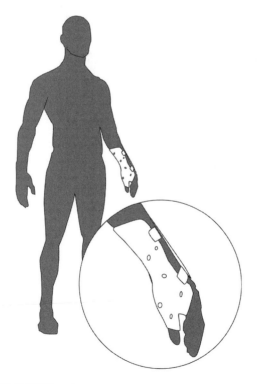

FIGURE 21.23 ■ WHO cock up.

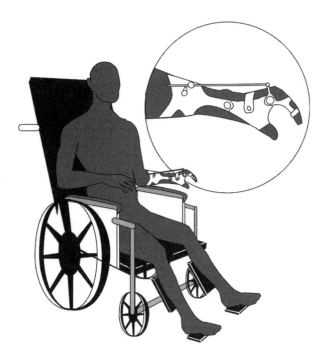

FIGURE 21.24 ■ WHO tenodesis.

a shoulder operated cable system or other external power source (eg, FES, compressed air) to create wrist extension. Myo-orthoses provide a user friendly and reliable switch operated FES facilitated tenodesis function primarily indicated for C5 quadriplegia.

ELBOW WRIST HAND ORTHOSIS (EWHO) AND ELBOW ORTHOSES (EOS)

EWHOs provide several functions including (1) positioning the hand in space, (2) providing elbow flexion, (3) elbow, forearm or wrist contracture management, and (4) postoperative elbow, forearm, wrist, and hand stabilization/immobilization. The orthosis can be prefabricated or custom fabricated; static with a set position for all segments or dynamic with static progressive or dynamic joints or a hybrid of the construction types; and fabricated from many types of materials. EOs are commonly prescribed for protection of unstable elbow joints without forearm or wrist deficits.

SHOULDER ELBOW WRIST HAND ORTHOSIS

Shoulder-elbow-wrist-hand orthoses (SEWHOs) are often designed for the short-term static immobilization of the shoulder following

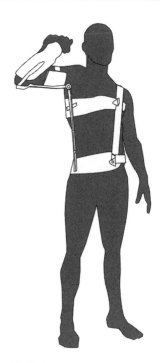

FIGURE 21.25 ■ SEWHO airplane.

postoperative reconstruction. One common static and prefabricated SEWHO, often referred to as an Airplane Splint, (Figure 21.25) immobilizes the shoulder in abduction and neutral rotation and with the elbow at 90 degrees so that the hand is placed out to the side and in front of the body. This position is difficult to maintain for prolonged periods. A dynamic type of SEWHO may be prescribed following brachial plexus injury and is designed to support the flaccid arm and may provide cable operated elbow flexion through a harness and powered by scapular abduction of the contralateral limb. The harness and cable control are similar to the Figure 21.8 harness and the cable system of an upper limb prosthesis.

Mobile Arm Support

Mounted to the back of the chair or wheelchair, the mobile arm support (MAS) or balanced forearm orthosis primarily supports the forearm and hand of the user. The MAS consists of a trough for the forearm often with a hand support (or may be modified for WHO use) and a set of hinged linkages with 2 or 3 segments allowing for gravity balanced arm horizontal abduction and adduction within a limited arc. Standard and elevating designs allow for movement at a predetermined height or variable height controlled with elastic bands. The orthosis is not managed (ie, attachment, adjustment, and maintenance) by the client but by an assistant and may be used only for specific activities such as eating, communication, and so on. The primary prescription criteria are partial upper limb paralysis particularly proximal weakness but with preserved elbow flexion power, for example C5 spinal cord injury. Wheelchair design and details of the back require assessment for mounting of the MAS and for proper sitting posture.

SPINAL AND CRANIAL ORTHOSES
Spinal orthoses are provided for a wide variety of diagnoses. The goals are to provide (1) abdominal support, (2) pain management, (3) control spine position (reposition flexible deformity, support and accommodate fixed deformity, and prevent the progression of deformity), and (4) control spine motion. These goals are primarily accomplished by the reduction of gross spinal motion, the stabilization of individual motion segments, and the application of forces to control the progression of vertebral column deformities. Spinal orthoses are generally categorized by the spinal segments, the gross spinal motions controlled, the level of customization and the materials used to fabricate the orthosis.

SACROILIAC ORTHOSES (SIOs) AND LUMBAR SACRAL ORTHOSES
SIOs are recommended for sacroiliac joint instability due to trauma, over-use or pregnancy. They provide stability by compression directly on the sacrum as the "keystone" of the pelvis, by circumferential compression of the entire pelvis, and by compression and support of lower abdominal muscles. Canvas or other flexible materials are commonly used and the orthoses are often prefabricated.

Lumbosacral orthoses (LSOs) are recommended to manage pathologies in the L2–S1 region. The anterior trimlines extend from the xiphoid process to the symphysis pubis and posteriorly from the inferior angle of the scapula to the sacrococcygeal junction. LSOs can be categorized as either semirigid or rigid. A corset style LSO (Figure 21.26) is a commonly prescribed semirigid spinal orthosis for the relief of low back pain. The corset may be made of fabric or other flexible materials with adjustable closures to ensure a snug fit and rigid horizontal stays or molded plastic inserts for additional stiffness. The corset increases abdominal compression to provide relief of stress on the posterior spinal musculature and thereby provides pain relief.

Rigid spinal orthoses are defined by the plane of motion that is most restricted by the orthosis. The Chairback and the Knight LSO (Figure 21.27) both control motion in the sagittal plane and are

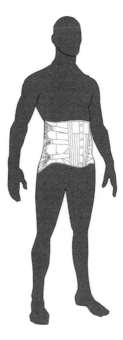

FIGURE 21.26 ■ LSO corset.

composed of a rigid posterior frame with a pelvic band, a thoracic band, and a pair of paraspinal uprights. In addition, they both have a corset front which creates abdominal compression to further support the lumbosacral spine. They differ in that the Knight LSO also provides restriction of frontal plane motion with the addition of a pair of lateral uprights. The Williams extension and coronal plane control LSO is constructed with a similar rigid posterior frame but, with (1) oblique bars replacing the paraspinal bars, (2) mobile attachments at the thoracic band and lateral bars, and (3) an inelastic pelvic strap. The design allows flexion of the lumbar spine and limits extension. The Williams LSO is prescribed for the treatment of spondylolisthesis. All 3 of these LSOs are traditionally constructed of leather covered metal bands and are custom fabricated. Prefabricated thermoplastic versions are available. Custom molded thermoplastic body jacket style LSOs are available and provide rigid tri-planar motion limitation due to the rigid materials and the intimacy of fit over the pelvis.

THORACIC LUMBAR SACRAL ORTHOSES

TLSOs are recommended to manage pathologies in the T3–S1 region. They have anterior trimlines that extend from the sternal notch to the

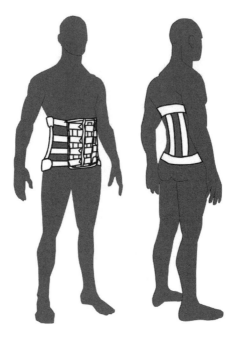

FIGURE 21.27 ■ LSO knight.

symphysis pubis and posteriorly from the spine of the scapula to the sacrococcygeal junction. TLSOs can be categorized as either semirigid or rigid. A corset style TLSO is a commonly prescribed semirigid spinal orthosis for the relief of lumbar and/or thoracic spine pain. Similar to the LSO corset, the TLSO corset relies on abdominal compression to provide relief of stress on the posterior spinal musculature and thereby provide pain relief. They differ in that the TLSO includes a posterior extension to the spine of scapula with shoulder straps used to create an extension force on the thoracic spine and limit flexion. Rigid TLSOs include the Taylor and Knight Taylor designs. Both are composed of a rigid posterior frame with a pelvic band, a thoracic band, a pair of paraspinal uprights, an interscapular band, and axillary straps for flexion and extension control. The Knight Taylor design includes all of the aforementioned components with the addition of lateral bars for coronal plane control. As in the LSO versions, leather covered metal bands are the traditional materials; however, foam covered thermoplastic versions are now common. A corset front is also

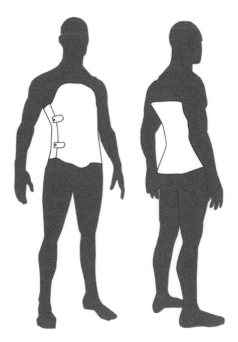

FIGURE 21.28 ■ TLSO body jacket.

used to create abdominal compression to further support the spine. Custom molded thermoplastic body jacket style TLSOs (Figure 21.28) are available and provide the most effective rigid tri-planar motion limitation due to their rigidity and the intimacy of fit over the pelvis and trunk. The body jacket style TLSOs can be fabricated as bivalve or anterior over-lap style for donning. Hyperextension style TLSOs including the Jewett are specifically designed for T10–L2 anterior compression fractures and are designed to prevent flexion and allow extension of the thoracolumbar spine. They are generally a rigid, pre fabricated frame design using a classic 3 point pressure system with body contact via a sternum pad, pubic pad, and a thoracolumbar pad. TLSOs for the management of scoliosis (Figure 21.29) have the primary goal of preventing the progression of the spinal deformity. They achieve this goal through (1) end point control, (2) transverse loading, (3) curve correction, and (4) the combined effect. These techniques are all done in an effort to increase the critical loading capabilities of the spinal column. There are several versions of low profile TLSOs designed for scoliosis management including Boston,

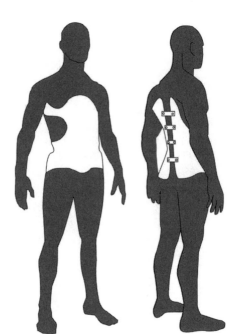

FIGURE 21.29 ■ TLSO scoliosis.

Rosenberger, Miami, Lyonnaise, and Wilmington. Compliance with wearing times and routine follow-ups for adjustments are critical to curve stabilization.

CERVICAL THORACIC LUMBAR SACRAL ORTHOSES

Cervico-thoracic-lumbo-sacral orthoses (CTLSOs) such as the Minerva provide control of the entire spine for stabilization following multilevel trauma or post-surgical reconstruction. The Minerva style orthosis can be entirely custom fabricated or can be a combination of custom fabricated TLSO with a prefabricated cervical extension. The Milwaukee CTLSO is prescribed for the treatment of idiopathic scoliotic curves with an apex at T7 or superior or for cases of Scheuermann's kyphosis. The Milwaukee consists of a custom molded pelvic section, metal frame superstructure, neck ring, and lateral straps and pads.

CERVICAL ORTHOSES

Cervical orthoses (COs) can be generally categorized as flexible, semirigid, or rigid. They provide control primarily of sagittal plane motion (flexion more than extension) and to a lesser extent frontal plane

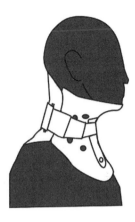

FIGURE 21.30 ■ CO Philadelphia.

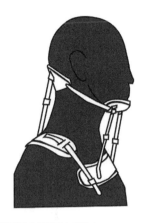

FIGURE 21.31 ■ CO 4 poster.

motion (lateral flexion) but do not limit transverse plane rotation movements well. The soft foam collar is a simple, prefabricated, flexible CO often prescribed as a general kinesthetic reminder. The Philadelphia collar and similar orthoses (Figure 21.30) are popular semirigid COs for use with stable mid-cervical injuries or used after weaning out of a more rigid orthosis. Poster style rigid COs (2 and 4) (Figure 21.31) are described based on the number of rigid bars or posts used to support the head on the shoulders and upper thorax. They are used primarily for sagittal plane control either with a stable spine following trauma or postoperatively when rigid fixation is required in the C3–C6 region of the cervical spine.

CERVICAL THORACIC ORTHOSES
Cervicothoracic orthoses (CTOs) are used to extend the region of immobilization to the lower cervical and upper thoracic levels and are indicated for pathologies in the C1–T2 region. CTOs control flexion more effectively than extension due to the longer mechanical anterior lever arms. They are commonly prescribed for stable fractures, flexion injuries in the C3–T1 region, extension injuries in the C3–C5 region, general postoperative stabilization, and after weaning out of HALO use. The Sternal Occipital Mandibular Immobilizer (SOMI) is an example of a CTO and is an alternative to the poster style CO. It is preferred when donning in supine is required as there are no posterior bars. The SOMI specifically limits flexion and is most effective in the C1–C5 region.

The Halo (Figure 21.32) is a rigid CTO used for unstable cervical injuries and particularly for upper cervical spine instability (occiput-C2).

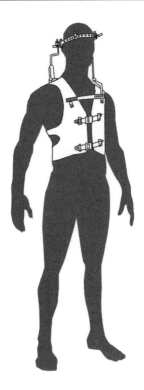

FIGURE 21.32 ■ Halo.

The halo ring is fixed into the skull with 4 screws and into 2 or 4 bars which then attach to a rigid vest for shoulder and upper thorax loading.

Amputees Sample Order Set

Jarrod Friedman

Diagnosis: *BKA or AKA*

Admit to: Acute rehabilitation unit (Amputee)

Condition: Stable

Allergies: List known drug or other allergies

Precautions: Fall precautions

Vital Signs: q 8 to 12 hours

Activity: Initially WC level, if appropriate ambulation with crutches or walker (Rolling or Pickup)

Diet: Regular or cardiac or renal dependent on PMhx

IV Fluids: None

Nursing: Routine and incision dressing changes q shift initial if drainage, q12 otherwise.

Therapies
    Physical Therapy: 2 to 3 hr/d: Strengthen and ROM of residual limb and UE, conditioning
    Occupational Therapy: Evaluation for equipment needs
    Prosthetic:
        Prosthetic evaluation
        Stump prep with rigid removal dressing or stump shrinker or ace wrap.
    Speech: Not needed normally but consider evaluation if appropriate
    Psychology: Evaluation variable dependent surrounding issues
    Vocational Rehabilitation: May be appropriate on outpatient once stable.
    Social Work: Discharge planning and family organization and communication

Modalities: See modality section. Heat or ice common prn.
    Chronic amputee: TENS, Laser, US, Infrared and others sometimes used.

Prophylaxis
    Contracture Prevention:
    BKA

    ■ Extension platform under distal limb when in wheelchair or seated
    ■ No pillows under the knee. May place pillow distally to maintain full knee extension while in bed.
    ■ ROM 0-110 to full ROM daily—or thrice daily
    ■ Quadriceps strengthening.

    AKA

    ■ Lying on stomach approx 20 minutes minimum thrice daily to prevent hip flexion contracture
    ■ Hip extensor and abductor and adductor strengthening
    ■ Hip ROM TID with ensuring extension and adduction and abduction is maintained.

Skin: Monitor stump and sacral region, educate on pressure relief.

Pain
■ Once cleared by the surgical team residual limb self-massage and skin mobilization, decreases risk of pain from scar restriction and may decrease neuroma encapsulation and subsequent pain.

DVT: Pneumatic compression devices on contralateral lower extremity
■ Heparin 5000 q 12 hours
■ Enoxaparin

Bowel

Gastritis
- H2 blocker
- proton pump inhibitor

Constipation (especially, if on opiods for pain management):
- Stool softeners once or twice daily
- Senna 1 to 2 by mouth daily
- Bisacodyl suppositories as needed if no bowel movement in 2 to 3 days

Medications
- **Pain Medications**
  Key is to ensure that patient has good pain control so they will participate in therapies and minimize risk of chronic pain. If needed, ensure medication is given prior to therapy to foster participation.

  Phantom Pain
  - Gabapentin 100 mg or 300 mg tabs titrate q2 days(1–3) until up to 1800 mg/d or
  - Amitriptyline 25 to 75 mg po qhs or
  - Duloxetine 30 to 60 mg po q 12 hours or
  - Pregabalin 50 to 75 mg po q 12 hours

Bone Pain
  Short Acting
  - Oxycodone 5 or 10 mg tabs po q 6 to 8 hours prn breakthrough pain or
  - Oxycodone/Acetaminophen (Percocet®) 5/325 mg to 10/325 mg 1 to 2 po q 68 hours prn breakthrough pain or
  - Hydrocodone/acetaminophen (Vicodin®) 5/500 or 7.5/650 mg 1 to 2 po q 8 hours prn breakthrough pain

  Long Action: Use with caution indicated if pain is uncontrolled while using short acting opioids throughout the day.
  - Morphine sulfate extended release (MS contin®, Kadian®, Avinza®) 15 mg po qd to q 12 hours or
  - Methadone 2.5 mg to 5mg po q12 hours or
  - Oxycodone extended release (Oxycontin®) 10 mg po q 12 hours or
  - Fentanyl patches (Duragesic®) 12 mcg/hr or 25 mcg

  Skin/Incisional Pain
  - Scar and incision light massage once healed or healing to prevent long term pain issues.

Labs: baseline Labs, CBC with diff, BMP, Alb or Pre-Alb (nutrition monitoring)

Length of Stay: 7 to 14 days

Goals

1. Ambulation with temporary prosthesis

2. Don and Doff prosthesis

3. Incision care

4. Pain control

5. Strengthening of lower extremities, muscles adductors and abductors, hip flexors, gluteus medius, hamstring, and quadriceps.

6. Cardio-pulmonary conditioning.

■ REFERENCES

1. Centers for Medicare and Medicaid Services. Local Coverage Determinations (LCD) for Lower Limb Prosthesis [#L11464]. Medicare Coverage Database. http://www.medicarenhic.com/dme/medical_review/mr_lcds/mr_lcd_current/L11464_2010-01-01_PA_2010-04.pdf

2. Gailey R, Roach K, Applegate E, et al. The amputee mobility predictor: an instrument to assess determinants of lower-limb amputee's ability to ambulate. *Arch Phys Med Rehabil.* 2002; 83: 615–627.

3. Kuiken T. Targeted Reinnervation for Improved Prosthetic Function. In: Bussell M, Kraft G, eds. New Advances in Prosthetics and Orthotics. *Physical Medicine and Rehabilitation Clinics of North America.* Philadelphia, PA: Saunders; 2006: 1–13.

■ ADDITIONAL READINGS

1. Smith G, Michael J, Bowker J, eds.*Atlas of Amputations and Limb Deficiencies: Surgical, Prosthetic, and Rehabilitation Principles.* 3rd ed. American Academy of Orthopedic Surgeons; 2004. 6300 North River Road Rosemont, IL 60018.

2. Hsu J, Michael J, Fisk J, eds. *AAOS Atlas of Orthoses and Assistive Devices.* 4th ed. American Academy of Orthopedic Surgeons, Mosby Elsevier; 2008. 1600 John F Kennedy Blvd. Ste 1800 Philadelphia, PA 19103–2899.

3. Cuccurullo S. ed. *Physical Medicine and Rehabilitation Board Review.* Demos Medical Publishing; 2004.

4. Braddom R, Buschbacher R, Chan L, et al, eds. *Physical Medicine & Rehabilitation.* 3rd ed. Saunders Elsevier; 2007.

22

Spinal Cord Injury Rehabilitation

Jarrod David Friedman

■ SPINAL CORD INJURY EPIDEMIOLOGY

According to the National Spinal Cord Injury Statistical Center 12 000 new spinal cord injuries (SCIs) occur in the United States every year. The vast majority are men under the age of 40. The most common cause of SCI is motor vehicle collisions. Over the age of 45, the most common cause is falls. Violence (primarily gunshot wounds) accounts for 15% of the SCIs in the United States. The racial/ethnic distribution of SCI cases and other demographic characteristics are detailed in Table 22.1.

The most common levels of injury are C5 for complete SCI and T12 for incomplete injuries. Most injuries occur from C4 to C7, T4 to T6 and at the thoracolumbar junction (T10–L1). Non-traumatic causes of SCI are detailed in Table 22.2.

SCI CLASSIFICATION

The American Spinal Injury Association (ASIA) has established examination guidelines that are currently the universal standard for the examination and evaluation of SCI patients. This assessment involves the evaluation of both the sensory and motor system in a uniform fashion. The initial examination should be performed within the first week post injury. For prognostic purposes, the ASIA evaluation should be repeated when the patient is out of spinal shock (reflexes return). Repeat testing is recommended since patient effort and condition at examination can vary and for improving reliability. Multiple evaluations done over several days are considered superior to one single examination.

The ASIA classification and examination has 3 basic components:

1) SENSORY

The sensory system is evaluated using both pin prick and light touch on the right and left sides. Scoring is described in Table 22.3. A physician should perform *pin prick* evaluation using a standard unused safety pin. The sharp edge is used to determine a patients' ability to sense the sharp and the dull safety cover of the pin if the patient is able to sense dull sensation. Physicians should perform a *light touch* evaluation with a wisp of cotton. The control for examination is the face, unless facial injury is noted or suspected.

TABLE 22.1 ■ Epidemiology of traumatic SCI.

INCIDENCE	
	12 000 new cases per year or 40 case per million population
PREVALENCE	
	Approximately 262 000 people currently living with SCI in the United States
ETIOLOGY	
	• MVA 41% • Falls 27% • Violence 15% • Sports 8% • Other 9%
AGE (AVERAGE)	
	28.7 (1973–1979) 40.2 (since 2005)
SEX	
	80.8% Male
LEVELS	
	• C5 Most Common Level • T12 Most Common Level amongst paraplegics
RACE (SINCE 2005)	
	• Caucasian 66.2% • African–American 27.0% • Hispanic–American 7.9% • Asian–American 2%

Data from Annual Report for Spinal Cord Injury Model Systems Public Version 2009, National Spinal Cord Injury Statistical Center, University of Alabama at Birmingham, February 2010.

TABLE 22.2 ■ Non-traumatic causes of SCI.

• Spinal stenosis

• Cancer—most commonly breast, lung, or prostate

• Transverse myelitis

• MS

• Syringomyelia

• Vascular ischemia (thoracoabdominal aneurysms can result in injury to the artery of Adamkiewicz causing T12–L1 ischemic injury.)

TABLE 22.3 ■ Sensory scoring system.

Score	Description
NT	Not Testable: used when a level cannot be tested due to secondary factors (cast, cognitive impairment, or other factors)
0	Inability to register a difference between sharp and dull on pin prick or unable to sense light touch
1	Ability to register a difference but the sharp is not as precise as that noted on the face. Regarding light touch face is more precise than testing area.
2	Patient notes sensation is the same on their face and on the dermatomal level being tested.*

*If hyperesthesia is present the level is given a grade 1 and not 2.

2) MOTOR

The motor system is evaluated based on assessment of specific myotome groups with the patient in a supine position. At levels where motor testing is not feasible (thoracic), the motor is assumed to correspond to the sensory examination. Motor scoring is detailed in Table 22.4.

The most caudal myotome tested with manual muscle test findings equal to or greater than 3/5 with the segment proximal noted to be normal (5/5) is the motor level. For levels where there is no motor testing, the level would correspond to the last normal sensory level.

3) ANAL SPHINCTER

The sphincter is tested for voluntary anal contraction through digital examination and is graded as present or absent.

ASIA IMPAIRMENT SCALE

The sensory, motor, and anal sphincter contraction evaluation provides key information used to determine the patients' relative impairment levels and the ASIA Impairment Rating. Table 22.5 describes the multiple levels and scores that are determined through the examination. The ASIA impairment scale ranges from A to E with A indicating the most severe findings and E representing a normal exam. Details for scoring are described in Table 22.6.

■ SPINAL CORD INJURY SYNDROMES (FIGURE 22.1)
BROWN-SEQUARD SYNDROME

Incomplete SCI as a result of damage to the lateral half of the spinal cord (hemisection) resulting in damage to the corticospinal

TABLE 22.4 ■ Motor scoring system.

Score	Description
NT	Not Testable: used when a level cannot be tested due to secondary factors (cast or other immobilization, spasticity or contracture)
0	Absent
1	Palpable or visible contraction
2	Active movement, full range of motion with gravity eliminated
3	Active movement, full range of motion against gravity
4	Active movement full range of motion against gravity and some resistance
5	Active movement full range of motion against gravity and normal resistance
5*	Muscles by examiners judgment has NL strength but factors preclude full ROM or NL function.

TABLE 22.5 ■ Various SCI impairment levels.

Sensory Level	Is the most caudal dermatome level with both pin prick and light touch scoring 2/2.
Motor Level	The most caudal myotome tested whose manual muscle test was noted to be equal to or greater than 3/5 with the segment proximal noted to be normal (5/5) on testing.
Neurologic Level of Injury (NLI)	The most caudal level where motor and sensory are intact.
Sensory Index Score (112 maximum)	Summary of all the sensory scores for both light touch and pin prick.
Motor Index Score (100 maximum)	Summary of motor testing 25 points for each limb and 100 for all 4 extremities.
Zone of Partial Preservation (ZPP)	The segments below the NLI with noted preservation of sensory or motor findings reserved for complete SCI.

tracts and dorsal column, which cross at the level of the brain stem leading to a loss of proprioception and motor function (paralysis) ipsilateral to the lesion. The spinothalamic tracts cross at the spinal level resulting in loss of pain and temperature sensation on the contralateral side.

TABLE 22.6 ■ ASIA impairment scale.

Grade	Description	Injury Type
ASIA A	*Complete injury*	*Sensory and motor complete*
ASIA B	*Incomplete injury* with no motor function preserved below the NLI but some sensory including Sacral 4–5 preservation is present.	*Sensory incomplete Motor complete*
ASIA C	*Incomplete injury* with sensory sacral sparing and motor function preserved below the NLI. This may be >3 levels below the NLI but <50% of the muscles below the NLI have motor score of ≥3.	*Sensory incomplete Motor incomplete*
ASIA D	*Incomplete injury* with sensory sacra sparing and motor function preserved >3 levels below the NLI and greater then >50% of the muscles below the NLI must have a motor score of ≥3 or Voluntary anal contraction is present.	*Sensory incomplete Motor incomplete*
ASIA E	Normal: Motor and sensory functions are normal.	*Normal*

ANTERIOR CORD SYNDROME
Damage to the anterior two-thirds of the spinal cord as the result of disruption in blood flow to the anterior spinal artery. This can occur as a result of trauma, embolus, hypotension, or arterial occlusion. On rare occasions, it can occur as a result of aortic clamping during surgery. Patients present with absence of motor and pain sensation below the level of the injury. Blood supply through the posterior spinal artery spares the dorsal columns resulting in normal proprioception below the level of the injury.

CENTRAL CORD SYNDROME
The most common of the SCI syndromes occurring primarily in older individuals. This injury is typically the result of a cervical hyperextension injury usually in the presence of spondylosis and is characterized by disproportionately weak upper extremities compared to lower extremities. Sensory loss below the level of the injury is variable.

CONUS MEDULLARIS INJURY
A syndrome characterized by a mixed upper motor neuron and lower motor neuron presentation. Clinical findings include areflexic bowel

Central cord syndrome

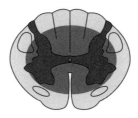

Anterior cord syndrome

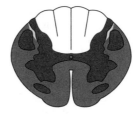

Brown-sequard syndrome

Cortico-spinal tract

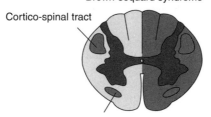

Anterior spino thalamic tract

FIGURE 22.1 ■ Common incomplete SCI syndromes. Adapted from Wikipedia.

and bladder and sensory loss in a saddle distribution with or without lower extremity weakness.

CAUDA EQUINA SYNDROME
This is not a true SCI but involves damage to multiple lumbosacral nerve roots that form the cauda equina and thus upper motor neuron signs are absent. Clinical presentation is similar to conus medullaris injury with bowel and bladder involvement. Asymmetric pain and sensory loss are usually present in the distribution of the nerve roots involved. Reflexes are absent distal to the injury level.

PROGNOSIS AFTER SCI

For the purpose of determining prognosis, examinations at or within 24 hours of injury are not as accurate as those done at 72 hours. Evaluation of pin prick has better reliability than light touch examination and return of pin prick sensation is the best sign of recovery enabling better predictability.

The review of a patient's reflexes can help determine prognosis. In incomplete SCI, deep tendon reflexes tend to have larger amplitudes compared to complete injuries.

The presence of an abnormal plantar response at 72 hours has a high correlation with complete SCI and portends a poor prognosis. Presence of a crossed adductor response (contralateral adduction and internal rotation to a patellar tap or knee jerk), which is absent in complete injuries, correlates with a greater likelihood of motor recovery in the lower extremities. The absence of the bulbocavernosus reflex within 72 hours after injury suggests a lower motor neuron injury.

Most upper extremity recovery occurs in the first 2 to 6 months post injury with greatest gains occurring in the first 3 months. Motor recovery can continue up to and into the second year post injury; with average functional plateau for complete and incomplete at 12 to 18 months and 9 to 12 months, respectively (1). Recovery potential based on initial motor scores is summarized in Table 22.7.

ACUTE SCI

In acute SCI, prehospital management includes standard ACLS protocols with care directed at ensuring proper spinal stabilization at the event scene. All patients should be assumed to have a SCI or bony instability until proven otherwise. The goal of initial stabilization is to minimize acute injury and prevent progression of direct injury and damage to the spinal cord from indirect causes. Direct and indirect causes of SCI are summarized in Table 22.8.

TABLE 22.7 ■ Review of observational reports on recovery.

Initial Motor Scores	Motor Recovery Potential
1–2/5	>95% reach 3/5
Key muscles and some immediate adjacent level with 0/5	50%–60% will reach 1/5
Adjacent muscles 1 level away from 0/5	Up to 25% can reach 3/5
Adjacent muscles 2 levels away from injury	<10% recover 1/5 strength

TABLE 22.8 ■ Examples of direct and indirect causes of SCI.

Direct	Indirect
Foreign Body (bullet, knife)	Hypo-perfusion
Bony compression	Metabolic overload
Tumor	Thrombus
Instability	Local toxic metabolites
Fracture	
Mass compression	

SCI Pearls
- Complete SCI usually recover one level distal to their initial NLI.
- Complete SCI above T9 normally do not regain lower extremity motor function.
- Complete SCI below T9, amongst these individuals 33% recover some lower extremity function.
- Nontraumatic SCI patients have shorter length of stay and lower incidence of spasticity, orthostasis, pressure ulcer, dysreflexia, DVT, and pneumonia
- More likely to continue to work if: young, lower level of injury, less severe injury, educated, driven, and married.
- Consider concomitant brain injury if there is new cognitive impairment, frontal signs, disparity of upper and lower body tone and spasticity, or paradoxical breathing.

NEUROGENIC SHOCK

Acute SCI interrupts the sympathetic nervous system below the level of injury resulting in vasodilatation. If the injury is proximal to the sixth level of the thoracic spine the result is cardiovascular disregulation with a significant loss in systemic vascular resistance. If the injury is proximal to the first thoracic level the patient loses the ability to have compensatory increases in their cardiac rate. These issues result in the classic SCI neurogenic triad; often coexisting with hypovolemia:

- Hypotension
- Bradycardia
- Hypothermia

SPINAL SHOCK

Spinal shock is the loss of spinal reflexes with flaccid paralysis, hypotonia, areflexia, with loss of bowel and bladder reflexes and sphincter control. The absence of muscle tone and normal vascular reflexes below the level of injury causes impaired blood-pressure control leading to orthostasis and orthostatic hypotension. Spinal shock is considered resolved when the distal reflexes start to return; delayed plantar reflex followed by the return of the bulbocavernosus reflex. The earlier the return of deep tendon reflexes the better the prognosis. Following resolution of spinal shock, patients can be noted to have the onset of spasticity, hyperreflexia, and clonus.

NEUROGENIC AND SPINAL SHOCK MANAGEMENT

A patient who is noted to be in shock should be treated with invasive monitoring, volume resuscitation, and vasopressors to maintain blood pressure. Invasive monitoring is important to prevent pulmonary edema and respiratory damage secondary to over-hydration. The uncontrolled sympathetic discharge in acute SCI can cause extravasation of fluid from pulmonary vasculature.

The disruption that occurs between the spinal cord and the sympathetic nervous system leads to bradycardia especially in the first several weeks post injury. In the initial stages of SCI management, monitoring bradycardia and providing supportive care is necessary. In some patients, especially those with injuries at the upper thoracic and cervical area, bradycardia may be serious enough to require transvenous pacing (temporary or permanent). It is important to remember that bradycardia in SCI patients is not a result of atrial dysfunction but a result of uninhibited vagal parasympathetic stimulation on the heart.

Hypotension occurring as a result of spinal and neurogenic shock can result in mean arterial pressure (MAP) around 55 and systolic blood pressure of 90 mmHg or lower. Cardiovascular support with intravenous fluids and pressors (eg, dopamine, ephedrine, florinef, and midodrine, among others) can be used to maintain a MAP above 85 and a systolic blood pressure above 110 mmHg. This is important to maintain spinal-cord perfusion.

While there is discussion of the use of hypothermia and even membrane stabilizing agents (gabapentin, 2001) (2) to slow the metabolism within the spinal cord, decrease progression of further spinal-cord damage and/or help mildly injured cells to recover; there is no definitive evidence available to demonstrate that these techniques result in improved long-term outcomes.

■ ACUTE SCI EVALUATION

x-ray: Used for initial screening of the spine and evaluation of bony structures.

CT scan: Allows for further evaluation of bony structure and central canal when fractures or abnormalities are suspected but not clearly visualized on x-ray. It is the evaluation of choice to determine bony encroachment within the spinal canal. Contrast can be used to evaluate for spinal cord and nerve compression.

MRI: Magnetic resonance imaging (MRI) can be used in the acute and subacute stages following SCI to evaluate spinal cord integrity, determine localization, and identify presence of intraspinal and extra spinal hemorrhage and edema. Several findings on MRI are associated with poor prognosis (3,4):

- Presence of spinal-cord hemorrhage
- Larger length of spinal-cord hemorrhage
- Greater expanse of edema proximal to distal
- Spinal cord compression
- Abnormalities are noted to expand more than one vertebral segment

MRI STIR: Imaging can be used to evaluate for edema within the cord in acute injury. Bony fracture can be visualized as a hyper-intense signal with the marrow.

T2 GRE: Is the best tool to evaluate for acute cord hematoma.

MRA: Used to evaluate for vertebral artery injury.

TREATMENT
METHYLPREDNISOLONE

Three separate trials of the National Acute Spinal Cord Injury Study (NASCIS) (5,6) looked at the effects of methylprednisolone after SCI. NASCIS 2 trial results demonstrated significant differences on outcomes when high-dose methylprednisolone was initiated within 8 hours of injury at 30 mg/kg bolus followed by 5.4 mg/kg/hr for 23 hours (7,8). NASCIS 3 reported improved benefit when methyl-prednisolone was extended to 48 hours post injury and initiated 3 to 8 hours post injury (6). Methylprednisolone administration is considered a treatment option in both the Neurosurgical Guidelines and the Spinal Cord Medicine Consortium Clinical Practice Guidelines (9,10). Emergency medical personnel usually have methylprednisolone available and immediate administration to patients with suspected injury is considered standard protocol (9,10,11,12). Use of methylprednisolone varies due to concerns regarding post infusion side effects. The NACIS' evidence is considered by some to be insufficient (especially for complete SCIs). Others are concerned about the side effects of steroids, specifically, steroid induced myopathy, which has been associated with both the 24-hour and the 48-hour protocols (13). Steroid utilization has also been shown to cause hyperglycemia, gastritis, and pneumonia in some patients who receive the 48-hour infusion. The 48-hour infusion has also been associated with increased risk of infection. The risk of side effects versus benefit needs to be considered (7).

COMMON MEDICAL COMPLICATIONS AFTER SCI
PULMONARY

The leading cause of mortality in the first year after SCI is pulmonary complications with all levels of injury being at risk (6,14). Contributing factors to pulmonary complications include atelectasis, hypoventilation, and inability or difficulty managing secretions. SCI injuries with damage at C1–3 will require 24-hour ventilator support post injury with a backup ventilator/portable ventilator and supportive devices. Those with SCI at C5 and below usually do not require long-term ventilation support. The requirements for patients with injuries at the fourth cervical level are variable.

Without the tone of the abdominal wall to provide support and assist in coughing and expiration, SCI patients generally have decreased expiratory capacity and may not be able to generate the peak cough expiratory flow (PCEF) of 5 to 6 liters or more, which is needed to clear secretions properly. Due to the segmental innervations of the intercostal muscles, patients with higher level injuries have more severe impairments of cough and exhalation. Spinal cord patients with high-level injuries eventually lose their expiratory reserve (vital capacity is equal to inspiratory capacity). Without proper PCEF secretions can accumulate and also impair ventilation and subsequent oxygen and carbon dioxide exchange. These factors can lead to infections of the lung and death.

Given the loss of expiratory ability, the need to perform pulmonary toileting and to teach assisted cough maneuvers is important to maintain good pulmonary hygiene, prevent infection, and other pulmonary complications.

ABDOMINAL BINDERS

It provides support to the abdominal cavity pushing against the abdominal contents and improving diaphragmatic support and positioning thus assisting in expiratory function and coughing especially while upright.

SECRETION MANAGEMENT

Secretion management is a very important component of SCI management. The basic types of secretion management assistance include: postural drainage, percussion, vibration, and cough assistance techniques or devices. All of these techniques are designed to help mobilize and loosen secretions. Prior to these therapies, bronchodilators administration can be considered to facilitate opening of the airways and improve drainage and/or expectoration of secretions.

There are 10 standardized positions for postural drainage (Figure 22.2). Commonly, patients are placed in a Trendelenburg position (head down) between 10 to 45 degrees to assist in drainage. This can be done independently or in conjunction with other modalities. If performed in the morning,

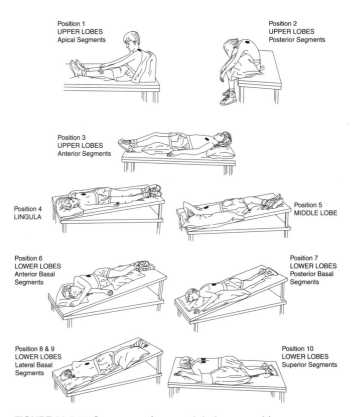

FIGURE 22.2 ■ Summary of postural drainage positions.

the benefits may continue into the night reducing overall secretion accumulation. Precautions must be employed due to the potential for position associated increases in blood flow return which can lead to cardiovascular complications given the inability to regulate sympathetic and parasympathetic responses. If patients have active infections, extra caution should be used due to risk for increases in flow of secretions from diseased to healthy lobes of lung.

Chest percussion therapy can be performed manually or with machine assistance by trained physical or respiratory therapists. During the expiratory phase, a therapist or mechanical device (at 5 Hz) rhythmically strikes the chest wall in the area where drainage assistances is desired. Manual chest percussion is performed by hand while mechanical percussion involves the use of specially designed machines for time periods that vary dependent upon individual tolerance (1–5 minutes).

Vibration therapy is used throughout the respiratory cycle not just the expiratory phase. The machine runs at 10 to 15 Hz for similar time frames as mechanical percussion. These machines can be more costly; but in patients with a high volume of secretions and/or poor clearance prevention of complications justifies its use.

Insufflation–exsufflation devices are highly effective in the removal of secretions. Positive pressure is provided during inspiration resulting in insufflation. This increases the patient's vital capacity which must be a minimum of 1200 to 1500 ml to allow for an effective cough (PCEF of at least 5–6 L/sec). The insufflations are provided through masks or directly into endotracheal or tacheostomy tubes. The insufflations are followed by a negative-pressure/controlled suction also called exsufflation. This mechanical technique creates a PCEF of 7 to 11 L/s, which is necessary for proper clearance of secretions. Oral suctioning is used to remove secretions in the oral cavity and posterior oropharynx. Suctioning of airway secretions must be performed using a sterile technique and with caution due to propensity for cardiac abnormalities, pulmonary edema, increased intracranial pressure, tracheal, and/ or mucosal damage.

ACTIVE-ASSIST COUGH

A manually assisted cough is performed with the application of an external force to various sites of the trunk during a cough or the expiratory phase. This requires the assistance of another individual (clinician, nurse, or personal assistant) to facilitate the cough and expiration. Active-assist cough maneuvers include side-lying abdominal thrust assist, costophrenic assist, anterior chest compression assist, or counter-rotation assist. Contraindications include rib fractures, recent abdominal or thoracic surgery, ileus, or the presence of inferior vena cava filters (which can be dislodged by these maneuvers).

SELF-ASSIST COUGH

A self-assisted cough is also possible. To perform this type of cough, the head and trunk are quickly flexed starting from an initial position of relative extension. Contraindications are similar to those for active assist cough.

CARDIOVASCULAR

The interruption in the mechanics of the cardiovascular system in acute and chronic SCI is critical and can lead to several medical problems ·   ling secondary injury and/or death. Common cardiovascular seque- ̃CI are summarized in Table 22.9.

     'ents who have an injury above the T7 level will have disrup-   ɔrmal cardiovascular control and of the interactions between

TABLE 22.9 ■ Cardiovascular issues in spinal cord injury.

Cervical and Thoracic	Lumbar
Orthostatic hypotension	Orthostatic hypotension
Distal Venous Blood Pooling (increased DVT risk)	Distal Venous Blood Pooling(increased DVT risk)
Bradycardia	
Autonomic dysreflexia	

the parasympathetic and sympathetic nervous systems. In SCI, the sympathetic nervous system customary inhibitory feedback mechanisms are impaired with function present only at the local level with parasympathetic response maintained. As a result of the parasympathetic and sympathetic nervous system dysregulation, SCI at T6 or above results in autonomic dysreflexia (see Appendix 3).

Injury at T5 or above results in impaired adrenal function causing dysregulation of adrenaline release.

T1 to T4 are the spinal levels that provide innervation to the myocardium and AV nodes. Injuries at T1 or above result in disconnection between the central nervous system and sympathetic nervous system.

Initially, SCI patients have hypotension and bradycardia; occurring during the first several weeks post injury and stabilizing over time with appropriate management. SCI patients have lower MAP and lower systolic blood pressures. The MAP post injury is usually between 55 to 65 mmHg with systemic pressures at 90 to 100 mmHg due to decreased resting systemic vascular resistance. Bradycardia is also common immediately post injury and may continue for up to 8 weeks post injury, especially in cervical and high-thoracic SCI.

TREATMENT FOR COMMON CARDIOVASCULAR ISSUES

Orthostatic Hypotension is common after SCI. Many patients adapt over time to this sequela (several weeks to months). External vascular support of the arterial and venous system with compression stocking, bilateral lower extremity compression wrapping, and abdominal binders is recommended. The principle is to provide support to the venous system, prevent excessive pooling of blood in the lower extremities, and improve venous return. During physical therapy sessions a tilt table can be used for short periods of time to facilitate adaptation to the SCI and reduce orthostatic episodes. Initial treatment duration is 5 to 10 minutes. Patients should be monitored for tolerance and medical stability with particular focus on changes in alertness, dizziness, shortness of breath, headaches, nausea, hypotension, changes in heart rate, or respiratory rate.

If any of these occur the tilt table session should be discontinued. If a tilt table is not available, physical therapists can work with the patient by progressively elevating the head of the bed, as tolerated, and by having the patient sit on the edge of the bed or in a wheelchair. These techniques can also be implemented by other team members to improve tolerance and foster adaptation.

Oral or intravenous fluids with or without oral salt supplementation can be used to treat orthostatic hypotension. Vasopressors (eg, midrodine) can also be administered in severe cases but are not recommended for night time or bedtime use as there is a risk of hypertension when in a supine position. Mineralorticoids, such as florinef, have been used to increase sodium reuptake while at the same time indirectly increasing intravascular fluid. These agents should be used with caution due to the risk for hypernatremia and hypokalemia. Monitoring of serum electrolytes is recommended during treatment.

Patients with severe bradycardia and hypotension should be evaluated by cardiology for cardiac pacemaker candidacy.

Autonomic Dysreflexia (AD) occurs when exposure to noxious stimuli results in disinhibited stimulation of the sympathetic nervous system in patients with injuries at T6 or above. The hallmarks of AD are bradycardia and relative hypertension (20–40 mmHg above baseline). Noxious stimulation below the level of the lesion leads to uncontrolled sympathetic discharge. Sympathetic outflow continues, uninhibited, until the noxious stimulus is eliminated. Peripheral vasculature will constrict resulting in increased venous return which in turn elevates blood pressure. Increases in venous return trigger carotid baroreceptors, activate vagal circuitry, and thus, bradycardia ensues.

Treatment of AD requires immediate elimination of the noxious stimulus. Most important is the prevention of cardiac arrhythmias, seizures, ischemic/hemorrhagic stroke, retinal hemorrhages, pulmonary edema, and death.

Signs of AD

- Flushing and sweating above the level of lesion (parasympathetic signs).
- Piloerection below the level of injury (sympathetic signs).
- Paroxysmal hypertension 20 to 40 mmHg above baseline.
- Headache or nasal congestion
- Bradycardia
- Anxiety

Common Causes

- Obstructed, twisted, or kinked indwelling urinary catheter
- Distended bladder

■ Distended or impacted rectal vault or bowel

■ Urinary tract infection

■ Fracture

■ Ingrown toenails

■ Other noxious stimuli (heterotopic ossification, pain, pressure ulcer, and acute abdominal pathology, among others)

Treatment

Immediately
■ Loosen clothes
■ Release abdominal binder
■ Remove compression stockings

Secondary
■ If an indwelling urinary catheter is present, inspect the tubing carefully for twists or kinks and flush to determine if obstruction is present.
■ Perform bladder scanning to evaluate for distension.
■ In the absence of an indwelling urinary catheter, catheterize the bladder while using lidocaine gel to prevent further noxious irritation.
■ Perform a rectal exam. If rectal vault is full of stool, perform manual evacuation.
■ Check skin and digits for any visible abnormality or possible noxious cause (ie, ingrown nail).

■ If no cause is found or systolic blood pressure is above 150 mmHg, consider using a short acting anti-hypertensive agent.
  ■ Nitropaste ½ to 1 inch is preferred since it is easy to remove once noxious stimulus is removed.
  ■ Other choices
    ■ Nifedipine 10 mg PO, may repeat q 30 to 60 minutes as needed.
    ■ Clonidine patch 0.1 can also be used in cases of sustained hypertension. Clonidine is a good alternative since the patch can be removed after the AD episode is treated. Patients should be monitored since rebound tachycardia is possible.
  ■ Severe cases
    ■ Hydralazine (intravenous or oral) 10 to 20 mg
    ■ Nitroprusside IV

■ Patients can develop temporary hypotension which should be managed as follows:
  ■ Trendelenburg positioning
  ■ Intravenous fluids
  ■ Removal of topical antihypertensives.

DEEP VEIN THROMBOSIS (DVT)

Endocrine changes along with venous pooling increase the potential for systemic venous thrombosis. The use of low molecular weight heparin is preferred over unfractionated heparin in SCI patients. While comparison showed equal rates of DVT, the incidence of pulmonary embolism and bleeding was higher in patients using unfractionated heparin (15). Treatment is recommended for a total of 6 to 8 weeks post injury. In high-risk patients, those with confirmed DVT, or those who have contraindications to anticoagulation, inferior vena cava (IVC) filter placement should be considered. It is important to remember that IVC filters do not prevent DVT. In addition, manual-assisted cough maneuvers cannot be performed after placement.

BLADDER

SCI patients will typically have an indwelling urinary catheter at the time of admission to a rehabilitation hospital or unit. A bladder program is initiated when the patient is medically stable and no longer requires intravenous fluids or antibiotics and/or monitoring of input and output (9). The goal of bladder management is to prevent high volumes within the bladder, which increases the risk of urinary reflux to the kidney, resulting in kidney damage and/or infection.

During the spinal shock period, the bladder is flaccid often with some preservation of sphincter tone. As reflexes return, patients with injury above the conus medullaris (upper motor neuron injury) will have continued sphincter tone or heightened tone. Bladder reflexes usually return as spinal shock resolves leading to bladder contractions in association with increasing urine volumes. These contractions, which are the result of parasympathetic input from the S2–4 ganglion via the pelvic nerve, are normally opposed by inhibition of contraction or bladder relaxation a result of sympathetic stimulation (T10–L2) or beta adrenergic stimulation via the hypogastric nerve. Stimulation of bladder contraction and inhibition of bladder contraction occur normally with simultaneous relaxation or contraction of the bladder neck and sphincter, respectively. In some SCI patients, this process does not occur, known as bladder-sphincter dysynergia. Dysynergia creates a high-pressure system, which places the patient at risk for reflux of urine into the ureters and subsequently into the kidneys. Chronic retrograde flow of urine into the kidneys can lead to renal failure. Proper bladder management seeks to maintain low bladder volumes to prevent secondary complications.

An indwelling catheter serves to continually drain the bladder maintaining a low-pressure system. Clean intermittent catheterization (CIC) is the preferred method for bladder management in SCI patients. Level of injury and hand dexterity should be considered when making a decision regarding how to best manage the bladder; indwelling catheter versus CIC. With the use of assistive devices, males with injuries at C6 or below and females with injuries at C7 or below can perform CIC. Urinary volumes should be kept below 500 ml each time catheterization is performed. Consumption of oral fluids should be adjusted to ensure volumes are kept within this range, especially overnight. In the inpatient setting bladder scanning can provide important clinical information to enable the physician to determine the proper frequency of catheterization and whether oral fluid intake needs to be adjusted. It is important to consider that during the acute post injury period large volumes of intravenous fluids are given that may accumulate in the interstitial space (ie, third space accumulation). As SCI patients are mobilized during rehabilitation, fluid will normally shift from the intersitial space into the blood vessels. Thus, SCI patients tend to require more frequent catheterization during the first 2 weeks of their rehabilitation course than they will need later on.

Other considerations for bladder management include sphincterotomies, ventral continent stomas, and suprapubic catheters. These options can provide independence for patients when intermittent catheterization is not possible or for those who have difficulty accessing the perineum for catheterization.

Urinary bacterial colonization is common in SCI patients. Prophylactic antibiotics for prevention of urinary tract infection are not recommended (16). Treatment should be implemented only after confirmation of a symptomatic infection. Clinical signs of infection include development of autonomic dysreflexia, cloudy or malodorous urine, fever, lethargy, and general malaise. Infections with stone forming organisms (most prominently proteus, but also serratia and klebsiella) should be treated. Additional information on neurogenic bladder management is presented in Chapter 11.

GASTROINTESTINAL

Impaired or disrupted innervation of the small and large intestine and anal sphincter results in a lower motor neuron syndrome in injuries to the cauda equina or upper motor neuron bowel in SCI at or above the conus medullaris. This results in increased bowel transit time placing patients at increased risk for ileus and peristalsis changes. Monitoring for signs of abdominal distention, decreased or absent bowel sounds, changes in bowel activity, nausea, vomiting, or abdominal pain is necessary, and symptoms should prompt further evaluation. Abdominal x-rays series, ultrasound for identification of gallstones or pancreatic cysts, along with liver and pancreatic blood panels should be considered when symptoms are present.

Prophylactic treatment is highly recommended with H2 blocker or proton pump inhibitors (17). The typical treatment span should be limited to less than 4 weeks (unless other factors are present) to reduce the risk of *clostridium difficile* infections (18). The reader can refer to Chapter 13 for details on neurogenic bowel management.

■ OTHER ISSUES

Heterotopic Ossification (HO) is the abnormal formation of a new bone around joints and within muscles. Common sites include hips, shoulder, elbow, and knees. It is most likely to occur within the first 6 months after SCI. Evaluation includes x-rays of the affected area(s) and monitoring of serum alkaline phosphatase levels. Triple-phase bone scan can be used when there is high level of suspicion and x-rays are negative since it can detect HO within the first 1 to 2 weeks.

Hypercalcemia: Immobilization hypercalcemia occurs due to increased osteoclastic activity and bone resorption in the immobilized limbs. Initially bone resorption will result in hypercalciuria. If the kidney is unable to keep up with excretion of serum calcium, hypercalcemia will develop. Patients with SCI, especially males, are at high risk for hyper-calcemia secondary to higher bone density and larger bone mass. This commonly occurs between 2 weeks and 6 months after injury with achievement of calcium steady state within 6 months from the time of injury. Bone density scans after 6 months usually reveal decreased bone density below the level of the injury. Evaluation of parathyroid, thyroid, and vitamin D levels should be performed along with initial serum calcium levels. Common signs and symptoms of hypercalcemia include lethargy, fatigue, nausea, anorexia, muscle cramps, polydipsia, and polyuria. Initial treatment should include aggressive intravenous hydration with or without the addition of diuretics such as furosem-ide. An indwelling catheter is useful during treatment. In severe cases, those with levels lesser than 12.0 mg/dl, therapy with intravenous bisphosphonates should be considered.

Osteoporosis: SCI patients will lose close to 25% of their bone mass within 3 months post injury and 33% by 14 months post injury due to increased osteoclastic activity and decreased osteoblastic activity. This leads to initial loss of trabecular bone; loss of cortical bone occurs over time. Bone density should be evaluated periodically using tra-ditional methods. Treatment should include calcium and Vitamin D supplementation and weight-bearing exercises. Bisphosphonates should be considered for confirmed osteoporosis.

Skin Care/pressure ulcers: Pressure relief is a critical aspect in manage-ment of those with SCI. Knowledge and monitoring of sites prone to skin breakdown is extremely important (heels, hips, occiput, sacrum, shoulders, and spine of scapula). As soon as spine stabilization is verified, a turning schedule (every 2 hours) should be initiated (28).

Use of heel, occipital, and sacral protection is recommended along with careful monitoring of these areas and education in high-risk patients. Pressure areas can also include the ischium, lateral malleoli, and superior calf in wheelchair users. SCI patients should perform weight shifts every 15 minutes or off loading every 15 minutes for 45 seconds to ensure proper blood flow to weight-bearing areas. This can be accomplished manually or by using wheelchairs with tilt-in-space capabilities.

THERMOREGULATION

SCI disrupts some of the body's thermoregulation mechanisms including shivering, vasoconstriction, and vasodilation by disrupting connection with the hypothalamus.

Patients with spinal injury are prone to episodes of hypothermia and hyperthermia. It is not uncommon for patients to experience a lower temperature below the level of the lesion. Environmental changes are necessary to maintain adequate temperature control.

■ FUNCTIONAL OUTCOMES AFTER SCI

C4 is a key level for independent respiratory function potentially allowing SCI patients to breathe without mechanical ventilation.

C5 adds key muscles for shoulder function and elbow flexion along with partial innervation of brachialis and brachioradialis. This allows for mobility independence with the use of power wheelchairs with specialized controls and feeding with adaptive equipment.

C6 preservation enables patients to perform active wrist extension and subsequently tenodesis grip. The tendons of the thumb, index, and finger flexors will shorten and wrist extension results in opposition of the thumb and index finger. This movement is key for tasks requiring finer control of the hand such as clean intermittent catheterization. Patient with this level of injury can be independent with manual wheelchair mobility and with bladder care.

C7 preservation of the triceps function allows for elbow extension. Patients can perform weight shifts, transfers, and some meal preparation independently in addition to the functions mentioned above.

C8 preservation allows dexterous use of the hands. Patients with this level of injury are able to perform self-care activities and mobility using a manual wheelchair independently.

High thoracic levels. Patients with high thoracic injuries are able to be independent with all self-care including bladder and bowel management, feeding, transfers, and wheelchair mobility.

Low thoracic levels: These patients have complete independence in basic care along with high-level wheelchair activities. It is possible for these patients to have the ability to ambulate household distances with knee-ankle-foot orthoses (KAFOs) and forearm crutches and/or walkers.

Lumbar 1–2 levels: Patients with high lumbar injuries have preserved quadriceps and hip flexor function, which enables ambulation for short distances with ankle-foot orthoses AFOs or KAFOs with assistive devices.

Lumbar 3–4 levels: Patients can perform knee extension and some ankle dorsiflexion. Patients should be able to ambulate both household and community distances, but will require (AFOs) and assistive devices.

Lumbar 5 and below: Patients should be completely independent in all activities although bladder function may be affected.

■ REFERENCES

1. Ditunno JF, Flanders A, Kirshblum S, Graziani V, Tessler A, et al. Predicting outcome in traumatic SCI. In: Kirschblum S, Campagnolo DI, DeLisa JA, eds. *Spinal Cord Medicine.* Philadelphia, PA: Lippincott Williams & Wilkins; 2002: 108–122.

2. Friedman, Somal, Gittler. Dysesthetic pain as a predictor of motor recovery in incomplete SCI [Abstract]. *Archives of Physical Medicine and Rehabilitation.* 82(9):1291.

3. Shepard MJ, Bracken MB. Magnetic resonance imaging and neurological recovery in acute spinal cord injury: observations from the National Acute Spinal Cord Injury Study 3. *Spinal Cord.* 1999;37(12):833–837.

4. DeVivo M, Stover S. Long-term survival and causes of death. In: Stover S. et al. eds. *Spinal Cord Injury Clinical Outcomes From the Model Systems.* Gaithersburg, MA: Aspen; 1995:289–316.

5. Bracken MB, Shepard MJ, Holford TR, et al. Administration of methylprednisolone for 24 or 48 hours or tirilazad mesylate for 48 hours in treatment of acute spinal cord injury. Results of the third national acute spinal cord injury randomized controlled trial. National Acute Spinal Cord Injury Study. JAMA. 1997;277:1597–1604.

6. Coleman WP, Benzel D, Cahill DW, et al. A critical appraisal of the reporting of the National Acute Spinal Cord Injury Studies (II and III) of methylprednisolone in acute spinal cord injury. *J Spinal Disord.* 2000;13(3):185–199.

7. Nesathurai S. Steroids and spinal cord injury: revisiting the NASCIS 2 and NASCIS 3 Trials. *J Trauma.* 1998;45(6):1088–1093.

8. Hugenholtz H. Methylprednisolone for acute spinal cord injury: not a standard of care. *CMAJ.* 2003;168(9):1145–1146.

9. Consortium for Spinal Cord Medicine. *Early Acute Management in Adults With Spinal Cord Injury: A Clinical Practice Guidelines for Health-Care Providers.* Washington, DC: Paralyzed Veterans of America; 2007.

10. Management of acute central cervical spinal cord Injuries. Neurosurgery. 2002;50(3)(suppl):S166–S172.

11. Discussion with Jeffrey Sternlicht MD, Chairman of Emergency Medicine, Greater Baltimore Medical Center, Towson, MD.

12. Eck JC, Nachtigall D, Humphreys SC, Hodges SD. Questionnaire Survey of spine surgeons on the use of methylprednisolone for acute spinal cord injury. Spine. 2006;31:E250–E253.

13. Qian T, Guo X, Levi AD, Vanni S, Shebert RT, Sipski ML. High-dose methyl-prednisolone may cause myopathy in acute spinal cord injury patients. *Spinal cord.* 2004;43:199–203.
14. Jackson AB, Gromes TE. Incidence of respiratory complications following spinal cord injury. *Arch Phys Med Rehabilitation* 1994;75:270–275.
15. Consortium for Spinal Cord Medicine. *Prevention of Thromboembolism in Spinal Cord Injury.* 2nd ed. Washington, DC: Paralyzed Veterans of America; 1997.
16. Morton SC, Shekelle PG, Adams JL, et al. Antimicrobial prophylaxis for urinary tract infection in persons with spinal cord dysfunction. *Arch Phys Med Rehabil.* 2002;83:129–38.
17. Simon RK, Hoyt DB, Winchell RJ, Holbrook T, Eastman AB. A risk analysis of stress ulceration after trauma. *J trauma* 1995;39:289–293.
18. Dial S, Delaney JA, Barkun AN, Suissa S. Use of gastric acid suppressive agents and the risk of community-acquired Clostridium difficile-associated disease. *JAMA.* 2005;294:2989–2995.

Stroke Rehabilitation

Richard D. Zorowitz

■ INTRODUCTION

Stroke remains one of the most common rehabilitation problems in the world today. Stroke comprises over half of the neurologic admissions to community hospitals and is a leading cause for long-term disability (1). There are 795 000 new or recurrent cases of stroke reported annually (2). Of these, 50% had some hemiparesis, 30% were unable to walk without some assistance, 26% were dependent in activities of daily living, 19% had aphasia, and 26% were institutionalized in a nursing home (3). The estimated cost of care and earnings lost due to stroke in 2009 totaled $73.7 billion (2).

There is strong evidence that intensive poststroke rehabilitation significantly improves functional outcomes. For every 100 patients receiving organized inpatient multidisciplinary rehabilitation, extra 5 returned home independently (4). Patients receiving specialized stroke services, including rehabilitation services, had a significantly greater probability to survive and live at home up to 10 years after their strokes (5-7). Patient satisfaction is significantly better when clinicians comply with stroke rehabilitation guidelines, even after controlling for patient functional outcome (8).

However, effective stroke rehabilitation does not depend exclusively on the types of therapies a stroke survivor receives. Evidence-based treatments have demonstrated that the risk of stroke recurrence can be significantly reduced. There are also a number of pharmacological treatments based on small studies that suggest that functional outcomes from stroke can be improved when combined with intensive rehabilitation. Finally, consensus-based opinions among rehabilitation professionals have guided clinicians in standards of care when evidence from formal trials is absent. This chapter combines all levels of evidence to formulate practical orders that optimize medical and rehabilitation care of the stroke survivor.

■ SECONDARY STROKE PROPHYLAXIS
ANTIPLATELET AND ANTICOAGULANT AGENTS

Every stroke survivor admitted for rehabilitation must be considered for secondary prophylaxis of stroke. Stroke survivors with noncardioembolic ischemic stroke or transient ischemic attack (TIA), monotherapy consisting of aspirin 50 to 325 mg by mouth daily or clopidogrel 75 mg by mouth daily, or the combination of aspirin 25 mg and extended-release dipyridamole 200 mg by mouth twice daily are acceptable options for initial therapy to reduce the risk of recurrent stroke and other cardiovascular events (9). The combination of aspirin and extended-release dipyridamole is recommended over aspirin alone, but should be titrated using one tablet of aspirin/extended-release dipyridamole with aspirin 81 mg for 7 days to reduce the risk of headache. Combination therapy of aspirin and clopidogrel is not routinely recommended for secondary prophylaxis, unless there is a specific indication (ie, coronary stent or acute coronary syndrome) as the addition of aspirin to clopidogrel increases the risk of cerebral hemorrhage.

In most stroke survivors with cardioembolic ischemic stroke (eg, atrial fibrillation, acute myocardial infarction and left ventricular thrombus, dilated cardiomyopathy, valvular heart disease), anticoagulation with adjusted-dose warfarin (target INR, 2.5; range, 2.0–3.0) is recommended (10). Stroke survivors with an acute myocardial infarction and confirmed left ventricular mural thrombus should be treated with oral anticoagulation for at least 3 months and up to 1 year. A stroke survivor with rheumatic mitral valve disease with or without atrial fibrillation should add aspirin 81 mg by mouth daily to anticoagulation therapy. A stroke survivor with ischemic cardiomyopathy should add aspirin (preferably in the enteric-coated form) in doses up to 162 mg by mouth daily together with oral anticoagulant therapy. A stroke survivor with a mechanical prosthetic heart valve despite adequate therapy with oral anticoagulants should be treated with adjusted-dose warfarin (target INR, 3.0; range, 2.5–3.5) along with aspirin 75 to 100 mg by mouth daily. If the stroke survivor is unable to take oral anticoagulants, aspirin 325 mg by mouth daily is recommended. A stroke survivor with mitral valve prolapse, mitral valve calcification, or aortic value disease may be treated with antiplatelet therapy only. A stroke survivor without atrial fibrillation who has mitral regurgitation resulting from mitral valve calcification may be treated with either antiplatelet or warfarin therapy. Antiplatelet agents should not be routinely added to warfarin because of the additional risk of bleeding.

When patients taking antithrombotic agents suffer a hemorrhagic stroke, the decision to restart antithrombotic therapy depends upon the risk of recurrent hemorrhage, the risk of arterial or venous thromboembolism, and the overall state of the patient. If the hemorrhagic stroke survivor who requires warfarin has a very high risk of thromboembolism, warfarin therapy may be restarted 7 to 10 days after the onset of the hemorrhage (11). If the stroke survivor has a lower risk of cerebral infarction (eg, atrial fibrillation without prior ischemic stroke) and a higher risk of amyloid angiopathy (eg, elderly patients with lobar hemorrhage), or if overall neurological function is very poor, an antiplatelet agent may be chosen over warfarin to prevent recurrence of an ischemic stroke.

ANTIHYPERTENSIVE AGENTS

Hypertension is the most important treatable risk factor in ischemic stroke. In hemorrhagic stroke, treating hypertension is the most important step to reduce the risk of recurrent intracerebral hemorrhage (11). Because elevation in blood pressure following a stroke is likely a physiological response to brain ischemia (12), aggressive antihypertensive management should begin approximately 7 to 10 days poststroke, unless early treatment is indicated. In hemorrhagic stroke, hypertension should be treated early to prevent vasogenic edema due to the disruption of the blood–brain barrier in the ischemic area around the hemorrhage (13).

Health benefits have been associated with average blood pressure reductions of 10/5 mm Hg, and normal BP levels have been defined as less than 120/80 mm Hg by JNC-7 (14). (Class IIa, Level of Evidence B). However, absolute target blood pressures should be individualized in stroke survivors since it is unclear below what blood pressure cerebral perfusion may be compromised. At present, available data support the use of a diuretic agent or the combination of a diuretic and an angiotensin-converting enzyme inhibitor (ACEI) (10). The choice of specific drugs and targets should be based on specific patient characteristics (eg, extracranial cerebrovascular occlusive disease, renal disease, cardiac disease, and diabetes mellitus). In addition, lifestyle modifications (eg, sodium restriction and weight loss) should be included as a part of a comprehensive antihypertensive program.

ANTIHYPERLIPIDEMIA AGENTS (STATINS)

Hyperlipidemia is not as well established as a risk factor for recurrent stroke. However, a recent study demonstrated that statin therapy was effective for stroke survivors and without known coronary heart disease to reduce the risk of cardiovascular events and recurrent stroke (15). As a result, stroke survivors with elevated cholesterol, comorbid coronary artery disease, or evidence of an atherosclerotic origin should be managed according to National Cholesterol Education Program (NCEP) III guidelines (16), which include lifestyle modification, dietary guidelines, and medication recommendations. In stroke survivors with or without coronary heart disease or symptomatic atherosclerotic disease, statin therapy with a target LDL-C level of 100 mg/dL is recommended. In stroke survivors who are at very high risk or have multiple risk factors, statin therapy with a target LDL-C level of 70 mg/dL is recommended. Stroke survivors with low HDL cholesterol may be considered for treatment with niacin or gemfibrozil.

ANTIHYPERGLYCEMIC AGENTS

Diabetes is a significant risk factor for stroke. However, data are sparse regarding the secondary stroke prevention of survivors with diabetes. Nevertheless, glucose control is recommended to near-normoglycemic levels among diabetic stroke survivors to reduce microvascular and possibly macrovascular complications (10). The goal for hemoglobin A1c should be less than 7%.

In addition to glucose control, more rigorous control of blood pressure and lipids should be undertaken in diabetic stroke survivors. While all major classes of antihypertensive agents are suitable for blood pressure control in this population, ACEIs and angiotensin receptor blockers are recommended as first-choice medications because they are more effective in reducing the progression of renal disease. With respect to hyperlipidemia, LDL cholesterol (LDL-C) targets are recommended as low as 70 mg/dL.

LIFESTYLE CHANGES

Secondary stroke prevention also depends upon significant lifestyle changes. Stroke survivors who smoke, have heavy alcohol consumption, or use illicit drugs (eg, cocaine) should be counseled to stop the use of these substances. Stroke survivors should be encouraged to reduce weight through reduced caloric intake, increased physical activity, and behavioral counseling to a body mass index of 18.5 to 24.9 kg/m² and a waist circumference less than 35 inches for women, and 40 inches for men. Clinicians should encourage physical activity of at least 30 minutes of moderate-intensity physical exercise most days to reduce risk factors and comorbid conditions that increase the likelihood of recurrence of stroke. A supervised exercise program may be recommended (10).

■ SECONDARY STROKE COMPLICATIONS
CONTRACTURE PREVENTION

Because of the development of the flexor synergy pattern in the upper limb and the extensor synergy pattern in the lower limb, one must evaluate range of motion in the affected limbs frequently to prevent contractures. Range of motion exercises without traction should be performed to prevent brachial plexus or other nerve injury. A shoulder splint in 45 degrees of abduction may prevent positioning in adduction and internal rotation at night. A shoulder support during ambulation may prevent traction on the brachial plexus. An armrest in the wheelchair may help to position the arm in a more neutral position. A resting hand splint may help to stretch the wrist and finger muscles if tone begins to develop. A pressure-relief ankle–foot orthosis may prevent foot drop both in bed and in the wheelchair.

DEEP VENOUS THROMBOSIS AND PULMONARY EMBOLISM

Deep venous thrombosis (DVT) may occur in up to 20% to 75% of stroke survivors (17). Clinical signs and symptoms, such as pain, swelling, and warmth of the extremity, are at best marginally diagnostic. Prevention of DVT and pulmonary embolism (PE) is essential in ischemic and hemorrhagic stroke survivors with restricted mobility. Treatment includes heparin 5000 units every 8 to 12 hours, enoxaparin 30 mg subcutaneously every 12 hours, or enoxaparin 40 mg subcutaneously daily (18). For stroke survivors who have contraindications to anticoagulant therapy, intermittent pneumatic compression (IPC) devices, and elastic stockings are used. Prophylaxis may be discontinued once the patient is ambulating consistently in or out of the parallel bars (19).

Prophylaxis for DVT and PE is not contraindicated for hemorrhagic stroke survivors. Initially, IPC devices should be used. In stable patients, anticoagulant prophylaxis with heparin or enoxaparin may begin as early as the second day after the onset of the hemorrhage (18) but not later than the third or fourth day from onset (4). Hemorrhagic stroke survivors who develop an acute proximal venous thrombosis, particularly those with clinical or subclinical pulmonary emboli, should be considered for acute placement of a vena cava filter. The decision to add long-term antithrombotic therapy several weeks or more after placement of a inferior vena cava filter must take into consideration the etiology of the hemorrhage, associated conditions with increased arterial thrombotic risk (eg, atrial fibrillation), and the overall health and mobility of the patient.

CONSTIPATION

Strokes may disinhibit the reflex mechanisms for emptying the bowels, and sensation or cognitive impairments may prevent control of defecation. Diets should include adequate fluids and fiber. A bowel program may start with docusate 100 mg by mouth every 12 hours. If a laxative is needed, senna 17.2 mg by mouth at 12 p.m. may be started to target a bowel program for the evening hours. If a suppository or enema is required, it should be given in the evening after dinner to take advantage of the gastrocolic reflex.

BLADDER DYSFUNCTION

A variety of voiding disorders may be observed after stroke (20). Since many stroke survivors are transferred to the rehabilitation unit with indwelling catheters, a decatheterization protocol should be initiated immediately after admission. Once the catheter is removed, postvoid residuals (PVRs) by bladder scan or catheterization should be obtained at least every 8 hours to assess bladder emptying. If the bladder scan is greater than 400 cm^3, intermittent catheterization should be performed to prevent bladder stretching. If the patient voids, but PVR volumes are greater than 100 cm^3, pharmacologic therapy should be considered. As long as PVRs are abnormal or changes in medications are made, PVRs should be monitored to ensure that bladder function is normalizing. Associated conditions such as urinary tract infection, fecal impaction, and reduced mobility should be evaluated and treated (21). Toileting every 2 to 4 hours during the day, and fluid restriction after dinner may prevent incontinence in a majority of patients (22). External catheters may decrease the incidence of enuresis. Intermittent or indwelling catheterization may be necessary in stroke survivors with areflexic bladders.

PRESSURE SORES

Pressure sores result from both extrinsic (pressure, shear forces, friction, and moisture) and intrinsic (anemia, contractures, spasticity, diabetes, malnutrition [vitamins B, C, K; zinc], edema, and obesity) etiologies (23). In supine position, common locations of pressure sores include the heels, sacrum, and occiput. In sitting, they may occur in the ischial tuberosities. General measures to prevent pressure sores include adequate nutrition and hydration, as well as proper incontinence care. In bed, appropriate mattresses may distribute pressure, and pressure-relief ankle–foot orthoses may prevent ankle contractures as well as boots provide pressure relief to the heel and foot. If stroke survivors require assistance in bed mobility, they should be turned at least every 2 hours. In wheelchairs, patients should be issued appropriate cushions to distribute pressure, and if possible, should be taught techniques of pressure relief.

DYSPHAGIA

Swallowing dysfunction may occur in up to one-third of patients with cortical or brainstem lesions (24). Complications of poststroke dysphagia include malnutrition and aspiration. Symptoms associated with aspiration include dysphonia and an impaired gag reflex associated with impaired cough (25–28). If dysphagia is suspected, evaluation by a speech-language pathologist should take place as soon as possible.

DEPRESSION

Depression occurs in 25% to 79% of stroke survivors in the acute medical or rehabilitation setting, but less than 5% receive psychotherapeutic or medical intervention (29). Depression may be related to mourning the loss of function or to the alteration of function of catecholamine-containing neurons. Diagnosis is usually clinical, and treatment includes psychotherapy and medications. While there are no definitive studies to support nor refute the routine use of pharmacotherapeutic and psychotherapeutic treatments for depression after stroke (30), a neuropsychological evaluation should take place on admission or as soon as depression is suspected. If the diagnosis of major depression is confirmed, pharmacologic therapy with a serotonin-specific reuptake inhibitor should be initiated.

■ NEUROSTIMULANT THERAPY

Pharmacological interventions also may have a role in motor recovery. Methylphenidate, a mild central nervous system stimulant whose mode of action is not well understood, may decrease depression and improve function in the early stages after stroke (31). A meta-analysis of amphetamine treatment in stroke recovery demonstrated some evidence of significant changes in motor function, but no definite conclusions could be reached (32). Side effects with these drugs may include appetite suppression, hypertension, and cardiac arrhythmias.

Also, the seizure threshold may be reduced in those who have a history of epilepsy.

Other small studies have demonstrated the potential of some drugs to improve function after stroke. Fluoxetine may help to facilitate motor recovery independent of its effect as an antidepressant (33). A course of single-dose levodopa over 3 weeks demonstrated significant improvements in motor recovery (34). The use of amantadine significantly improved walking cadence and length of heel-to-toe movements (35). At the same time, drugs such as clonidine, prazosin, neuroleptics and other dopamine receptor antagonists, benzodiazepenes, phenytoin, and phenobarbital actually may impair motor recovery, although the reasons are not fully understood (36).

Stroke Sample Order Set

Richard D. Zorowitz

Diagnosis: Stroke, Cerebral Infarct, or Cerebral Hemorrhage

Admit to: Acute rehabilitation unit (stroke)

Condition: Stable

Allergies: List known drug or other allergies

Precautions: Fall precautions

 Aspiration precautions

Vital Signs: q8 to q12 hours

Activity: Initially, WC level, progress to ambulation with Walker (Rolling or Pickup), Quad cane, or Single-point cane

Diet: Regular, cardiac, or diabetic as applicable. Specify liquids consistency (thin, nectar, or honey) and solids consistency (regular, chopped, mechanical soft, pureed)

Nursing: Routine and incision dressing changes q shift initial if drainage, q12 otherwise.

Therapies
 Physical Therapy: Strengthen and ROM of affected limbs, transfers, static/dynamic Sitting/standing balance, transfers, ambulation, cardiopulmonary conditioning
 Occupational Therapy: Strengthen and ROM of affected upper limb, evaluation of functional cognition, functional transfers, activities of daily living, evaluation for adaptive equipment
 Speech-Language Pathology: Evaluation for speech-language disorder and/or cognitive-communication disorder; evaluation for swallowing disorder

Neuropsychology: Evaluation of cognitive disorder; evaluation of adjustment disorder

Social Work: Discharge planning and family organization and communication

Prophylaxis
Contracture Prevention:
Upper Limb
- ROM without traction to prevent contracture
- 45-degree shoulder-abduction sling for nighttime positioning
- Shoulder support for ambulation to prevent traction by gravity
- Armrest in wheelchair as needed.

Lower Limb
- Pressure-relief ankle–foot orthosis to prevent foot drop

DVT: Heparin 5000 q8 to q12 hours, or Lovenox 30 mg sq q12 hours, or Lovenox 40 mg sq daily

Constipation:
- Colace 100 mg po q12 hours
- Senna 17.2 mg po at 12p.m.
- Dulcolax 5 mg tabs per rectum every 1 to 2 evenings prn if no BM

Bladder Incontinence (also, decatheterization protocol)
- Remove indwelling catheter
- Post-void residuals (PVR) by bladder scan or catheterization every 6 hours if no void
- Intermittent catheterization every 6 hours for no void and bladder scan > 400 cc; or every 6 hours if void occurs and bladder scan > 100 cc

Medications
Stroke prophylaxis
Hypertenision
Hyperlipidemia
Stroke neurostimulants

Baseline Medications
Pain Medications:
Key is to ensure that patient has good pain control, so they will participate in therapies and minimize risk of chronic pain. Patient gets medication prior to therapy to ensure participation.
Muscle or Joint Pain:
Short-Acting (examples)
Oxycodone 5 or 10 mg tabs po q6 to q8 hours prn breakthrough pain

or

Percocet 5/325 to 10/325 mg 1 to 2 po q6 to q8 hours prn breakthrough pain or Vicodin 5/500 or 7.5/650 mg 1 to 2 po q8 hours prn breakthrough pain

Labs: CBC with differential, Basic Metabolic Profile, PT/INR
(if on anticoagulation), Albumin and Prealbumin (if needed for
nutritional reasons, eg, enteral feeds)
Length of Stay: 10 to 14 days

Goals

Increase range of motion and strength of affected muscles. Ambulation
with appropriate assistive device and orthosis (facilitatory and
compensatory strategies)

Activities of daily living with appropriate adaptive equipment (facilitatory
and compensatory strategies)

Compensatory strategies for speech-language and/or cognitive-
communication impairments (facilitatory and compensatory strategies)

Prevention of secondary complications: bowel, bladder, skin breakdown,
contractures

Cardiopulmonary conditioning.

■ ADDITIONAL READING

1. Stein J, Harvey RL, Macko RF, Winstein CJ, Zorowitz RD, eds. *Stroke Recovery and Rehabilitation*. New York, NY: Demos Medical Publishing; 2009.
2. Duncan PW, Zorowitz RD, Bates B, et al. Management of adult stroke rehabilitation care. A clinical practice guideline. *Stroke*. 2005;36:e100.
3. Office of Quality and Performance. Department of Veterans Affairs. Stroke rehabilitation VA/DoD clinical practice guidelines. *http://www.oqp.med.va.gov/cpg/STR/STR_base.htm*. Accessed December 31, 2008.
4. Teasell RW, Foley NC, Salter K, Bhogal SK, Jutai J, Speechley MR. EBRSR: evidence-based review of stroke rehabilitation. *http://www.ebrsr.com*. Accessed December 31, 2008.

■ REFERENCES

1. Centers for Disease Control and Prevention (CDC). Prevalence of disabilities and associated health conditions among adults: United States, 1999. *MMWR Morb Mortal Wkly Rep*. 2001;50: 120–125.
2. Lloyd-Jones D, Adams R, Brown TM, et al. 5. Stroke (Cerebrovascular disease). In: Heart Disease and Stroke Statistics - 2010 Update. A Report from the American Heart Association. *Circulation* 2010;121:e46-e215. DOI: 10.1161/CIRCULATIONAHA.109.192667. Accessed November 1, 2010.
3. Kelley-Hayes M, Beiser A, Kase CS, Scaramucci A, D'Agostino RB, Wolf PA. The influence of gender and age on disability following ischemic stroke: the Framingham study. *J Stroke Cerebrovasc Dis*. 2003;12:119–126.
4. Langhorne P, Duncan P. Does the organization of postacute stroke care really matter? *Stroke* 2001;32(1):268–274.
5. Indredavik B, Bakke F, Solberg R, Rokseth R, Haaheim LL, Holme I. Benefit of a stroke unit: a randomized controlled trial. *Stroke*. 1991;22(8):1026–1031.
6. Indredavik B, Bakke F, Slordahl SA, Rokseth R, Haheim LL. Stroke unit treatment improves long-term quality of life: a randomized controlled trial. *Stroke*. 1998;29(5):895–899.

7. Indredavik B, Bakke F, Slordahl SA, Rokseth R, Haheim LL. Stroke unit treatment. 10-year follow-up. *Stroke*. 1999;30(8): 1524–1527.

8. Reker DM, Duncan PW, Horner RD, et al. Postacute stroke guideline compliance is associated with greater patient satisfaction. *Arch Phys Med Rehabil*. 2002;83(6):750–756.

9. Adams RJ, Albers G, Alberts MJ, et al. Patients with stroke and transient ischemic attack. Update to the AHA/ASA recommendations for the prevention of stroke. *Stroke*. 2008;39;1647–1652.

10. Sacco RL, MD, Adams R, Albers G, et al. Guidelines for prevention of stroke in patients with ischemic stroke or transient ischemic attack. A statement for healthcare professionals from the American Heart Association/American Stroke Association Council on Stroke: co-sponsored by the Council on Cardiovascular Radiology and Intervention. *Stroke*. 2006;37: 577–617.

11. Broderick J, Connolly S, Feldmann E, et al. Guidelines for the management of spontaneous intracerebral hemorrhage in adults: 2007 update. A guideline from the American Heart Association/American Stroke Association Stroke Council, High Blood Pressure Research Council, and the Quality of Care and Outcomes in Research Interdisciplinary Working Group. *Stroke*. 2007;38:2001–2023.

12. Wallace JD, Levy LL. Blood pressure after stroke. *JAMA*. 1981;246(19):2177–2180.

13. Lavin P. Management of hypertension in patients with acute stroke. *Arch Int Med*. 1986;146(1):66–68.

14. US National Heart, Lung, and Blood Institute; National Institutes of Health. The seventh report of the Joint National Committee on Prevention, Detection, Evaluation, and Treatment of High Blood Pressure. Bethesda, MD: December, 2003. NIH Publication 03-5233.

15. Amarenco P, Bogousslavsky J, Callahan A III, et al; Stroke Prevention by Aggressive Reduction in Cholesterol Levels (SPARCL) Investigators. High-dose atorvastatin after stroke or transient ischemic attack. *N Engl J Med*. 2006;355:549–559.

16. US National Heart, Lung, and Blood Institute; National Institutes of Health. The Third Report of the National Cholesterol Education Program (NCEP) Expert Panel on Detection, Evaluation, and Treatment of High Blood Cholesterol in Adults (Adult Treatment Panel III). Bethesda, MD: 2001. NIH Publication 01-3670.

17. Turpie AG. Prophylaxis of venous thromboembolism in stroke patients. *Sem Thrombosis Hemostasis*. 1997;23(2):155–157.

18. Albers GW, Amarenco P, Easton JD, Sacco RL, Teal P. Antithrombotic and thrombolytic therapy for ischemic stroke. American College of Chest Physicians Evidence-Based Clinical Practice Guidelines (8th Edition). *Chest*. 2008;133:630S–669S.

19. Bromfield EB, Reding MB. Relative risk of deep venous thrombosis or pulmonary embolism post-stroke based upon ambulatory status. *J Neuro Rehab*. 1988;2(2):51–56.

20. Borrie MJ, Campbell AJ, Caradoc-Davies TH, Speers GFS. Urinary incontinence after stroke: a prospective study. *Age Ageing*. 1986;15:177–81.

21. Linsenmeyer TA, Zorowitz RD. Urodynamic findings of patients with urinary incontinence following cerebrovascular accident. *NeuroRehabil*. 1992;2(2):23–26.

22. Sogbein SK, Awad SA. Behavioural treatment of urinary incontinence in geriatric patients. *CMA J.* 1982;127:863–864.

23. Nurse BA, Collins MC. Skin care and decubitus ulcer management in the elderly stroke patient. *PM&R State of the Art Rev.* 1989;3(3):549–562.

24. Veis SL, Logemann JA. Swallowing disorders in persons with cerebrovascular accident. *Arch Phys Med Rehabil.* 1985;66(6):372–375.

25. Linden P, Siebens AA. Dysphagia: predicting laryngeal penetration. *Arch Phys Med Rehabil.* 1983;64:281–284.

26. Horner J, Massey EW. Silent aspiration following stroke. *Neurology.* 1988;38:317–319.

27. Horner J, Massey EW, Brazer SR. Aspiration in bilateral stroke patients. *Neurology.* 1990;40:1686–1688.

28. Horner J, Buoyner FG, Alberts MJ, Helms MJ. Dysphagia following brain-stem stroke. *Arch Neurol.* 1991;48(11):1170–1173.

29. Gordon WA, Hibbard MR. Poststroke depression: an examination of the literature. *Arch Phys Med Rehabil.* 1997;78(6):658–663.

30. Hackett ML, Anderson CS, House AO. Interventions for treating depression after stroke. In: *The Cochrane Library, Issue 1.* Chichester, West Sussex: John Wiley & Sons, Ltd; 2005.

31. Grade C, Redford B, Chrostowski J, Toussaint L, Blackwell B. Methylphenidate in early poststroke recovery: a double-blind, placebo-controlled study. *Arch Phys Med Rehabil.* 1998;79(9):1047–1050.

32. Martinsson L, Hårdemark H, Eksborg S. Amphetamines for improving recovery after stroke. *Cochrane Database Syst Rev.* 2007;(1):CD002090. DOI:10.1002/14651858.CD002090.pub2

33. Dam M, Tonin P, De Boni A, et al. Effects of fluoxetine and maprotiline on functional recovery in poststroke hemiplegic patients undergoing rehabilitation therapy. *Stroke.* 1996; 27(7):1211–1214.

34. Scheidtmann K, Fries W, Muller F, Koenig E. Effect of levodopa in combination with physiotherapy on functional motor recovery after stroke: a prospective, randomised, double-blind study. *Lancet.* 2001;358(9284):787–790.

35. Baezner H, Oster M, Henning O, Cohen S, Hennerici MG. Amantadine increases gait steadiness in frontal gait disorder due to subcortical vascular encephalopathy: a double-blind randomized placebo-controlled trial based on quantitative gait analysis. *Cerebrovasc Dis.* 2001;11(3):235–244.

36. Goldstein LB. Common drugs may influence motor recovery after stroke. The Sygen in Acute Stroke Study Investigators. *Neurology.* 1995;45(5): 865–871.

Traumatic Brain Injury Rehabilitation

Melanie Brown, Melissa Gong,
and Maria Eppig

■ INTRODUCTION

The term traumatic brain injury (TBI) refers to injury to the brain caused by an external force. Open TBI involves disruption of the dura mater, whereas the dura mater remains intact during a closed TBI. Primary causes of injury include diffuse axonal injury (DAI), petechial hemorrhages, contusions, and cranial nerve injuries. Secondary causes of injury following TBI may include intracerebral hemorrhage, intracerebral edema, hypoxia, excitotoxicity, and oxidant injury. During a TBI, the rapid acceleration and deceleration of the brain within the skull results in DAI within the brain. DAI may or may not be visible on neuroimaging studies. DAI may result in generalized deficits including loss of consciousness, coma, confusion, and incoordination (1).

It is estimated that 1.5 million people per year experience TBI in the United States. Three percent of these injuries are fatal. Ninety percent of these injuries are classified as mild. Falls are the leading cause of TBI, followed by motor vehicle collisions, and blunt trauma (including assaults and sports related injuries). Alcohol is involved in more than 50% of TBI cases (2).

The best Glasgow Coma Scale (GCS) score (see Appendix 5) within the first 24 hours following injury is used to classify TBI as mild (GCS 13–15), moderate (GCS 9–12), or severe (GCS 3–8) (1).

Older age, longer length of coma, and prolonged duration of posttraumatic amnesia have consistently been shown to be predictors of poor outcome following TBI. Following severe TBI (ie, Initial GCS <8), severe disability is unlikely (<10% chance) when coma lasts less than 2 weeks or when posttraumatic amnesia lasts less than 2 months. Good recovery is unlikely (<10% chance) when coma lasts longer than 4 weeks, posttraumatic amnesia lasts longer than 3 months, or patient is older than 65 years of age (2).

The Rancho Los Amigos Cognitive Scale (see Appendix 17) is used to describe the stages of cognitive recovery following TBI (1).

Severe TBI may result in coma. The term coma refers to a cognitive state in which there is a lack of wakefulness. The patient's eyes remain closed, and there is no electroencephalogram evidence of a sleep–wake cycle. A patient in a minimally conscious state demonstrates evidence of a sleep–wake cycle and awareness of environmental stimuli (eg, sustained visual fixation and pursuit, purposeful movements, emotional responses to salient stimuli, command following, and verbalization). Coma emergence programs are designed to encourage cognitive recovery by providing patients with a wide variety of environmental stimuli. Progression from coma to minimally conscious state is identified through multiple examinations at different times, by a variety of clinicians, with a variety of stimuli (3).

The majority of individuals who survive mild brain injuries (ie, concussions) recover well without residual cognitive deficits. Unfortunately, a significant minority develop postconcussive syndrome. Postconcussive syndrome is associated with physical, cognitive, and emotional problems including headaches, dizziness, fatigue, visual disturbances, light and noise sensitivity, cognitive impairments, depression, anxiety, and irritability. Symptom-based treatment may include analgesics, antidepressants, education, reassurance, and cognitive remediation (3).

■ THEORIES OF NEUROLOGIC RECOVERY
The leading theories of neurologic recovery following TBI involve central nervous system reorganization (neuroplasticity) through unmasking and sprouting. Unmasking theorizes that several potential synaptic pathways exist for the execution of a single neurologic function. During optimal brain activity, the most efficient (primary) synaptic pathway executes the neurologic function, and parallel pathways are masked. Following a TBI, a lesion may develop affecting the primary pathway, resulting in the unmasking of a less efficient parallel pathway, which then takes over execution of the neurologic function. Sprouting theorizes that when a lesion occurs, unaffected neurons in the surrounding area create new synapses that take over for the affected neuron (1).

Research data demonstrates that intensive therapy emphasizing cognition enhances cognitive recovery following TBI. Although research data is not definitive, widely used medications with theoretical potential to enhance cognitive recovery following TBI include dopamine agonists (ie, Amantadine and Bromocriptine) and acetylcholine agonists (ie, Methylphenidate and Modafinil) (1).

■ BEHAVIOR MANAGEMENT
Agitation, decreased arousal, and depressed effect are among the most common undesirable behaviors that interfere with functional recovery following TBI. Sources of agitation, decreased arousal, and depressed effect include the brain lesion itself, premorbid personality, withdrawal, hypoxemia, pain, overstimulation by staff and environment, sleep–wake cycle disturbance, medical issues (cardiac, pulmonary, infection),

medications, and physical restraints. It is important to measure the frequency of the target behavior to determine the efficacy of treatment interventions (4,5).

Agitation may be reduced by limiting environmental stimuli and by creating a structured daily routine. Medications such as Inderal, Trazodone, Seroquel, Depakote, and Tegretol are used to decrease agitation. Haldol and benzodiazepines have the potential to slow cognitive recovery, and should be avoided if at all possible. A stimulating and optimistic atmosphere may assist individuals with decreased arousal and depressed effect. Amantadine, Bromocriptine, Methylphenidate, and Modafinil are used to improve arousal and attention. Serotonin reuptake inhibitors have been shown to be safe and effective in the treatment of depression following TBI (4,5).

When managing undesirable behaviors, an organized approach to medication intervention is recommended. Start low and go slow. Provide an adequate therapeutic trial. Perform continuous reassessment (identify and measure the target behavior). Monitor drug–drug interactions. Change strategy if symptoms intensify (4,5).

■ MEDICAL COMPLICATIONS

Medical complications, including hydrocephalus, dysautonomia, hyponatremia, heterotopic ossification (HO), venous thromboembolism (VTE), aspiration pneumonia, and spasticity, may result in unexpected functional decline and instability following TBI (1).

Hydrocephalus is commonly caused by cerebral atrophy associated with ventricular dilation and results in progressive cognitive decline. Neuroimaging findings consistent with hydrocephalus include the absence of sulci, enlarged ventricles, and periventricular lucency (1).

Dysautonomia involves paroxysmal increases in heart rate, temperature, and blood pressure caused by surges of epinephrine and norepinephrine following TBI. Decerebrate and decorticate positioning can also occur. Centrally acting beta-blockers (eg, Inderal) are indicated for management of heart rate, temperature, and blood pressure. In addition, evidence supports the use of Bromocriptine in managing long-standing dysautonomia. Nitroprusside derivatives should be avoided, because they cause intracerebral vascular dilation, which may result in increased intracranial pressure. Hypotension has been associated with worse outcomes and should be avoided following TBI (1).

Hypotonic hyponatremia is common following TBI. It may be due to the syndrome of inappropriate antidiuretic hormone (SIADH) or cerebral salt wasting (CSW). In SIADH, hyponatremia is dilutional. It is due to excessive water retention by the kidneys without an inciting disturbance in sodium balance. It is characterized by higher than normal urine osmolality and low plasma osmolality. Antidiuretic hormone (ADH) is not appropriately suppressed in response to low plasma osmolality; thus, further water retention ensues. Treatment includes fluid restriction to approximately 1 L/d, sodium supplementation, and diuresis. Demeclocycline is reserved for chronic SIADH. In CSW, there is excessive sodium excretion, possibly secondary to impaired renal reabsorption. CSW is characterized by low urine and plasma osmolalities. CSW is treated with fluid repletion with hypertonic saline. Less commonly occurring is diabetes insipidus, where there is a lack of ADH secretion, which results in polydipsia and polyuria. Treatment is with Desmopressin (1).

HO, formation of lamellar bone in soft tissue, commonly involves the shoulder, elbow, and hip regions in TBI survivors. Risk factors include prolonged coma, spasticity, and bone fractures. Signs and symptoms include increased warmth and edema, decreased range of motion, and worsening contractures. Early detection of HO is with triple phase bone scan. Serum alkaline phosphatase is elevated in HO, but is a nonspecific finding. Creatine phosphokinase may be more valuable in the management of HO, because levels are elevated acutely, and decline when treatment for HO is successful. HO is treated with etidronate disphosphonate at 20 mg/kg/d for 2 weeks, followed by 10 mg/kg/d for 10 weeks and concurrent nonsteroidal anti-inflammatories (ie, Indomethicin). Surgical excision of HO is usually delayed until full maturation of the ectopic bone, which usually requires 12 to 18 months. Recurrence of HO is common (1).

TBI survivors are at increased risk for VTE. Deep vein thrombosis (DVT) is among the most commonly occurring forms of VTE. Signs and symptoms include pain in the extremity, warmth, and swelling. If a DVT is suspected, bilateral venous ultrasounds of the lower extremities should be obtained. VTE prophylaxis includes low molecular weight heparin at 40 mg once daily, unfractionated heparin 5000 units 3 times daily, or oral warfarin. When anticoagulation is contraindicated, pneumatic compression devices, compression stockings, and inferior vena cava filters may be used for individuals who develop a DVT (1).

Cranial nerve dysfunction and lack of coordination may result in dysphagia and aspiration pneumonia following TBI. Silent aspiration is common; therefore, modified barium swallow studies are more valuable than bedside swallow evaluations. One of the best treatments for swallowing dysfunction is to modify the consistency of food and drink. Using strategies such as a simple chin tuck, or elevating the head of bed during mealtime can also reduce aspiration risk (1). Formal evaluation by a speech-language pathologist is recommended if aspiration is suspected.

Spasticity is a velocity-dependent increase in muscle tone. Spasticity commonly develops in days to weeks following TBI. If spasticity develops, aggressive joint range of motion is indicated. Medications including Dantrium and Baclofen may be indicated if spasticity causes pain or interferes with functional activities. Centrally acting antispasmodics (eg, Valium and Flexeril) should be avoided due to cognitive side effects (1).

■ **PAIN MANAGEMENT**

Headaches and neuropathic pain syndromes are common following TBI. An appropriate diagnostic work up is necessary to identify potential sources of pain (eg, extension of intracranial hemorrhage, bone fracture, HO, thromboembolism, abscess, peripheral neuropathy, radiculopathy, etc). Due to cognitive side effects, it is best to avoid narcotics when managing post TBI pain. Less sedating analgesics such as acetaminophen, nonsteroidal antiinflammatories, and neurogenic agents (eg, Lyrica, Neurontin, Elavil) are better options for pain management following TBI.

■ **SEIZURE MANAGEMENT**

Posttraumatic seizures are classified as immediate, early, or late. Following TBI, immediate seizures occur within 24 hours, early seizures occur after 24 hours but within 7 days, and late seizures occur more than 7 days following TBI. The risk of late seizures increases with biparietal contusions, dural penetration with metal fragments, multiple intracranial surgeries, subdural hematoma with evacuation, midline shift greater than 5 mm, and multiple or bilateral cortical contusions. Seizure prophylaxis is recommended for all TBI survivors with a GCS less than 12. Seizure prophylaxis should be discontinued 7 days following closed TBI, if the survivor has only immediate seizures or if the survivor remains seizure free. TBI survivors who experience early or late seizures should be treated with antiepileptic medications for at least 12 months. Although phenytoin is commonly used for seizure prophylaxis in the acute phase, it may slow cognitive recovery. Consider other antiepileptic agents (eg, Keppra, Depakote, and Tegretol) when extended seizure prophylaxis is indicated (6–8).

■ **BOWEL AND BLADDER MANAGEMENT**

Incontinence is common following TBI. It has been associated with prolonged length of stay in acute rehabilitation and poor functional outcome.

Bowel incontinence may be due to an uninhibited neurogenic bowel, lack of awareness of the need to defecate, or the inability to communicate the need to defecate secondary to impaired cognition or aphasia. In order to minimize fecal incontinence, it is important to develop a daily bowel program that provides consistent timing of fecal evacuation. If dysphagia occurs and gastrostomy or jejunostomy feeding is required, high fiber supplementation or fiber-rich enteral feeds may be used to bulk the stool and prevent diarrhea. Stool softeners (eg, Colace) may be used to prevent constipation. Laxatives (eg, Senna) may be used to promote peristalsis and move fecal material through the colon. Suppositories (eg, Dulcolax or glycerin) may be scheduled daily for effective bowel evacuation.

Following TBI, urinary incontinence is most commonly related to neurogenic bladder dysfunction. In a healthy brain, the corticopontine mesencephalic nuclei allow bladder storage; the pontine mesencephalic pathway coordinates bladder contraction and sphincter relaxation; and the pelvic and pudendal nuclei mediate the parasympathetic micturation reflex. Disruption of any of these pathways may result in incontinence due to a hyperreflexic bladder wall with an uninhibited micturation reflex (9).

Initial treatment for urinary incontinence may include an indwelling catheter, which should be discontinued as soon as possible to prevent urinary tract infection and urethral erosion. Following catheter removal, postvoid residuals should be monitored every 6 hours to assess bladder emptying. Intermittent catheterization should be employed for postvoid residuals greater than 250 cm^3. Alpha adrenergic antagonists (eg, Flomax) can be used to aid in relaxation of the bladder neck. If bladder storage capacity is limited by hyperreflexia, anticholinergic medications (eg, Ditropan) may be indicated (9).

■ DISPOSITION
Recovery following TBI may continue for 3 to 24 months. Although resources to support physical recovery are commonly available, resources to support cognitive recovery may be extremely limited. Most insurers provide financial support for physical rehabilitation, but cognitive rehabilitation is excluded from many insurance policies. Because of cognitive deficits and safety concerns, TBI survivors may require 24-hour supervision for a prolonged period of time. Social workers and case managers are valuable advocates and can help identify the resources available to TBI survivors for community reentry.

TBI Sample Order Set

Melanie Brown

Diagnosis:	Traumatic Brain Injury
Admit to:	Acute rehabilitation unit (TBI)
Condition:	Stable
Allergies:	List known drug or other allergies
Precautions:	Fall precautions
Vital Signs:	q8 hours
Activity:	Out of bed with assistance.
Diet:	Regular vs modified consistency with or without supervision. (Pureed/Mechanical Soft, Thin/Thick Liquids)
IV Fluids:	None
Bowel:	Colace 100 mg BID Senna 2 tabs QPM Dulcolax suppository QHS as needed

Diagnosis:	Traumatic Brain Injury
Bladder:	Time void q4 hours while awake
	Bladder scan postvoid and record amount
	Bladder scan q6 hours if no void
	Straight cath for volume >250 cc
Skin:	Check skin daily for skin breakdown
	If immobile, reposition q2 hours.

DVT

Prophylaxis:	Lovenox 40 mg SQ Q Day
Pain	
Management:	As needed vs standing dose depending on cognition.
	Tylenol 650 mg q4 hours as needed vs Tylenol 1000 mg TID
	And/or Ibuprofen 600 mg TID with meals prn vs standing dose
	And/or Ultram 50 mg to 100 mg q6 hours prn
	And/or Lyrica 75 mg to 150 mg BID for neuropathic pain.
	Avoid narcotics due to cognitive side effects.
Physical Therapy:	1 to 2 h/d
	ROM, strengthening, bed mobility, sitting balance, transfers, standing balance, ambulation, stair ambulation, community ambulation, balance, endurance
Occupational	
Therapy:	1 to 2 h/d
	Upper extremity neuromuscular re-training, casting/splinting as needed for spasticity management, feeding, grooming, bathing, dressing, toileting, transfers, functional cognitive skills, visual–perceptual skills, household skills
Speech:	1 to 2 h/d
	Cognitive linguistic and communication skills
	Dysarthria and dysphagia evaluate and treat
Psychology:	Evaluate and treat for signs and symptoms of depression.
	Neuropsychological testing as appropriate.
Vocational	
Rehabilitation:	May be appropriate as an outpatient once stable.
Social Work:	Discharge planning and family organization and communication

Medications:

- **Baseline medications**
  In patients with decreased arousal avoid sedatives if possible.
  (eg, β-blockers, α-blockers, calcium channel blockers, anticholinergics, Dilantin, Haldol, Valium, etc)

- **Agitation Medications**
  Trazodone 50 mg q4 hours prn and 100 mg QHS
  And/or Seroquel 25 mg q8 hours prn and 50 mg QHS
  And/or Depakote 250 mg BID
  And/or Inderal 20 mg BID
  And/or Ativan 1 to 2 mg q6 hours prn severe agitation
  Avoid Haldol due to cognitive side effects

- **Arousal and Attention Medications**
  Ritalin 5 mg to 15 mg BID (7 AM and 12 PM)
  And/or Provigil 200 mg QAM
  And/or Amantadine 100 mg BID
  And/or Bromocriptine 5 mg BID (useful for speech initiation)

- **Depression Medications**
  Serotonin selective re-uptake inhibitors (eg, Zoloft 100 mg QHS, Lexapro 10 to 20 mg QHS)
  Note: Ritalin and Trazodone have antidepressant properties

- **Seizure Prophylaxis**
  Depakote 250 mg BID
  Or Tegretol 200 mg BID
  Or Keppra 500 mg BID
  Avoid Dilantin if possible.
  For patients with closed head injuries, consider discontinuing seizure prophylaxis after 7 days.

- **Spasticity Medications**
  Dantrium 25 mg to 100 mg BID (monitor liver function)
  Baclofen 10 mg BID to QID (as tolerated)
  Avoid Valium due to cognitive side effects

Labs: Baseline CBC, BMP, Alb or Pre-Alb, Mg, Phos
                 Baseline urinalysis and culture
                 Baseline EKG

Length of Stay: 7 to 14 days

GOALS

1. Maintain medical stability and prevent medical complications including thromboembolism, pneumonia, seizures, urinary tract infections, uncontrolled pain, contractures, and skin breakdown.

2. Establish safe and effective nutritional intake.

3. Achieve bowel and bladder continence.

4. Achieve safe and independent function including mobility and activities of daily living (feeding, grooming, bathing dressing, toileting, transfers, household skills, functional cognition, and visual–perceptual skills).

5. Establish effective memory, orientation, and communication strategies.

6. Establish consistent daily routine and sleep–wake cycle (avoid excessive stimulation).

7. Increase awareness of deficits.

8. Patient and caregiver education, training, and discharge planning.

■ REFERENCES

1. Cifu DX, Kreutzer JS, Slater DN, Taylor L. Rehabilitation after traumatic brain injury. In: Braddom RL, ed. *Physical Medicine and Rehabilitation.* 3rd ed. Saunders Elsevier; Philadelphia, PA 2007:1133–1174.

2. Brown AW, Elovic EP, Kothari S, Flanagan SR, Kwasnica C. Congenital and acquired brain injury. 1. Epidemiology, pathophysiology, prognostication, innovative treatments, and prevention. *Arch Phys Med Rehabil.*2008;89:S3–S8.

3. Kwasnica C, Brown A, Elovic E, Kothari S, Flanagan S. Congenital and acquired brain injury. 3. Spectrum of the acquired brain injury population. *Arch Phys Med Rehabil.*2008;89:S15–S20.

4. Flanagan SR, Kwasnica C, Brown AW, Elovic EP, Kothari S. Congenital and acquired brain injury. 2. Medical rehabilitation in acute and subacute settings. *Arch Phys Med Rehabil.* 2008;89:S9–S14.

5. Elovic E, Kothari S, Flanagan SR, Kwasnica C, Brown AW. Congenital and acquired brain injury. 4. Outpatient and community reintegration. *Arch Phys Med Rehabil.* 2008;89:S21–S26.

6. Anonymous. Antiseizure prophylaxis for penetrating brain injury. *J Trauma.* 2001;51:S41–S43.

7. Chang BS, Lowenstein DH. Practice parameter: antiepileptic drug prophylaxis in severe traumatic brain injury: report of the Quality Standards Subcommittee of the American Academy of Neurology. *Neurology.* 2003;60(1):10–16.

8. Teasell R, Bayona N, Lippert C, Villamere J, Hellings C. Post-traumatic seizure disorder following acquired brain injury. *Brain Inj.* 2007;21(2):201–214.

9. Chua K, Chuo A, Kong KH. Urinary incontinence after traumatic brain injury: incidence, outcomes and correlates. *Brain Inj.* 2003;17(6):469–478.

Wheelchair Prescriptions

Dorianne Rachelle Feldman,
Michael Lang Bushby, and Phong Kieu

■ INTRODUCTION

Prescription of assistive devices is a major component of rehabilitation. Of these devices, wheelchairs are one of the most essential; designed to fit and cater to the individual's specific needs. As "durable" medical equipment (DME), wheelchairs are intended to last for years, making the thoroughness of the evaluation process even more important. Wheelchairs function as the primary means of short- or long-term locomotion for patients who are nonambulatory or who have very poor endurance. Mobility may be an independent (active) or dependent (passive) process. Often, this is the only way for these individuals to partake in activities, which are necessary and meaningful. For the average manual wheelchair user, time spent in the wheelchair is estimated at 9.2 h/d (1).

Therefore, wheelchair prescription is an essential component of patient care for this population and works best when performed conjunctively by select health care professionals (physiatrist, specialized occupational and/or physical therapist, wheelchair vendors, and patient/family). This process must incorporate both a comprehensive evaluation and consideration of the wheelchair user(s) activity demands to preserve and ultimately promote functional independence and health.

■ WHEELCHAIR EVALUATION

Determining an appropriate wheelchair prescription requires an understanding of the fundamentals of wheelchair design including those factors that impact mobility and those that influence posture within the seating system. To ensure favorable results, a thorough evaluation process must be conducted to determine the clients' needs and goals, both short- and long-term.

Other factors to consider include body habitus, environments, impairments, comorbid medical conditions, endurance (both endurance for mobility and postural endurance), behavior, posture, balance, transfer status, muscle tone, range of motion, and financial resources among others.

It is often necessary to prioritize a patient's needs during an evaluation. No piece of equipment solves all client concerns, and compromise is often necessary. Patient involvement and education should be performed from the onset of the evaluation process and continue on through the time of delivery and shortly after to maximize patient satisfaction and understanding. To ensure accuracy of measurements and identify postural impairments, the wheelchair evaluation process should be conducted on the mat, both in the supine and seated positions (2). The mat assessment allows the examiner to determine general joint mobility, alignment/positioning including asymmetries, muscle length, and physical function (2,3).

It serves as a useful way to assess for deformities, both permanent (managed by adaptation) or malleable (managed through correction when possible) of the spine or pelvis. Careful measurement of patient body dimensions and appropriate prescription of wheelchair to meet body measurements is of primary importance during seating evaluation.

WHEELCHAIR DIMENSIONS

1. **Seat depth** is measured from the back of the buttocks to the popliteal region. Ideally, there should be approximately 1 to 2 inches between the popliteal space and the anterior aspect of the seating surface (4). When obtained correctly; forces are dispersed evenly through the pelvis and the femurs. If too shallow, the user is at risk for skin breakdown and maladaptive posturing (excessive hip abduction or flexion). In contrast, if too deep, there is a tendency for skin breakdown (popliteal fossa and calves) and posterior pelvic tilt positioning.

2. **Seat width** is measured as the distance from the most lateral aspect of one buttock to the other (at the widest point) and must guarantee appropriate support for the greater trochanters. It is generally recommended for the seat width to be around 1 inch greater than the pelvic width (4). If too wide, wheelchair propulsion is more challenging usually requiring greater than normal amounts of shoulder abduction. Conversely, a seat that is too narrow provides ineffective support/pressure relief and may lead to integumentary compromise in addition to compensatory, unwanted postural changes (pelvic rotation to remove pressure from the lateral hips). In addition to body dimensions, other factors impact clinical reasoning when determining an appropriate seat width for a patient. Of course, doorway clearance must be considered; particularly for negotiation of home and other environments.

3. **Lower leg length** is measured from the most posterior aspect of the heel to the popliteal region. It is critical that there is at least 2 inches between the ground and the foot rests for clearance (4). However, caution must be taken to avoid elevation of the distal femur. The rear portion of the footrest must be designed to promote front wheel (caster) mobility. Elevating or angled foot rests and seat height are adjusted for accessibility.

4. **Back height** is determined by measuring from the buttock to the inferior angle of the scapula. When the back is too high, scapulohumeral motion is restricted because the back of the chair extends

beyond the inferior angle of the scapula interfering with wheelchair propulsion. At times, a higher back may be preferred; as in cases of poor trunk control or in power or manual tilt and recline chairs, which require frequent seat to back angle changes.

In select, more involved clients these dimensions may be helpful (2):

1. Hip-to-occiput measurement: used for headrest positioning.

2. Chest depth: measurement taken for lateral thoracic supports or anterior thoracic support components.

3. Arm rests: placement and design can be variable based on client needs and can assist with postural alignment. Positioning is determined by measuring from the sitting surface to the elbow.

4. Trunk width at the inferior border of the ribs, at the nipple line, and at the acromion process: these measurements are particularly important when selecting appropriate back rests and lateral thoracic supports, and more so when fabricating custom seating components to accommodate for a severe postural deformity.

5. Knee width: in patients with significant hip abduction contractures, this measurement may differ significantly from hip width and be an important consideration in seating and positioning.

It is extremely important to consider how the wheelchair will be used to avoid prescription of a chair that is incompatible with a client's daily roles and environment. Additional considerations for wheelchair use include time spent in the chair, mobility needs, mode of transportation (automobile vs public transportation), the ability of the chair to allow for growth (pediatric population), patient age, and need for additional devices (ventilator, oxygen, and tank). It is also tremendously helpful to survey the family and/or caregivers.

For those spending long periods of time in a wheelchair, it's important to plan for the chair to support either independent or dependent pressure relief. It is critical to educate the client about the convenience and portability aspects of the intended wheelchair. Portability needs are variable depending on the client. Many clients prefer wheelchairs which can be folded for travel. In contrast, chairs with rigid frames can be placed in an automobile, albeit not without compromising vehicle seating capacity. However, folding frame chairs tend to be less stable than rigid frame chairs, and lose mechanical efficiency during manual propulsion due to the greater number of moving parts.

For pediatric patients, it is important that the wheelchair frame enables growth. Otherwise, replacement is required more frequently due to the child out-growing his/her chair.

Environmental considerations are also fundamental to the success of the wheelchair prescription. The environment includes not only the home, but also other settings such as one's school, religious institution, and community venues.

The wheelchair vendor-prescriber relationship is fundamental. Vendors serve as the primary point of contact after equipment has been fitted and delivered. As the patient's needs change and/or the wheelchair requires maintenance and/or repair, the vendor can assist in directing these services.

Medical factors also play a major role in the overall evaluation and prescription process. Of these, the most commonly addressed include muscle tone, range of motion, edema, strength/movement patterns, skin integrity/wound history and future risk for integumentary problems, cognitive status, weight, neurologic impairments (seizures, ataxia, and dystonia), behavior (self-injurious behavior, elopement risk), postural considerations (fixed vs flexible deformity, asymmetry, pelvic tilt, scoliosis, and contracture), pain, postural endurance/tolerance, sitting balance, transfers, and complexity of positioning relative to caregiver's ability to assist.

The standard wheelchair found most commonly in hospitals or institutions is ideal for temporary purposes but not typically custom-fitted and should not be considered for prolonged client use. These chairs are too heavy to support extensive self-mobility. Refer to Figure 25.1 for the major components of a standard wheelchair.

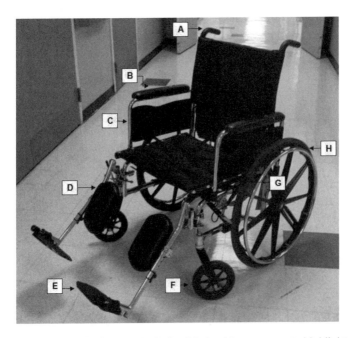

FIGURE 25.1 ■ Standard hospital wheelchair with components highlighted: (A) Push handles; (B) Arm rest; (C) Skirt Guard; (D) Leg rest; (E) Foot rest; (F) Castors; (G) Brake and brake handle; (H) Tire with push rim; (I) Axle.

■ MOBILITY

Manual wheelchairs are routinely assigned to both independent and dependent users. In contrast, power wheelchairs are usually chosen for those with more severe impairments, albeit those who do have the ability to be independent with alternate methods for propulsion. Figure 25.2 shows various mobility options.

MANUAL MOBILITY

Standard manual mobility is well-established and ordinarily quite successful (Figure 25.2a). However, some wheelchair users' mobility options are limited by pain, impaired cardiac/pulmonary status, and poor arm strength and trunk control (5,6).

A number of options exist for alternate manual mobility such as power-assist systems that augment the wheelchair users' physical effort (though adding to the overall weight of the chair), or locomotion generated by the wheelchair user through levers, rims, or by foot propulsion (7). Another factor to consider is whether a client who is at an independent level for long-distance propulsion should use power-assist technology—a system which may afford better protection against overuse upper extremity injuries (4,5). Power assist systems augment the user's physical efforts with motor-driven force and greatly reduce

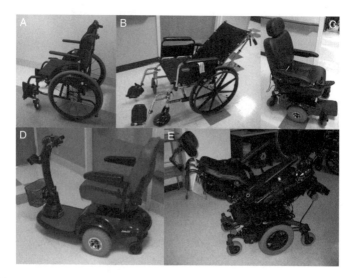

FIGURE 25.2 ■ Various manual and power wheelchairs available: (A) Light weight wheelchair with anti-tippers; (B) Reclining standard wheelchair; (C) Power wheelchair; (D) Power scooter; (E) Tilt-in-space power wheelchair.

the physical demand of prolonged self-mobility (5). However, they add weight to the wheels of the chair and require more upkeep than a standard wheelchair wheel.

POWERED MOBILITY

Since the advent of powered mobility approximately 59 years ago, options and means of transportation have improved considerably (8). There are several types of powered wheelchairs: standard, programmable, lightweight/portable, and customized/motorized. The power mobility evaluation process begins with selection of the most appropriate power base; rear-wheel, front-wheel, or mid-wheel drive. In rear-wheel drive wheelchairs, the rear wheels are larger increasing speed, navigation, and maneuverability; but due to the small front wheels negotiation of uneven terrain may be limited. They also have a larger turning radius creating mobility challenges in small areas. Front-wheel drive mechanisms afford greater control on irregular terrain since the small wheels are located posteriorly, but many users find front-wheel drive chairs awkward, particularly when turning, and at faster velocities the chair can "fish tail" (2).

In mid-wheel drive systems, the rear wheels are situated closer to the mid-point of the chair, increasing driving capacity in indoor as well as outdoor settings where obstacles are present and often, unpredictable (Figure 25.2c). Users must be cautious on rugged terrain so as not to catch the smaller front and rear wheels.

Once the base is selected, powered positioning components such as tilt, recline, lower extremity elevation, total seat elevation, and other more specialized features like standing and stair climbing can be considered. Specialized controls are another consideration at this stage, and may include standard wheelchair electronics (joystick), eye gaze systems, sip and puff systems, voice controls, head controls or specialized hand controls. If the patient intends to drive an automobile while in a wheelchair, seating, positioning, and input accessories must accommodate for leg clearance, steering, adaptive driving controls, and assistive technology/switch access.

Functional mobility and independence can also be augmented, particularly in older adults, by the use of a scooter. Scooters are widely prescribed and offer the user powered locomotion which is less expensive, uncomplicated, and travel compatible. Typically, scooters have either three or four wheels and are powered by a motor which is located posteriorly. Upper extremity strength, mobility, and coordination are necessary for transferring, steering, and breaking. Disadvantages include limited stability due to top-heaviness, larger turning radius, decreased accessibility (counters, sinks, and tables), and inability to accommodate positioning challenges (2).

A scooter is rarely a viable option for in-home mobility unless the home environment is specifically designed for that purpose (Figure 25.2d). Another consideration when using mobility options is the fact that additional training is generally required in order to ensure success, particularly in older adults (2,3).

Given the intricate and often novel control mechanisms, short-term equipment trials are recommended prior to submitting the final order to make certain that the proposed equipment functions as intended and meets the patient's goals. In this stage, relationships with vendors are critical.

■ FRAME DESIGN

Options for frame design include fixed back (frame set at approximately 90 degrees to seat), rear wheel posterior off-set, tilt, and recline mechanisms (9).

Tilt and recline systems will be covered in more detail when seating is reviewed. Figures 25.2b and 25.2e show images of recline and tilt systems, respectively. Fixed back chairs are more compact and lightweight. A posterior off-set rear wheel design (1¼ inch) is typically selected for bilateral above-knee amputee patients (9).

In this position, the center of gravity is optimized to account for the lighter load of the residual limbs and to prevent posterior tilting when traversing upward slopes and curbs. Given the wheel position relative to the user, anti-tipping devices are usually recommended and training is essential. Alternatively, the frame can be designed with a seat dump (frame height is higher in the anterior portion than the posterior) to prevent forward motion (7).

■ AXLE POSITION

The position of the axle is critical to the overall wheelchair and propulsion mechanics. An axle which is placed in a forward position enables backward tipping to negotiate curbs, but is less desirable for propulsion (seat more posterior in relation to pushrim). A high or low positioned axle inversely alters the seat height and typically requires commensurate caster modification.

■ TIRES

Tires are extremely important for locomotion and tracking and can be pneumatic with supplemental air needs or firm necessitating less upkeep. Wheels can be either plastic or metal with spokes and vary in size; many options exist for locking using handles of various configurations, lengths, and engagement maneuvers (push vs pull), as needed.

■ PUSHRIMS

Pushrims also play a major role in maneuverability and propulsion. Available materials include titanium, plastic, and foam with or without extension pieces. Similar to most wheelchair components, handrim styles and configurations can be chosen according to client specifications. Ratcheting handrims may be preferred in select cases of impaired manual dexterity.

As opposed to traditional pushrim(s) use, lever drive systems can be implemented unilaterally or bilaterally to facilitate transmission of forces via shoulder and elbow muscles from the lever(s) to the wheels. This mechanism is thought to decrease the energy expenditure, fatigue, and wear and tear on distal hand/wrist joints and muscles (7,10).

Whereas, 1-arm drive chairs are beneficial for those who have 1-sided deficits and who are only able to generate a propulsive force with the unimpaired side.

■ SEATING AND POSITIONING

Choices for wheelchair seating systems are among the most important considerations when choosing mobility equipment. In this step, a client's needs may be addressed in several ways to promote safety, augment function, alleviate discomfort, and prevent unnecessary medical complications, prescription errors, and client dissatisfaction.

The key to proper positioning is implementation; targeting specific body parts in a logical, sequential fashion. The alignment of the pelvis is most essential given the interdependence of the legs, trunk, head, and shoulder girdle/arms; efforts should proceed accordingly. Neutral positioning is recommended for the pelvis, shoulders, and head, which should also be erect (11). For the elbows and lower extremities, optimal positioning is pure flexion (90 degrees at hips, knees, and ankles) (4,11).

However, while the above is ideal for a patient whose trunk and limbs do not fit this pattern, it may be counterproductive to force body parts into a configuration that counteracts preexisting body alignment. It may even contribute to worsening of postural deformities and/or skin breakdown.

Reclining chairs allow the wheelchair back to be adjusted to various degrees in a posterior direction with regard to the seat to provide pressure relief and can be either full or semireclining; however, recline mechanisms add considerable weight to the overall chair. Also, there is an increased risk for shearing forces when maneuvering between the standard and reclining positions increasing the risk of skin breakdown; an important consideration for those with sensory deficits and poor postural control. Additionally, reclined positions tend to exacerbate posterior pelvic tilt and "sacral sitting" which can also lead to skin breakdown. Figure 25.2b shows an image of a reclining wheelchair.

A tilt system adjusts the wheelchair user's orientation in space while maintaining a fixed position (3).

At the same time, it automatically redistributes pressure from one area (the buttocks and posterior thighs) to another area (posterior trunk and head). Tilt can occur in either a forward or backward direction for positioning purposes (12), which is often a more desirable alternative for those with severe spinal curvatures, sensory impairment, inability to perform pressure relief and/or remain upright independently (2). Figure 25.2e shows the image of a tilting system.

COMPONENTS OF A SEATING SYSTEM

There are several positioning options including but not limited to cushions, backs, lateral thoracic supports, medial and lateral thigh supports/guides, abductor and adductor pads, as well as lap belts and thoracic supports. Material choices are extensive and should be selected wisely to accommodate seating and positioning specifications.

CUSHIONS

Cushions function to support body position, distribute pressure, and maintain alignment. When seated, the ischial tuberosities bear a large percentage of a patient's body weight, followed by the greater trochanters, sacrum, and finally the coccyx (13).

There are specialized techniques and a variety of options available for cushion selection and vendor collaboration is essential to this step. Wheelchair cushions may be air or gel filled or composed of foam, plastics, or composite materials. Figure 25.3 shows various types of cushions. Alternatively, cushions can contain combinations of some or all of these materials with options for customization based on individual client needs. Geometric patterns such as planar, angled, or contoured designs are often used to cradle the pelvis and femurs.

The following information is meant to provide a basic introduction to wheelchair cushion selection:

Foam cushions (Figures 25.3a and b) are utilized for uncomplicated positioning and pressure relief concerns. Poured or custom-molded foam is often considered for patients with significant orthopedic

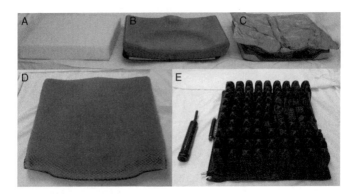

FIGURE 25.3 ■ Seat cushions: (A) Standard foam; (B) High density foam; (C) Gel cushion; (D) Honeycomb cushion; (E) Air cushion with pump.

deformities not suited for prefabricated equipment. Foam tends to be moderately heavy. Other characteristics include poor aeration and a short lifespan of approximately 1 to 2 years.

Air-filled cushions (Figure 25.3e) maximize pressure relief when fragile skin is a consideration and/or if lifestyle necessitates long periods of chair time. They offer dynamic support; a benefit for wheelchair users that adjust their positions frequently. The downfall is the need for extensive maintenance and risk for skin breakdown if over or under filled. Air-filled cushions can also be even more dynamic; consisting of several specifically placed air-filled chambers which serve to intermittently off-load the most pressure sensitive areas by allowing air to flow in and out accordingly.

Cushions with gel inserts (Figure 25.3c) afford excellent pressure relief, but provide poor ventilation and tend to trap heat and moisture, which tends to be quite bothersome in those with intact buttock sensation.

Plastic or composite "honeycomb" cushions (Figure 25.3d) are a good option for patients with incontinence, as they are generally washable and allow good air exchange. However, positioning capacity is rather limited precluding use in those requiring intensive correction.

Anti-thrust cushions often composed of foam or composite materials are generally used to control extensor tone. These cushions have trim lines, which are higher, anteriorly creating an inherent extension, which serves to restrict sliding.

Options also exist for custom fabrication, creating custom molds to accommodate more severe postural deformities that are not well-managed by off-the-shelf cushions.

WHEELCHAIR BACK SUPPORTS

Wheelchair backs may be soft or rigid, curved or planar and exist in many heights. Cutouts, integrated lateral thoracic, or lumbar supports, or even multiple-angular adjustments are possible to accommodate significant, fixed deformities. These items may be purchased in standard sizes or custom molded for exact fit.

The following are important considerations when selecting a wheelchair back:

1. Back height: the wheelchair back, as previously described, is usually placed with the top edge one to two inches below the inferior angle of the scapula for those independent with mobility, to prevent the back of the chair from impeding scapular movement. Higher backs are generally chosen for those dependent for mobility, such as in tilt or recline chairs and for those who have poor functional trunk control and/or significant orthopedic deformities.

2. Contour backs: are available in many different shapes or styles (planar or curved). Planar backs or mildly curved backs allow closer placement of lateral thoracic supports and limit thoracic kyphosis and scapular protraction. Curved backs also improve comfort in those with existing deformities and/or dependent alignment needs.

3. Fabric versus solid backs: fabric backs are lighter than solid backs and often have adjustable tension, affording mild to moderate trunk support. Fabric backs are appropriate for light-duty wheelchairs and those with limited support needs.

ADDITIONAL POSITIONING COMPONENTS:
Often, supplementary positioning components are required to optimize patient comfort and alignment (4):

1. Lateral thoracic supports

2. Headrests

3. Pelvic guides

4. Removable or permanent lateral (placed on the outside of the thighs to limit adduction)

5. Medial thigh pads (placed between knees to restrict abduction)

6. Medial and lateral thigh supports/guides which restrict hip joint motion (abduction/external rotation and abduction/internal rotation, respectively)

7. Lap belts

8. Anterior thoracic supports

9. Axillary straps

10. Footrests

11. Calf pads/panels

■ **OTHER CONSIDERATIONS**
It is possible to accessorize the wheelchair in different ways depending on a particular client's needs and lifestyle. Baskets, brakes/locks of variable shapes, lengths, and sizes, lap trays, baggage rests/transport devices, receptacles for drinks/assistive devices, attachments for knapsacks/bags, fasteners (tie-downs), and harnesses/straps (upper body, waist) including vests and jackets are items that are available for this purpose.

■ **SPECIAL TECHNIQUES**
There are various pressure-monitoring devices on the market (eg, sphygmomanometer mediated) which aid in cushion selection. An increasingly popular technique is pressure mapping, which can be used to optimize wheelchair seating both as an instructional and diagnostic tool (3).

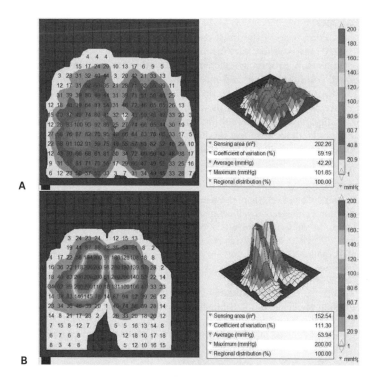

FIGURE 25.4 ■ Pressure mapping showing areas of increased pressure to assist in cushion molding; (A) Normal pressure mapping without areas of increased pressure; (B) Increased pressure along the ischeal tuberosities.

Several techniques exist for mapping based on feedback from sensors which monitor the amount of pressure displaced by a given cushion which is placed under the buttocks. A digital reading of pressure information is generated and displayed on a computer screen. Pressure mapping is an excellent complement to the standard mat evaluation and increases the likelihood that skin integrity will be protected by a given cushion. Pressure mapping is illustrated in Figure 25.4.

■ EQUIPMENT PROCUREMENT

Standards for reimbursement and medical necessity determination differ depending on the payor source and location. Successful procurement of DME, in this case wheelchairs and seating, often necessitates documentation in a letter format. Letters of medical necessity should discuss the medical diagnosis, comorbidities, and background circumstances including functional status, reason intended equipment is needed as opposed to something less expensive and consequences of not rendering.

■ SUMMARY

Wheelchairs are one of the most essential assistive devices and serve as the primary means of mobility for many users whether for short- or long-term purposes. A proper wheelchair prescription necessitates a careful, organized, comprehensive, and interdisciplinary approach involving not only the appropriate health care professionals, but also the client, family, and/or caregivers. To perform this well, special attention must be given to the evaluation, seating, and mobility process in the context of the client's personal goals, demands, and medical condition(s). Otherwise, mobility, functional status, quality of life, and health may be compromised.

■ REFERENCES

1. Yang YS, Chang GL, Hsu MJ, Chang JJ. Remote monitoring of sitting behaviors for community-dwelling manual wheelchair users with spinal cord injury. *Spinal Cord.* 2009;47(1):67–71.

2. Sabol TP, Haley ES. Wheelchair evaluation for the older adult. Clin Geriatr Med. 2006;22(2):355–75, ix.

3. Hastings JD. Seating assessment and planning. Phys Med Rehabil Clin N Am. 2000;11(1):183–207, x.

4. Koontz, A. et al. Prescription of Wheelchairs and Seating Systems. In: Physical Medicine and Rehabilitation. Braddom RL. ed.3rd ed. Edinburgh, UK: Elsevier Saunders; 2007.

5. Cooper RA, Fitzgerald SG, Boninger ML, et al. Evaluation of a pushrim-activated, power-assisted wheelchair. Arch Phys Med Rehabil. 2001;82(5): 702–708.

6. Veeger HE, van der Woude LH, Rozendal RH. Effect of handrim velocity on mechanical efficiency in wheelchair propulsion. Med Sci Sports Exerc. 1992;24(1):100–107.

7. Cooper, R.A. et al. Seating, Assistive Technology, and Equipment. In: Stroke Recovery and Rehabilitation.Stein, J. et al. eds. New York: Demos; 2009.

8. Woods B, Watson N. A short history of powered wheelchairs. Assist Technol. 2003;15(2):164–180.

9. Spiegler JH, Goldberg MJ. The wheelchair as a permanent mode of mobility a detaild guide to prescription. I. frame, armrests and brakes. Am J Phys Med. 1968;47(6):315–316.

10. van der Woude LH, Dallmeijer AJ, Janssen TW, Veeger D. Alternative modes of manual wheelchair ambulation: an overview. *Am J Phys Med Rehabil.* 2001;80(10):765–777.

11. Trefler E, Taylor SJ. Prescription and positioning: Evaluating the physically disabled individual for wheelchair seating. *Prosthet Orthot Int.* 1991;15(3):217–224.

12. Michael SM, Porter D, Pountney TE. Tilted seat position for non-ambulant individuals with neurological and neuromuscular impairment: a systematic review. *Clin Rehabil.* 2007;21(12):1063–1074.

13. Ferguson-Pell MW. Seat cushion selection. *J Rehabil Res Dev Clin Suppl.* 1990;(2)(2):49–73.

26

Wound Care

Zachary Martin

■ **WOUND HEALING**

The management of chronic wounds is gaining increased attention due to growing awareness of the high cost and morbidity of poorly healing wounds and a better understanding of the pathophysiology of wound healing. As health care providers dedicate themselves to practicing the science of wound care, outcomes will improve. In addition to a greater understanding of the fundamentals of wound healing, there are many emerging technologies that can be helpful to the practitioner treating refractory wounds.

Despite the heavy investment in advanced treatment modalities, good wound care starts with the basics.

■ **WHAT IS A CHRONIC WOUND?**

Chronic wounds are wounds that fail to heal along the normal healing pathway. In order to treat chronic wounds, it is important to recall the normal healing cascade that takes place in a healthy host with an acute injury.

Normal wound healing is a very complex and dynamic process. A simplified description generally divides this process into three overlapping phases: (1) inflammatory, (2) proliferative, and (3) remodeling.

1. Inflammatory phase. Some authors subdivide the inflammatory phase into a hemostatic and inflammatory phase. Immediately following an injury, blood and platelets enter the wound to stop the bleeding. Platelets secrete (among many things) histamine, platelet derived growth factor, and transforming growth factor. This causes vasodilation and an influx of neutrophils and macrophages. From days 2 to 4, the macrophages continue to secrete growth factors to promote fibroblast influx into the wound which signals the ending of the inflammatory phase and beginning of the proliferative phase.

2. Proliferative phase. The proliferative phase is dominated by the fibroblast and begins about 3 to 5 days after injury and continues for approximately 3 weeks. This is the period when angiogenesis and collagen deposition occurs. Granulation tissue appears in the wound and epithelialization can be observed.

3. Remodeling phase. The remodeling phase begins around 3 weeks and can continue for a year after injury. During this time, type III collagen is replaced by type I collagen which crosslinks, and increases the tensile strength of the wound (1). Chronic wounds are considered healed once epithelialized; however, the tissues will continue to evolve until the remodeling phase is complete.

Once a chronic wound has been identified, the process of returning the patient to the normal healing pathway can begin. As in most areas of medicine, proper treatment requires an initial accurate diagnosis. In almost all cases, a careful history and physical exam should result in a solid diagnosis. One can classify most wounds appropriately by their anatomic location and the patient's past medical history. The diagnosis should go beyond the simple identification of a pressure ulcer and should include an understanding of the underlying anatomic structure that is contributing to the wound as well as any contributing pathophysiology.

The diagnosis should be accompanied by an assessment of the wound bed. The presence of necrosis, exudate, purulence, or granulation tissue should be noted. The viable tissue at the base of the wound should be characterized. Does the wound extend into dermis, subcutaneous fat, paratenon, muscle, tendon, periosteum, or bone? The periwound tissue should also be assessed for signs of cellulitis, maceration, callus, or epiboly (rolled skin edges).

If the wound is on the lower extremity, the arterial and venous systems should be assessed. The clinician will need to determine whether history and physical exam alone is sufficient. Often noninvasive arterial Doppler studies will be necessary to adequately evaluate the lower extremity circulation. Studies have shown that the presence of a palpable pulse does not exclude the possibility of early peripheral arterial disease (PAD) (2).

Offloading is a critical early step in managing chronic wounds. This may require sitting restrictions, frequent repositioning, or nonweight bearing status. Pressure may play a role in less obvious ways from splints, wheelchair leg supports, and poor fitting shoes. It can be helpful to examine the footwear of patients with pedal wounds. Failure to identify the underlying pressure contributing to the wound will result in treatment failure and probably worsening of the wound.

Once a diagnosis has been made and adequate perfusion has been established, wound bed preparation can begin. Debridement can be performed surgically with scalpels, currettes, or hydrosurgery. Alternative forms of debridement include mechanical with dressing changes, chemical with enzymatic agents, or biological with maggots. If feasible, surgical debridement is often preferred. Sharp debridement allows for rapid wound bed preparation and assessment of the depth of injury. Frequent

TABLE 26.1 ■ Barriers to wound healing.

Intrinsic	Extrinsic
Edema	Pressure
Malnutrition	Infection
Ischemia	Poor Wound care
Radiation injury	
Fibrosis	

sharp debridements are associated with a faster rate of healing (3). There may be cases where surgical debridement is not practical or tolerated. These are the preferred times to use enzymatic debridement. Mechanical debridement with wet–dry saline dressings have largely fallen out of favor because it is painful and requires the dressing to dry which violates the principle of maintaining a moist wound bed. Maggot therapy is still used in select cases. It is recognized as a way to relatively painlessly and efficiently remove devitalized tissue from a wound. Although maggots are a legitimate form of wound bed management, the logistics and need for proper disposal of the maggots makes maggot therapy impractical for most medical settings in the United States.

In addition to identifying the cause of injury and preparing the wound bed, the physician managing a complex wound will need to identify any intrinsic or extrinsic barriers to healing (Table 26.1).

■ **INTRINSIC FACTORS**
EDEMA
Lower extremity edema will predispose the patient to developing wounds and inhibit the diffusion of oxygen to the skin. Thus it must be controlled in order to assist healing. Edema management involves excluding or managing venous disease and deep venous thromboses (DVTs) and initiating leg elevation, diuretics, and compression therapy when appropriate. Prior to instituting compression therapy adequate arterial inflow should be assured. Layered compression should start at the toes and extend up to the knee, to avoid creating swelling distal to the wraps. Typically layered compression wraps are used while the patient is healing a wound. After healing, the patient is transitioned into compression stockings at a pressure of 25 to 35 mm Hg. Lower pressure stockings are less ideal but may have a role when the patient does not tolerate higher levels of compression or only has very mild disease.

NUTRITION
The nutritional status of the patient should be assessed. Patients with significant wounds and under stress should receive 30 to 35 kcal/kg/d. This should include 1.25 to 1.5 gm/kg of protein. A well balanced diet

should be encouraged with oral supplements provided as needed. Vitamin and mineral supplements should be given if vitamin deficiency is suspected or dietary intake is poor. Zinc and vitamins A, B complex, and C are particularly important.

Ischemic and radiated tissues may require advanced treatments including revascularization procedures or hyperbaric oxygen (HBO) therapy. The management of wounds associated with PAD is discussed later in the chapter.

■ EXTRINSIC FACTORS

Ensuring that the wound care is conducive to healing and addressing issues like infection and pressure are critical to success. Once the wound etiology has been determined, and the wound bed prepared, the dressings can be selected. The goal of the dressing should be to keep the wound bed moist and the periwound tissue dry. In the outpatient setting, the frequency of dressing changes should be determined by the needs of the wound and the patient's resources. Clean, improving wounds can be dressed anywhere from daily to weekly, depending on the drainage and the patients' needs. Patients requiring compression therapy over wounds tend to have their dressings changed every 3 to 7 days. However, early on in therapy, daily wraps may be required. Dressing selection is a dynamic process and the clinician will need to adjust the treatment plan as the wound evolves. Most dressing changes are performed in a clean but not sterile environment. The wound needs to be cleaned of loose exudate and slough. There is little evidence to recommend a particular type of wound cleanser. Saline, sterile water, or tap water can all reasonably be used at the discretion of the health care provider depending on the circumstances (4). Some patients may report more comfort with one technique over the other.

Once the wound is clean, the dressing can be applied. One of the most frequently prescribed wound dressings is hydrogel and gauze daily. This combination keeps the wound moist, is generally well tolerated and is easy to apply. This is adequate for most wounds with mild drainage. When a more absorbent dressing is needed, hydrofibers or alginates can be selected. If tendon, bone or vital structures are exposed in the wound, special attention should be paid to ensure that they do not desiccate between dressing changes. When bacterial colonization is a concern, a silver impregnated dressing may be considered. Silver dressings tend to be more expensive and so rational use of the products is urged. Like systemic antibiotics, it is appropriate to select a stop date so that patients are not left on silver dressings for unnecessary lengths of time. Cytotoxic agents like iodine, peroxide, and Dakin's solution at standard concentrations should be avoided. Their use may be appropriate in rare, isolated short-term applications when managing gross wound contamination is prioritized over promoting wound healing.

Wound bed infection can be difficult to determine on clinical exam alone. Wounds that are not responding to local care should be reassessed for possible infection. Not all patients with clinically significant bacterial contamination will present with typical signs of infection (i.e. fever, erythema, warmth, and leukocytosis). Wound bed infections have been defined by a colonization of greater than 100,000 organisms per gram. Ideally, quantitative cultures should be obtained; however, these tests are not available to all clinicians. As an alternative, semi-quantitative wound swabs have shown some clinical utility (5). Judicious use of antibiotics is appropriate in patients with a significant clinical suspicion of wound bed infection. As with treating most other infections, antibiotics use should be focused and time limited. The clinician will need to determine whether a wound bed infection should be treated with topical or systemic antimicrobials.

■ SPECIFIC WOUNDS
PRESSURE ULCERS

Pressure ulcers occur in the sensory- and mobility-impaired patient. Tissue injury typically occurs over bony prominences. Tissue injury is caused by increased pressure on the overlying skin and fat. Areas of high pressure (eg, the ischium in a sitting patient) can be injured in as little as 2 hours, whereas lower pressure sites can tolerate longer periods of weight bearing. Thus offloading must be individualized to the wound. Once identified, these ulcers should be classified by their anatomic location.

Staging should be done according to the National Pressure Ulcer Advisory Panel (NPUAP) criteria (Table 26.2) (6).

In addition to staging the wound, the patient's sitting and weight-bearing history should be obtained. Offloading should be done with the specific anatomic location of the wound in mind. It may be useful to refer patients for pressure mapping. Tetraplegics should be prescribed tilting wheelchairs to allow them to relieve pressure while sitting. For large or worsening wounds, complete offloading may be necessary initially; however, once the wound is stabilized short periods of weight bearing can often be tolerated if adequately padded and time-limited. Moisture and friction will also contribute to wound formation and should be minimized.

Bone infection can be assessed by several methods. If after clinical exam, sedimentation rate, white blood cell count, and plain film xray, osteomyelitis is not evident but still suspected MRI's, bone scans or bone biopsies may be needed. When practical, bone biopsies not only assist in the diagnosis, but also aid in the treatment as bone cultures can be obtained at the same time. MRI is surpassing the bone scan as the preferred modality when advanced imaging is needed. The management of wound associated osteomyelitis is variable. Patients who are

TABLE 26.2 ■ Pressure ulcer stages revised, national pressure ulcer advisory panel.

Stages

Suspected Deep Tissue Injury:

Purple or maroon localized area of discolored intact skin or blood-filled blister due to damage of underlying soft tissue from pressure and/or shear. The area may be preceded by tissue that is painful, firm, mushy, boggy, warmer, or cooler as compared to adjacent tissue.

Further description:
Deep tissue injury may be difficult to detect in individuals with dark skin tones. Evolution may include a thin blister over a dark wound bed. The wound may further evolve and become covered by thin eschar. Evolution may be rapid exposing additional layers of tissue even with optimal treatment.

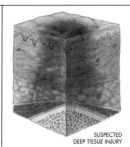

SUSPECTED
DEEP TISSUE INJURY

Stage I:
Intact skin with nonblanchable redness of a localized area usually over a bony prominence. Darkly pigmented skin may not have visible blanching; its color may differ from the surrounding area.

Further description:
The area may be painful, firm, soft, warmer, or cooler as compared to adjacent tissue. Stage I may be difficult to detect in individuals with dark skin tones. May indicate "at risk" persons (a heralding sign of risk).

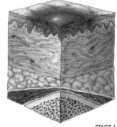

STAGE 1

Stage II:
Partial thickness loss of dermis presenting as a shallow open ulcer with a red pink wound bed, without slough. May also present as an intact or open/ruptured serum-filled blister.

Further description:
Presents as a shiny or dry shallow ulcer without slough or bruising.* This stage should not be used to describe skin tears, tape burns, perineal dermatitis, maceration, or excoriation.

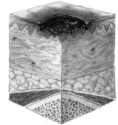

STAGE 2

Stage III:
Full thickness tissue loss. Subcutaneous fat may be visible but bone, tendon, or muscles are not exposed. Slough may be present but does not obscure the depth of tissue loss. May include undermining and tunneling.

Further description:
The depth of a stage III pressure ulcer varies by anatomical location. The bridge of the nose, ear, occiput, and malleolus do not have subcutaneous tissue and stage III ulcers can be shallow. In contrast, areas of significant adiposity can develop extremely deep stage III pressure ulcers. Bone/tendon is not visible or directly palpable.

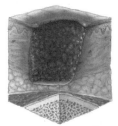

STAGE 3

Stage IV:
Full thickness tissue loss with exposed bone, tendon, or muscle. Slough or eschar may be present on some parts of the wound bed. Often include undermining and tunneling.

Further description:
The depth of a stage IV pressure ulcer varies by anatomical location. The bridge of the nose, ear, occiput, and malleolus do not have subcutaneous tissue and these ulcers can be shallow. Stage IV ulcers can extend into muscle and/or supporting structures (eg, fascia, tendon, or joint capsule) making osteomyelitis possible. Exposed bone/tendon is visible or directly palpable.

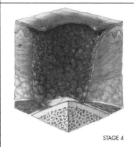

STAGE 4

Unstageable:
Full thickness tissue loss in which the base of the ulcer is covered by slough (yellow, tan, gray, green, or brown) and/or eschar (tan, brown, or black) in the wound bed.

Further description:
Until enough slough and/or eschar is removed to expose the base of the wound, the true depth, and therefore stage, cannot be determined. Stable (dry, adherent, intact without erythema or fluctuance) eschar on the heels serves as "the body's natural (biological) cover" and should not be removed.

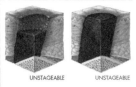

UNSTAGEABLE   UNSTAGEABLE

*Bruising indicates suspected deep tissue injury. Adpated with permission from Ref. (6).

acutely ill with leukocytosis, fever, and elevated sedimentation rates tend to require long-term, culture-specific antibiotics. However, it is not clear that chronically exposed bone in the absence of acute illness should be treated with systemic antibiotics in all instances. Surgical removal of devitalized or friable bone should be performed; however, it may not be practical to remove all of the involved bone. If the goal is to eradicate bone infection then consideration should be made to providing permanent soft-tissue coverage over the bone so that at the completion of antibiotics the wound is covered with durable soft tissue.

Flap repair for pressure ulcers should be considered for patients whose wounds are unlikely to heal in a timely fashion with good durable tissue. Appropriate surgical candidates respond to local care, comply with the offloading regimen and are motivated to participate in a postoperative program to protect the flap and prevent recurrences. These patients should be assessed for underlying osteomyelitis which can be treated prior to or in conjunction with the definitive surgical repair. Patients should be aware that there are a limited number of local flaps available at each wound site and therefore should only pursue treatment when they are absolutely committed to the treatment course which typically involves surgery followed by 3 to 6 weeks of strict offloading.

Wounds that fail to respond on a weekly basis should be reassessed for adequate offloading, proper dressing selection and infection. Many times patients will report that they are being compliant with their offloading, not realizing that a certain position or activity is contributing to their wound. Large stage 4 wounds may stall after a long period of steady improvement. After ensuring adequate wound bed preparation, offloading and infection control, the patient should be referred to a plastic surgeon for evaluation for flap reconstruction.

DIABETIC FOOT ULCERS

The cause of DFUs (diabetic foot ulcers) is often multifactorial. These patients tend to have vascular disease, neuropathy, and impaired granulocytic and chemotaxic activity (7). Initial attention should be paid to assessing the peripheral pulses. Noninvasive arterial studies can be helpful in determining the presence of PAD. Ankle-Brachial indices (ABIs) can be falsely elevated due to calcified vessels. Toe pressures often provide better information. Acute infection should also be addressed and systemic antibiotics used when necessary (Figure 26.1). The depth of the wound and presence of pus should be determined. Wounds that probe to bone may have concomitant osteomyelitis and further work-up is indicated. Once the tissues involved have been determined, then the wound should be graded according to Wagner's Grading (8) (Table 26.3).

Much like pressure ulcers, an underlying bony prominence can often be identified (i.e. metatarsal head). Identifying pressure points will help in selecting the appropriate offloading device. A consultation with a certified

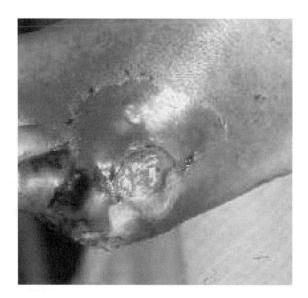

FIGURE 26.1 ■ DFU with eschar and associated cellulitis.

TABLE 26.3 ■ Wagner's Grading of foot lesions.

Grade 0	No open lesion
Grade 1	Superficial ulcer
Grade 2	Deep ulcer (extending to tendon, bone or joint capsule)
Grade 3	Involving deeper structures with evidence of abscess, tendonitis or osteomyelitis
Grade 4	Gangrene of some portion of the toes or forefoot
Grade 5	Gangrene involving most or all of the foot

Adapted with permission from Ref. (8).

pedorthotist can be very helpful in this regard. The patient's diabetes must be under good control. A hemoglobin A1C can provide insight into the patients' blood sugar control over time. A goal of less than 6.5% to 7% is suggested by leading organizations (9). Poorly controlled diabetics are at risk of poor wound healing, infection, and major amputation.

VENOUS STASIS ULCERS
These wounds generally occur between the mid-calf to just below the malleoli. Venous stasis ulcers (VSUs) typically result from chronic dysfunction of the venous system due to factors related to valvular dysfunction,

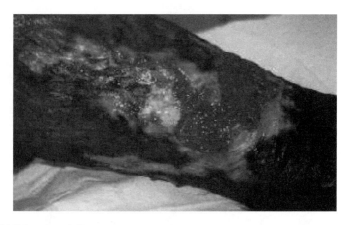

FIGURE 26.2 ■ VSU with granulating bed.

heart failure, chronic deep venous thromboses, and/or poor calf muscle pump function. Over time, chronic venous insufficiency leads to fibrosis of the subcutaneous tissues.

Venous ulcers tend to have irregular borders and granulating wound beds (Figure 26.2).

These patients may benefit from venous ultrasound work-up to evaluate for valvular incompetence or prominent venous perforators which may be amenable to saphenous stripping or perforator ligation which can improve healing and decrease the risk of recurrence (10).

Edema management in these patients is critical. Once adequate arterial inflow is determined, layered compression wraps should be used to decrease lower extremity swelling (11). Leg elevation and life-style modification is often necessary. Fluid management for patients with a component of heart failure may also be necessary. Patients with a history of VSUs often require chronic compression to prevent recurrences.

ARTERIAL ULCERS

PAD ulcers tend to be sharply demarcated and poorly granulating (Figure 26.3). They are often painful. The vascular work-up is critical for these patients. Often these patients will report a history of intermittent claudication or rest pain. If the patient has significant arterial disease, a vascular surgery consult should be obtained. Revascularization, in general, should precede major debridement. The perfusion of the limb continues to improve for about 3 to 4 weeks after revascularization (12). If the wound is acutely infected it may not be possible to postpone debridement until after revascularization. ABIs are an appropriate initial diagnostic test for patients suspected of PAD. ABIs of 0.9 to 1.1 are

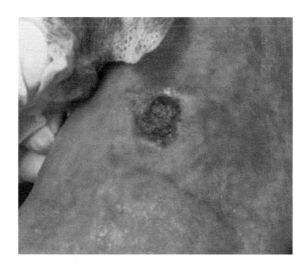

FIGURE 26.3 ■ Arterial ulcer on the dorsum of the foot.
Source: The Foot and Ankle Online Journal 1 (9): 2.

considered normal. Diabetics and patients with heavily calcified vessels may have falsely elevated ABIs. An ABI of 0.5 or less suggests a foot ulcer is unlikely to heal without vascular intervention. Ratios greater than 1.3 should be considered as potentially falsely elevated. Toe-Brachial Indices can be useful when ABIs are falsely elevated as digital pressures tend to be less affected by medial calcification (13).

Once the perfusion status has been assessed and addressed, wound care can proceed using the same principles outlined previously.

■ ADVANCED TREATMENT MODALITIES
For wounds that do not respond to conventional treatments, these advanced modalities may be useful. These tend to either be cost- or time-intensive treatments and should be used selectively to improve their cost-effectiveness. The following is a brief overview of a few commonly used therapies.

Sub-Atmospheric Dressings or negative pressure wound therapy (NPWT). These dressings have been shown to promote granulation tissue formation, control wound drainage and edema, stimulate wound perfusion, and promote wound healing (14). They should be considered for large wounds, deep wounds or those not responding to conventional treatment. Necrosis and infection should be resolved prior to their use and caution should be taken in anticoagulated patients in those patients with potentially exposed vascular structures. Typically a NPWT dressing will be changed every 48 to 72 hours. Disadvantages of NPWT are that it requires a patient to be attached to a pump (however mobile), the machine or dressing can fail requiring an unscheduled dressing change, and a small percentage of patients will find NPWT to be too painful.

HBO has been found to be clinically helpful in advanced Wagner's grade DFUs, radiated tissues, refractory osteomyelitis, and failing flaps and grafts. Its use can be considered in cases where local reversible hypoxia is contributing to the wound and where ischemia is not surgically correctable. Transcutaneous oxygen measurements can be obtained to determine whether the local tissues are ischemic and whether they might respond to HBO. These treatments can be very time consuming (for the patient) and expensive. A typical outpatient hyperbaric center will treat patients for 2 hours a day, 5 days a week for 4 to 8 weeks depending on their diagnosis. The most common complications include barotrauma to the ears and seizures due to oxygen toxicity.

Cellular therapy. This is a broad category and includes growth factors, cryopreserved human skin allografts, and cellular synthetic skin substitutes like Apligraft (comprised of human fibroblasts and keratinocytes) and Dermagraft (a biodegradable mesh seeded with human fibroblasts). These therapies tend to be expensive but can be cost-effective when used on appropriately selected patients. These tend to be patients who have failed to improve despite standard wound care and are cleared of infection.

Acellular therapy can consist of decellularized allogeneic or xenogeneic tissue or other biomaterials. These can be appropriate for replacing areas of deficient collagen or promoting cellular ingrowth by providing a collagen scaffold. They may also be used to cover and protect underlying structures and may decrease wound pain.

■ CONCLUSION

Wound healing is a highly complex process that involves an orderly sequence of cellular events. Chronic wounds fail to follow this orderly sequence for a variety of reasons. The care of chronic wound patients requires a proper diagnosis and intervention. Initially it may be necessary to evaluate wounds on a weekly basis to ensure that they are responding to treatment. Once steady improvement is observed and the wound is objectively improving, less frequent exams are appropriate. Wounds can be documented by simply measuring length, width, and depth. Although this is often adequate, these measurements may miss small improvements in an irregularly shaped wound. Newer photographic systems provide greater detail by measuring the complete surface area. It is important to have an objective way of measuring and documenting progress. When wounds fail to respond (i.e. show no consistant signs of improvement), the treatment plan should be adjusted. A chronic wound can be successfully healed by following a systematic evaluation and management strategy.

■ REFERENCES

1. Gabriel A, Mussman J, Rosenberg LZ, de la Torre JI. Wound healing, growth factors. *http://emedicine.medscape.com/plastic_surgery#wound*. Accessed June 14, 2010.

2. Collins T, Suarez-Almazor M, Peterson NJ. An absent pulse is not sensitive for the early detection of peripheral arterial disease. *Fam Med*. 2006; 38:38–42.

3. Steed DL, Donohoe D, Webster MW, Lindsley L. Effect of extensive debridement and treatment on the healing of diabetic foot ulcers. Diabetic Ulcer Study Group. *J Am Coll Surg*. 1996;183(1):61–64.

4. Fernandez R, Griffiths R, Ussia C. Water for wound cleansing. *Int J Evid Based Healthc*. 2007;5:305–323

5. Ratliff CR, Getchell-White SI, Rodeheaver GT. Quantitation of bacteria in clean, nonhealing, chronic wounds. *Wounds*. 2008;20(10):279–283. *http://www.medscape.com/viewarticle/582541*. Accessed June 15, 2010.

6. National Pressure Ulcer Advisory Panel (NPUAP). *http://www.npuap.org/pr2.htm*. Accessed June 15, 2010.

7. Singer AJ, Clark RAF.Cutaneous wound healing. *N Engl J Med*.1999;341 (10):738–746.

8. Wagner FW Jr. The dysvascular foot: a system for diagnosis and treatment. *Foot Ankle*. 1981;2(2):64–122.

9. Clark N. Defending ADA's A1c Target. *Doc News*. 2005; 2.

10. O'Donnell T Jr. The present status of surgery of the superficial venous system in the management of venous ulcer and the evidence for the role of perforator interruption. *J Vasc Surg*. 2008;48(4):1044–1052.

11. Laura Bolton. Compression in Venous Ulcer Management. *J Wound Ostomy Continence Nurs*. 2008;35(1):40–49. Copyright 2008, by the Wound, Ostomy and Continence Nurses Society. ISSN publication 1071–5754.

12. Caselli A, Latini V, Lapenna A, et al. Transcutaneous oxygen tension monitoring after successful revascularization in diabetic patients with ischaemic foot ulcers. *Diabet Med*. 2005;22(4):460–465. Published Online: January, 2005.

13. DeAnna Holtman NP, Vivian Gahtan MD. Peripheral arterial perfusion: is it adequate for wound healing? *Wounds*. 2008;20(8):230–235.

14. Niezgoda JA, Mendez-Eastman S. The effective management of pressure ulcers. *Adv Skin Wound Care*. 2006;19(suppl 1):3–15.

Appendix 1   *Amputation Level and Energy Expenditure of Mobility*

Prosthetic Ambulation/Mobility Type	Energy Expenditure (% increase above walking)
Wheelchair	9
Transtibial	25
Transtibial (bilateral)	41
Crutch (axillary, without prosthesis)	59
Transfemoral	65
Transfemoral (bilateral)	272

■ REFERENCES

Gonzalez EG, Corcoran PJ, Reyes RL. Energy expenditure in below-knee amputees: correlation with stump length. *Arch Phys Med Rehabil*. 1974;55:118.

Huang CT, Jackson JR, Moore NB, et al. Amputation: energy cost of ambulation. *Arch Phys Med Rehabil*. 1979;60(1):22.

Traugh GH, Corcoran PJ, Reyes RL. Energy expenditure of ambulation in patients with above-knee amputations. *Arch Phys Med Rehabil*. 1975;56:69.

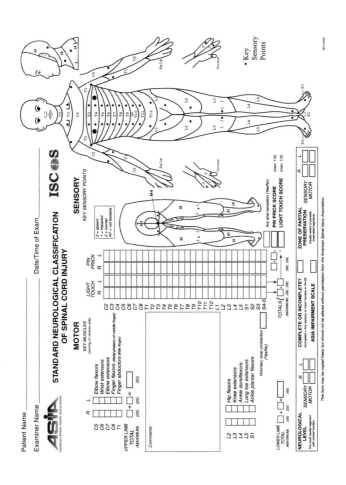

MUSCLE GRADING

0   total paralysis

1   palpable or visible contraction

2   active movement, full range of motion, gravity eliminated

3   active movement, full range of motion, against gravity

4   active movement, full range of motion, against gravity and provides some resistance

5   active movement, full range of motion, against gravity and provides normal resistance

5* muscle able to exert, in examiner's judgement, sufficient resistance to be considered normal if identifiable inhibiting factors were not present

NT not testable. Patient unable to reliably exert effort or muscle unavailable for testing due to factors such as immobilization, pain on effort or contracture.

ASIA IMPAIRMENT SCALE

☐   A = **Complete:** No motor or sensory function is preserved in the sacral segments S4-S5.

☐   B = **Incomplete:** Sensory but not motor function is preserved below the neurological level and includes the sacral segments S4-S5.

☐   C = **Incomplete:** Motor function is preserved below the neurological level, and more than half of key muscles below the neurological level have a muscle grade less than 3.

☐   D = **Incomplete:** Motor function is preserved below the neurological level, and at least half of key muscles below the neurological level have a muscle grade of 3 or more.

☐   E = **Normal:** Motor and sensory function are normal.

CLINICAL SYNDROMES (OPTIONAL)

☐   Central Cord
☐   Brown-Sequard
☐   Anterior Cord
☐   Conus Medullaris
☐   Cauda Equina

STEPS IN CLASSIFICATION

The following order is recommended in determining the classification of individuals with SCI.

1. Determine sensory levels for right and left sides.

2. Determine motor levels for right and left sides.
    Note: in regions where there is no myotome to test, the motor level is presumed to be the same as the sensory level.

3. Determine the single neurological level.
    This is the lowest segment where motor and sensory function is normal on both sides, and is the most cephalad of the sensory and motor levels determined in steps 1 and 2.

4. Determine whether the injury is Complete or Incomplete (sacral sparing).
    If voluntary anal contraction = No AND all S4-5 sensory scores = 0 AND any anal sensation = No, then injury is COMPLETE. Otherwise injury is incomplete.

5. Determine ASIA Impairment Scale (AIS) Grade:

    Is injury **Complete?**   If **YES,** AIS=A Record ZPP
    ↓ NO   (For ZPP record lowest dermatome or myotome on
                              each side with some (non-zero score) preservation)

    Is injury
    motor incomplete?   If **NO,** AIS=B
    ↓ YES   (Yes=voluntary anal contraction OR motor
                              function more than three levels below the motor
                              level on a given side.)

    Are at least half of the key muscles below the (single) neurological level graded 3 or better?

    NO   YES
    ↓   ↓
    AIS=C   AIS=D

    If sensation and motor function is normal in all segments, AIS=E
    Note: AIS E is used in follow up testing when an individual with a documented SCI has recovered normal function. If at initial testing no deficits are found, the individual is neurologically intact; the ASIA Impairment Scale does not apply.

Autonomic Dysreflexia Treatment Algorithm

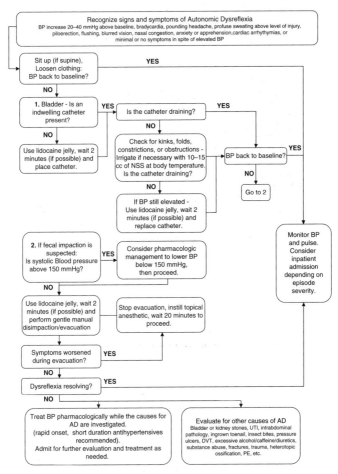

AD-Autonomic dysreflexia; BP-Blood pressure

Based on the published recommendations by the Consortium for Spinal Cord
Medicine: *Acute Management of Autonomic Dysreflexia: Individuals with Spinal Cord Injury Presenting to Health Care
facilities*. Paralyzed veterans of America, 2001.

Bowel Care Agents/Laxatives (Lower Motor Neuron Bowel)

Treatment	Type	Mechanism	Drug Interactions	Contraindications	Adverse Side Effects
Methylcellulose (Citrucel®) Psyllium (Metamucil®) Polycarbophil (FiberCon®) Guar Gum (Benefiber®)	Bulking agents	Contains natural fiber that increases content of feces, pulls water into the colon, and promotes bacterial growth	May decrease absorption and effects of salicylates, nitrofurantoin, tetracyclines, diuretics, coumadin, tegretol	Documented hypersensitivity; fecal impaction, intestinal obstruction, or undiagnosed abdominal pain	Gas Bloating Cramping
Manual disimpaction	Technique	Manual stool removal	none		Autonomic dysreflexia
Upper Motor Neuron Bowel					
Polyethylene glycol (Miralax®)	Osmotic	PEG is not absorbed and continues to hold water by osmotic action through the small bowel and the colon, resulting in mechanical cleansing.		Documented hypersensitivity; fecal impaction, intestinal obstruction, or undiagnosed abdominal pain	

Sodium phosphates (Fleet Phospho-Soda®) Magnesium hydroxide (Milk of magnesia) Magnesium citrate (Citroma®)	Saline laxatives	The active ingredients in saline laxatives are magnesium, sulfate, citrate, and phosphate ions. These ions draw water into the intestines. The additional water softens the stool, increases pressure within the intestines, and increases intestinal contractions.		Patients with impaired kidney function should not use laxatives containing magnesium or phosphate salts. Patients who need to limit their sodium intake, such as those with congestive heart failure, kidney disease, and high blood pressure, should not use laxatives that contain sodium.
Docusate (Colace®)	Stool softener	Surface-active agent emollient that prevents hardening of the feces by adding moisture to the stool	Decreases effects of warfarin and increases effects of phenolphthalein & mineral oil	Documented hypersensitivity; fecal impaction, intestinal obstruction, or undiagnosed abdominal pain

(Continued)

Bowel Care Agents/Laxatives (Lower Motor Neuron Bowel) (*Continued*)

Treatment	Type	Mechanism	Drug Interactions	Contraindications	Adverse Side Effects
Senna (Senokot®, Ex-Lax®)	Stimulant	Natural vegetable derivative that causes neuroperistaltic stimulation; acts on Auerbach's plexus	Decreases effects of anticoagulants	Documented hypersensitivity; fecal impaction, intestinal obstruction, or undiagnosed abdominal pain	Prolonged use can cause the colon lining to become darker than normal (melanosis coli) due to the accumulation of melanin Chronic, long-term use of stimulant laxatives can lead to loss of colon function (cathartic colon). After years to decades of frequent use of stimulant laxatives, the nerves of the colon slowly disappear, the colon muscles wither, and the colon becomes dilated. Consequently, constipation becomes increasingly worse and unresponsive to laxatives.

Bisacodyl suppository (Dulcolax®, Correctol®)	Oil-based stimulant	Direct stimulation of colonic mucosa to produce peristalsis. Stimulates rectocolic reflex	Decreases effects of warfarin and antacids	Documented hypersensitivity; fecal impaction, intestinal obstruction, or undiagnosed abdominal pain
Magic Bullet™ Suppository (polyethylene glycol-based bisacodyl)	PGB stimulant	Direct stimulation of colonic mucosa to produce peristalsis. Stimulates rectocolic reflex		
Digital stimulation	Technique	Stimulates rectocolic reflex		Autonomic dysreflexia

Brain Injury Assessment

Glasgow Coma Scale

Eye Opening (E)	Verbal Response (V)	Motor Response (M)
4 = Spontaneous eye opening	5 = Normal conversation	6 = Normal
3 = Opens to voice	4 = Disoriented conversation	5 = Localizes to pain
2 = Opens in response to pain	3 = Words, but not coherent	4 = Withdraws to pain
1 = No eye opening	2 = No words only sounds	3 = Flexion to painful stimuli (Decorticate posture)
	1 = No sounds	2 = Extension to painful stimuli (Decerebrate posture)
		1 = No movement
Total Score = E + V + M		

Adapted from Teasdale G, Jennett B. Assessment and prognosis of coma after head injury. *Acta Neurochirgica* 1976;34:4555.

Severity of Traumatic Brain Injury Based on GCS

Classification	GCS Score	Description
Mild	13–15	At lowest point after resuscitation and no brain injury abnormalities on neurologic examination. **Uncomplicated or low risk:** Normal CT scan of the brain. **Complicated or high risk:** CT scan of the brain reveals trauma.
Moderate	9–12	Grade at lowest point after resuscitation.
Severe	3–8	Grade at lowest point after resuscitation.

Concussion Grading

Grade	Criteria
I	Transient confusion
	No loss of consciousness
	Concussion symptoms or mental status abnormalities resolve in < 15 min.
II	Transient confusion
	No loss of consciousness
	Concussion symptoms or mental status abnormalities last >15 min.
III	Any loss of consciousness
	Seconds or minutes

When to Return to Play—Colorado Medical Society Guidelines

Grade of Concussion:	Return to play only after being asymptomatic with normal neurologic assessment at rest with exercise:
Grade 1 concussion	15 min or less
Multiple Grade 1 concussions	1 wk
Grade 2 concussion	1 wk
Multiple Grade 2 concussions	2 wk
Grade 3—brief loss of consciousness (seconds)	1 wk
Grade 3—prolonged loss of consciousness (minutes)	2 wk
Multiple Grade 3 concussions	1 month or longer, based on decision of evaluating physician

Source: Report of the Quality Standards Subcommittee, 1997.

Appendix 6

Dose Equivalents of Opioid Analgesic Drugs

Drug	Dose	
	Oral	*Parenteral*
Recommended for Routine Use		
Step 2 Opioids		
Codeine	100 mg every 4 h	50 mg every 4 h
Dihydrocodeine	50–75 mg every 4 h	N/A
Hydrocodone	15 mg every 4 h	N/A
Oxycodone	7.5–10 mg every 4 h	N/A
Step 3 Opioids		
Morphine	15 mg every 4 h	5 mg every 4 h
Oxycodone	7.5–10 mg every 4 h	N/A
Hydromorphone	4 mg every 4 h	0.75–1.5 mg every 4 h
Fentanyl	N/A	50 µg/hr every 72 h
Not Recommended for Routine Use		
Propoxyphene		N/A
Meperidine		50 mg every 2 h
Methadone		5 mg every 6 h
Levorphanol		1 mg every 6–8 h
Oral opiates begin relief at 30 min and last approximately 4 h		
IV opioids begin relief at 5 min and last 1–2 h		

Adapted with permission from Cuccurullo SJ. *Physical Medicine and Rehabilitation Board Review.* New York: Demos Medical Publishing, 2010.

Appendix 7 — *Activity Status Index*

Activity	Weight (Approximate METS)
Can you …	
1. take care of yourself, that is, eating, dressing, bathing, or using the toilet?	2.75
2. walk indoors, such as around your house?	1.75
3. walk a block or 2 on level ground?	2.75
4. climb a flight of stairs or walk up a hill?	5.50
5. run a short distance?	8.00
6. do light work around the house like dusting or washing dishes?	2.70
7. do moderate work around the house like vacuuming, sweeping floors, or carrying in groceries?	3.50
8. do heavy work around the house like scrubbing floors, or lifting or moving heavy furniture?	8.00
9. do yard work like raking leaves, weeding, or pushing a power mower?	4.50
10. have sexual relations?	5.25
11. participate in moderate recreational activities like golf, bowling, dancing, doubles tennis, or throwing a baseball or football?	6.00
12. participate in strenuous sports like swimming, singles tennis, football, basketball, or skiing?	7.50

Adapted from Hlatky MA, Boineau RE, Higginbotham MB, et al. A brief self-administered questionnaire to determine functional capacity (Duke Activity Status Index). *Am J Cardiol* 1989;64(10):651–654, with permission from Elsevier Ltd.

Entrapment Neuropathies of the Upper Extremities

Syndrome	Entrapment Location	Clinical Features	EMG Findings
Carpal tunnel syndrome (Median neuropathy at the wrist)	Wrist–Carpal tunnel	Numbness or paresthesias Digits 1–3 Wrist pain Phalen's sign (+) Tinel's sign (+) at wrist	• Sensory latency of >3.7 msec • ≥ 0.4 msec difference between median nerve and radial or ulnar nerve • Motor latency of more than 4.0 msec • Incremental change of 0.4 msec in the palmar serial sensory study
Ulnar neuropathy at the elbow	Cubital tunnel elbow	Paresthesias involving 4th and 5th fingers Elbow pain radiating toward the hand Prolonged elbow flexion worsens symptoms Tinel's sign (+) at elbow Wartenberg's sign (5th digit abduction) Froment's sigh (+)	• Delay of at least 10 msec affected arm relative to the unaffected arm. • Abnormal CV across elbow

Ulnar neuropathy at the wrist	Guyon's canal wrist	Paresthesias involving 4th and 5th fingers No loss of dorsal hand sensation (dorsal cutaneous branch leaves main trunk 5–8 cm proximal to Guyon's canal)	• Delay of at least 10 msec affected arm relative to the unaffected arm. • Normal CV across elbow forearm
Posterior interosseous nerve (Radial tunnel syndrome)	Entrapment at the supinator muscle, arcade of Frohse, radiohumeral band, or the tendon of the extensor carpi radialis brevis	tenderness over the nerve in extensor muscle group ~3 cm distal to the elbow Pain on resisted supination and extension of the middle finger Finger drop in severe cases	• Electromyographical abnormalities in the muscles distal to the entrapment • Findings on the supinator important to determine site of entrapment.
Neurogenic thoracic outlet syndrome		Tingling in the hands with shoulder abduction or elevation Weakness of all the intrinsic muscles of the hand and sensory loss over the ulnar side of the hand and forearm	• Most commonly normal in patients with intermittent symptoms.

Bayramoglu M. Entrapment neuropathies of the upper extremity. *Neuroanatomy.* 2004;3:18–24.
Dawson D. Entrapment neuropathies of the upper extremities. *NEJM.* 1993;329(27):2013–2018.

FIM® Instrument

LEVELS		
	7 Complete Independence (timely, safely) 6 Modified Independence (device)	**NO HELPER**
	Modified Dependence 5 Supervision (subject = 100%) 4 Minimal Assistance (subject = 75%+) 3 Moderate Assistance (subject = 50%+) **Complete Dependence** 2 Maximal Assistance (subject = 25%+) 1 Total Assistance (subject = less than 25%)	**HELPER**

	ADMISSION	DISCHARGE	FOLLOW-UP
Self-Care			
A. Eating			
B. Grooming			
C. Bathing			
D. Dressing: Upper Body			
E. Dressing: Lower Body			
F. Toileting			
Sphincter Control			
G. Bladder Management			
H. Bowel Management			
Transfers			
I. Bed, Chair, Wheelchair			
J. Toilet			
K. Tub, Shower			
Locomotion	W Walk / C Wheelchair / B Both	W Walk / C Wheelchair / B Both	W Walk / C Wheelchair / B Both
L. Walk, Wheelchair			
M. Stairs			
Motor Subtotal Rating			
Communication	A Auditory / V Visual / B Both	A Auditory / V Visual / B Both	A Auditory / V Visual / B Both
N. Comprehension			
O. Expression	A Auditory / V Visual / B Both	A Auditory / V Visual / B Both	A Auditory / V Visual / B Both
Social Cognition			
P. Social Interaction			
Q. Problem Solving			
R. Memory			
Cognitive Subtotal Rating			
TOTAL FIM® RATING			

NOTE: Leave no blanks. Enter 1 if patient is not testable due to risk.

Stance Phase Deviations

1. Foot Slap

   ■ When: heel strike to foot flat (initial contact to loading response)

   ■ What: rapid plantarflexion at heel strike with audible contact of forefoot and floor; can be unilateral or bilateral; may progress to foot drop if concentric control is lost due to fatigue

   ■ Anatomic causes

       □ Poor eccentric dorsiflexor control

   ■ Orthosis prescription

       □ AFO with dorsiflexion assist (posterior leaf or joints) or plantar flexion stop

       □ Myo-Orthosis if peripheral nerve is intact (Bioness L300® or WalkAide®)

2. Toes First

   ■ When: heel strike to foot flat (initial contact to loading response)

   ■ What: plantarflexed foot at heel strike causing toes to make first floor contact; may create ankle instability; if persists may create a leg length discrepancy; may also be associated with knee hyperextension.

   ■ Anatomic causes

       □ Weak dorsiflexors

       □ Plantarflexion contracture (pes equinus)

       □ Plantarflexor tone/extensor pattern

       □ Heel pain

       □ Hip and knee flexion contracture

       □ Severe leg length discrepancy

   ■ Orthosis prescription options

       □ AFO with dorsiflexion assist (posterior leaf or joints) or plantar-flexion stop

       □ Myo-Orthosis if peripheral nerve is intact (Bioness L300® or WalkAide®)

       □ Heel lift to accommodate for plantarflexion contracture

3. Ankle Instability

- When: all of stance phase possible

- What: excessive medial or lateral foot contact; inverted or everted foot; foot may contact the ground in a position and remain or contact neutral and move into the unstable position; inverted and PF foot is common with extensor tone patterns

- Anatomic causes

  □ Weak evertors or invertors

  □ Spastic evertors or invertors

  □ Contracture of ankle, subtalar, or forefoot

  □ Severe knee varus or valgus

- Orthosis prescription options

  □ Thermoplastic AFO with solid ankle or joints

  □ Metal AFO with T-strap

4. Excessive Knee Flexion at Heel Strike

- When: heel strike to foot flat (initial contact to loading response)

- What: excessive knee flexion/buckling at heel strike; lack of plantarflexion at ankle forces knee motion to accommodate and get foot flat; may lead to falls; worse on decline; patient will accommodate with shortened step length; less apparent with bilateral arm support (ie, walker or crutches)

- Anatomic causes

  □ Weak quadriceps

  □ Knee flexion contracture

  □ Hamstring spasticity/flexor pattern

  □ Knee pain

  □ Ankle dorsiflexion contracture

- Orthosis prescription options

  □ KAFO with locking mechanism

  □ KAFO with ankle joint that allows plantarflexion or is positioned in slight plantarflexion

  □ Soft heel or SACH heel shoe

5. Hip (Leg) External Rotation at Heel Strike

- When: heel strike to foot flat (initial contact to loading response)

- What: leg externally rotates from the hip joint at heel strike; lack of plantarflexion and knee flexion forces hip to accommodate; may be mild; patient will accommodate with shortened step length.

- Anatomic causes
  - ☐ Weak hip internal rotators and extensors
  - ☐ Knee extension contracture and dorsiflexion contracture
- Orthosis prescription options
  - ☐ Allow ankle to plantarflex (AFO or KAFO)

6. Knee Hyperextension

- When: midstance to heel off (midstance to preswing)

- What: knee extends past neutral with force and lack of control as the ground reaction force moves from posterior to anterior of the knee joint center of rotation; may be a progressive deformity and painful.

- Anatomic causes
  - ☐ Knee joint hypermobility
  - ☐ Knee extensor tone
  - ☐ Weak quadriceps; may be an active stabilizing effort
  - ☐ Plantarflexion weakness or contracture
  - ☐ Severe contralateral leg length discrepancy
- Orthosis prescription options
  - ☐ Knee orthosis if no ankle involvement
  - ☐ KAFO
  - ☐ AFO with set in slight dorsiflexion
  - ☐ Heel lift to accommodate for plantarflexion contracture or leg length discrepancy

7. Anterior Trunk Bending

- When: midstance to toe off (midstance to preswing)

- What: patient leans forward as weight is transferred to the leg; flexion at the hip and spine; may be associated with reliance on bilateral arm assistive device; short contralateral step length

- Anatomic causes
  - ☐ Hip flexion contracture
  - ☐ Weak quadriceps creating unstable knee; may use arm/hand to stabilize knee
  - ☐ Knee flexion contracture creating unstable knee
  - ☐ Low back pain
- Orthosis prescription options
  - ☐ Stabilize knee with knee orthosis, KAFO or AFO set in slight PF or with floor reaction design

8. Posterior Trunk Bending

- When: midstance to toe off (midstance to preswing)

- What: patient leans backward as weight is transferred to the leg; extension at hip and spine; may be bilateral and seen during static standing and also with use of bilateral arm assistive device

- Anatomic causes

  □ Weak hip extensors

- Why orthotic

  □ Existing HKAFO users add a hip extension stop

9. Lateral Trunk Leaning

- When: midstance (midstance)

- What: shift of trunk laterally; hip abduction or adduction, lateral trunk flexion or lateral shift of shoulders; may be very mild and well practiced; may be associated with posterior trunk leaning

  □ Trendelenburg (lean towards swing leg; uncompensated)

  □ Gluteus medius lurch (lean towards stance leg; compensated)

- Anatomic causes

  □ Weak hip abductors

  □ Painful hip joint

  □ Unstable hip joint

  □ Abduction contracture

  □ Severe leg length discrepancy

- Orthosis prescription options

  □ For existing KAFO users, consider a hip joint

  □ For existing KAFO or HKAFO users, check medial clearance

  □ Heel lift to accommodate leg length discrepancy

  □ Cane may reduce or eliminate

10. Wide Base Gait

- When: stance phase

- What: hip abduction; unilateral or bilateral

- Anatomic causes

  □ Abduction contracture; unilateral or bilateral

  □ Poor balance

  □ Severe leg length discrepancy

- Orthosis prescription options
    - ☐ For existing HKAFO users, check hip joint alignment
    - ☐ For existing KAFO or HKAFO users, check medial clearance
    - ☐ Heel lift to accommodate leg length discrepancy

11. Excessive Knee Flexion at Heel Off

- When: midstance to toe off (midstance to preswing)

- What: inadequate transition from midstance as the ground reaction force moves from posterior to anterior of the ankle axis; drop off at the end of stance; excessive dorsiflexion and knee flexion at end of stance; loss of the anterior lever arm

- Anatomic causes
    - ☐ Weak plantarflexors
    - ☐ Achilles rupture
    - ☐ Dorsiflexion contracture
    - ☐ Knee flexion contracture
    - ☐ Forefoot pain

- Orthosis prescription options
    - ☐ AFO with DF stop, floor reaction style is an option
    - ☐ Shoe with stiff sole or an extended steel shank added to shoe

Swing Phase Deviations

12. Foot Drop

- When: swing phase

- What: excessive plantarflexion during swing phase; may be associated with other deviations such as toes' first initial contact, ankle instability, steppage, and other long swing leg problems

- Anatomic causes
    - ☐ Weak dorsiflexors
    - ☐ Plantarflexion contracture
    - ☐ Plantarflexor tone/extensor pattern

- Orthosis prescription options
    - ☐ AFO with dorsiflexion assist (posterior leaf or joints) or plantarflexion stop
    - ☐ Myo-Orthosis if intact peripheral nerve (Bioness L300® or WalkAide®)

13. Steppage

- When: mid and late swing

- What: excessive hip and knee flexion; compensation for foot drop; is the most subtle of the available compensations and will usually be learned if patient has strength to do it

- Anatomic causes

  □ Compensation for foot drop—see 12

- Orthosis prescription options

  □ See 12 d.

14. Circumduction

- When: swing phase

- What: leg swings outward in a semicircular arc motion during swing phase and returns to midline for stance phase

- Anatomic causes

  □ Foot drop

  □ Knee extension due to contracture/fusion

  □ May be a compensation for a locked knee orthosis (KO, KAFO, HKAFO)

  □ Compensation for a long leg during swing phase when steppage is not possible, that is, weak hip flexors

- Orthosis prescription options

  □ AFO for correction of foot drop

  □ Unlock knee of orthosis; stance control orthotic knee joints, posterior offset with floor reaction

  □ Lift to contralateral shoe

15. Hip Hiking

- When: swing phase

- What: leg is elevated to clear the ground by lateral trunk flexion; "hiking" the pelvis and limb with lateral trunk flexors.

- Anatomic causes

  □ Same as 14 c and are often combined

- Orthosis prescription options

  □ Same as 14 d.

16. Vaulting

- When: mid-swing

- What: stance limb plantarflexion creates a functional leg length discrepancy allowing the swing side limb to advance in knee extension and/or ankle plantarflexion; very rapid pace is possible.

- Anatomic causes

  □ Compensation for long leg during swing, particularly when knee flexion is not possible or not desired

  □ Foot drop

  □ Hip fusion

- Orthosis prescription options

  □ Same as 14 d and gait training.

Posterolateral Approach	Anterolateral Approach
Avoidance of excessive hip flexion, adduction past neutral, internal rotation	Avoidance of hip hyperextension, adduction past neutral, external rotation

1. Do not bend knees more than 90°.
  • Suggest the use of a raised toilet seat
  • Avoid low and soft chairs
  • Avoid excessive trunk bending (do not bend to pick objects from the floor)
	1. Do not attempt to move the affected leg by lifting the hip without assistance (hyperextension avoidance).

2. Do not cross the legs at any time.
  • Sleep with abduction pillow
  • Avoid side sleeping
	2. Do not cross the legs at any time.
	  • Sleep with abduction pillow
	  • Avoid side sleeping

3. Do not turn the affected leg in (internal rotation at the hip)	3. Avoid turning the affected leg out (external rotation)

Mechanical Ventilation and Tracheostomy

Mechanical ventilation is the process of using an external device to assist in ventilation. The most common ventilation used is positive pressure airway ventilation, which can be applied using nasal, oral, or tracheal airways. Negative pressure ventilation has also been used but is not as common today except when exsufflation assistance is necessary to aid in secretionclearance. Some of the complications that can result from mechanical ventilation include barotrauma, dysrhythmias, secretion accumulation, and pulmonary infections.

Positive pressure ventilations are again the most commonly used. They can be set by volume or pressure. This meaning that volume preset airway ventilators deliver a preset volume of air with each breath. This volume will be delivered regardless of lung compliance or resistance. This type of ventilator is commonly used in emergency needs and home care.

Ventilators that use pressure-preset control will deliver air into the lung until preset pressure limit has been reached. While this will prevent excessive intra-airway pressure and subsequently barotraumas, it also means that the tidal volume is variable. However, these types of ventilators can compensate for airway leakage such as that which occurs around a tracheostomy site and will ensure that an adequate volume of air is delivered even with airway leakage. Many volume preset ventilators can also be set for pressure limits and subsequently mimic the function of pressure preset ventilators.

Three basic modes exist in assisted ventilation: AMV (assisted or control mechanical ventilation), CMV (controlled mechanical ventilation), or IMV (intermittent mandatory ventilation).

AMV: This is mechanical ventilation where the patient triggers a ventilator-delivered breath. This is done by a sensory within the ventilator that can be set to a predetermined level usually 2 to 3 cm of effort which when reached will trigger the ventilator to deliver a preset tidal volume of air. There is normally a control that ensures a minimal respiratory per minute is delivered even if the patient does not initiate. The advantages are that a patient can obtain higher than minimal respiratory rate when needed to meet activity and physiologic demands and can ensure respiratory needs are also met during periods such as sleep. Patients do not fight the ventilator on this type of setting and also minimizes issues such as hyperventilation, hypocapnia, or respiratory alkalosis, barotrauma when the settings are done properly.

CMV: This mechanical ventilation delivers a predetermined tidal volume at a predetermined rate. The patient is unable to initiate breathing and if any ability to control respiratory function is present, this type of setting can lead to issues like "fighting the ventilator." This is where the patient is doing the opposite action as the ventilator, and it can result in barotrauma and other complications.

IMV: This type of mechanical ventilation can be set to ensure a specific rate and tidal volume of air is delivered every minute, and the patient is still able to initiate their own breathing spontaneously. Unlike CMV where patients will fight the ventilator if they initiate a breath, no such events occur with IMV. This type of ventilation is useful when weaning a patient as it allows for the slow decrease in minute ventilation as the patients' respiratory strength and function improves. This is not commonly used in patients with myocardial disease as this technique requires greater oxygen consumption compared to AMV. Patients with central neurologic impairments and impaired central neurologic function or depressed respiratory drive IMV, is not the method of choice. IMV has the ability to be placed in a mode called synchronized IMV or SIMV. This is where the ventilator synchronizes with a patients' initiation of breathing. This technique will prevent an issue called stacking of spontaneous breaths on mandatory breaths. IMV and SIMV are not commonly used in home ventilator units.

Basic Ventilator Settings

AMV (assist control ventilation)	Recommend for home ventilator units (2–3 cm is nl setting for trigger)	Requires patients to have the ability to initiate breathing.
CMV (controlled mechanical ventilation)	High cervical spine injury or patients with no ability to initiate breath also used when unconscious, apneic, or lack of ability to initiate or control breathing.	Does not allow for patient to initiate breathing.
IMV (intermittent mandatory ventilation)	Not traditionally used at home. Used in pts fighting vents, have some ability to initiate or control breathing, failed other setting secondary to issues of decreased cardiac output in PPV, easy to use during weaning.	Higher work and oxygen consumption compared to AMV, not used in patients with depressed cardiac output during PPV or those with impaired or reduced respiratory drive or central neurologic impairment.
TV (tidal volume)	10–15 ml/kg (ideal body weight)	In SCI injury, 15 ml/kg is recommended.[i]
RR (respiratory rate)	12 breath/min	Variable depending on desired PaCOs or pH. Increased rate results in a decrease in $PaCO_2$
FiO$_2$ oxygen concentration	100%	Goal is FiO$_2$ 40%–50% will still providing adequate oxygenation.

Basic Ventilator Settings (*Continued*)

PaO$_2$ (arterial oxygen)	Desire >60 mmHg not less	SaO$_2$ >90%
PEEP (positive end expiratory pressure)	Initial 5 cm H$_2$O. Increase in 2–5 cm units.	Used to prevent closure of small airways and help maintain PaO$_2$ >60 or SaO2 >90%.
Global goal	Use the minimum FiO$_2$ to maintain PaO$_2$ >60% and a TV and RR to maintain pH and PaCO$_2$.	

Criteria for Transition to Home Ventilation

Clinical	Physiologic	Caregiver
Stable	ABG PaO$_2$ >60 mmHg on FiO$_2$ <40%	Committed
No dyspnea or tachypnea issues	PEEP <10 cm H$_2$O	Must understand ventilator basic
No cardiac dysrythmias	Not on IMV	Ensure vent and IPPV are functional at night.
Minimal secretions and ability to clear secretions consistently with or without assistive device	Physiologically stable Stable acid–base balance Stable metabolic status	
No significant aspiration	No acute infection	
Intact gag and cough reflex	Lung resistance and compliance stable	

WEANING TECHNIQUES

The basic principle of weaning off a ventilator is progressive withdraw of support while ensuring medical stability with monitor of pulse oximetry, arterial blood gases, and vital capacity. Consultation with pulmonary or respiratory team is reasonable and appropriate to assist or manage the weaning process. Managing the patient's anxiety is critical during the weaning process. If anxiety develops, the weaning process should be modified or stopped (see Table below). Many SCI patients do not have the capability to perform assisted breathing during symptomatic episodes or to help ensure pulse oximetry remains above 90%. There are certain times when the weaning should be terminated. Please refer to the table below for details. SCI can benefit from a gradual reduction in the utilization of IMV, SIMV, or AMV through elimination of the guaranteed rate control and support. This allows the patient to slowly take over the breathing process.

Criteria to Terminate Mechanical Ventilation Weaning Trials

Cardiovascular	
Blood pressure changes of	Sys Change ±20 mmHg or Dias bp decrease of 10 mmHg or more
Heart rate	HR change of 20 beats or more per minute or 20% above baseline or HR > 120 BPM.
Rhythm	Any rhythm change or cardiac arrhythmia
Respiratory	
RR	>30 or a change of 10/min from baseline
Clinically	The patient is noted to be extremely fatigued, when neurologic changes occur, working too hard for each breath, or using muscles which are not normally used.

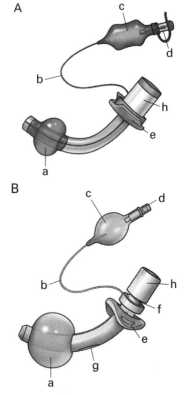

FIGURE 1 ■ Single lumen (A) and double lumen with inner cannula (B) plastic tracheostomy tubes. Tracheostomy parts: (a) cuff (b) inflation line (c) pilot balloon (d) luer valve (the syringe is attached here to inflate or deflate the cuff) (e) neck flange (f) disposable inner cannula (g) fenestration (h) connector.

TRACHEOSTOMY TUBES (FIGURE 1)

Metal Versus Plastic: Metal (usually stainless steel) tracheostomy tubes are reusable and cause less tissue reaction compared to plastic tracheostomy tubes. Plastic tracheostomy tubes are disposable and have a cuff option while metal tracheostomy tubes do not.

Cuff-Inflated Versus Cuff-Deflated: Cuff allows for a seal between the upper aerodigestive tract and the trachea, and prevents superior loss of air during ventilation. An inflated cuff does not allow for vocalization using speaking valves. Swallowing function can be affected in some cases with cuffed tracheostomy tubes.

Fenestrated Versus Nonfenestrated: Fenestrated tracheal tubes have an inner and outer cannula. The outer cannula has an opening cut to the side that allows for increased airflow to the upper airway so a patient can speak, breathe, and cough. It is important to ensure that the fenestrations do not touch the tracheal wall as tissue will grow into the fenestrations. Fenestration is used for patients who have the ability to spontaneously breathe for at least 2 hours off a vent and can swallow without aspiration. Stereotypically, SCI high cervical spinal cord patients will use nonfenestrated tracheal tubes to protect the airway.

Speaking Valves (Figures 2 and 3): These are 1-way valves made of plastic that can be fitted on to tracheostomy tubes and can be used in line with the ventilator. The valve opens on inspiration and close on expiration forcing the air across the vocal cords (Passy-Muir speaking valve or Olympic Trach-talking).

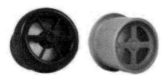

FIGURE 2 ■ Example of speaking valve (left) and in-line ventilator speaking valve (right).
Source: Photos courtesy of Passy-Muir, Inc., Irvine, CA.

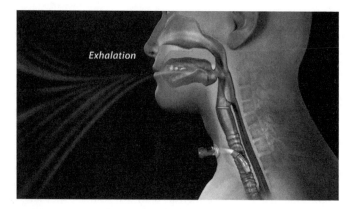

FIGURE 3 ■ Speaking valve in place. The valve allows inhalation through the tracheostomy tube, then redirects exhalation through the upper airway for vocalization.
Source: Photo courtesy of Passy-Muir, Inc., Irvine, CA.

ⁱ Consortium for Spinal Cord Medicine. *Respiratory Management Following Spinal Cord Injury: A Clinical Guideline for Health-Care Professionals.* Washington, DC: Paralyzed Veterans of America; 2005.

Appendix 13

Mini-Mental State Examination

Instructions: Ask the questions in the order listed. Score one point for each correct response within each question or activity.

Max.	Questions
5	"What is the year? Season? Date? Day of the week? Month?"
5	"Where are we now: State? County? Town/city? Hospital? Floor?"
3	The examiner names three unrelated objects clearly and slowly, then asks the patient to name all three of them. The patient's response is used for scoring. The examiner repeats them until patient learns all of them, if possible. Number of trials: _____
5	"I would like you to count backward from 100 by sevens." (93, 86, 79, 72, 65, . . .) Stop after five answers. Alternative: "Spell WORLD backwards." (D-L-R-O-W)
3	"Earlier I told you the names of three things. Can you tell me what those were?"
2	Show the patient two simple objects, such as a wristwatch and a pencil, and ask the patient to name them.
1	"Repeat the phrase: 'No ifs, ands, or buts.'"
3	"Take the paper in your right hand, fold it in half, and put it on the floor." (The examiner gives the patient a piece of blank paper.)
1	"Please read this and do what it says." (Written instruction is "Close your eyes.")
1	"Make up and write a sentence about anything." (This sentence must contain a noun and a verb.)
1	"Please copy this picture." (The examiner gives the patient a blank piece of paper and asks him/her to draw the symbol below. All 10 angles must be present and two must intersect.)

| 30 | TOTAL |

(Adapted from Rovner & Folstein, 1987)

Instructions for administration and scoring of the MMSE

Orientation (10 points):

■ Ask for the date. Then specifically ask for parts omitted (e.g., "Can you also tell me what season it is?"). One point for each correct answer.

■ Ask in turn, "Can you tell me the name of this hospital (town, county, etc.)?" One point for each correct answer.

Registration (3 points):

■ Say the names of three unrelated objects clearly and slowly, allowing approximately one second for each. After you have said all three, ask the patient to repeat them. The number of objects the patient names correctly upon the first repetition determines the score (0–3). If the patient does not repeat all three objects the first time, continue saying the names until the patient is able to repeat all three items, up to six trials. Record the number of trials it takes for the patient to learn the words. If the patient does not eventually learn all three, recall cannot be meaningfully tested.

■ After completing this task, tell the patient, "Try to remember the words, as I will ask for them in a little while."

Attention and Calculation (5 points):

■ Ask the patient to begin with 100 and count backward by sevens. Stop after five subtractions (93, 86, 79, 72, 65). Score the total number of correct answers.

■ If the patient cannot or will not perform the subtraction task, ask the patient to spell the word "world" backwards. The score is the number of letters in correct order (e.g., dlrow=5, dlorw=3).

Recall (3 points):

■ Ask the patient if he or she can recall the three words you previously asked him or her to remember. Score the total number of correct answers (0–3).

Language and Praxis (9 points):

■ Naming: Show the patient a wrist watch and ask the patient what it is. Repeat with a pencil. Score one point for each correct naming (0–2).

■ Repetition: Ask the patient to repeat the sentence after you ("No ifs, ands, or buts."). Allow only one trial. Score 0 or 1.

- 3-Stage Command: Give the patient a piece of blank paper and say, "Take this paper in your right hand, fold it in half, and put it on the floor." Score one point for each part of the command correctly executed.

- Reading: On a blank piece of paper print the sentence, "Close your eyes," in letters large enough for the patient to see clearly. Ask the patient to read the sentence and do what it says. Score one point only if the patient actually closes his or her eyes. This is not a test of memory, so you may prompt the patient to "do what it says" after the patient reads the sentence.

- Writing: Give the patient a blank piece of paper and ask him or her to write a sentence for you. Do not dictate a sentence; it should be written spontaneously. The sentence must contain a subject and a verb and make sense. Correct grammar and punctuation are not necessary.

- Copying: Show the patient the picture of two intersecting pentagons and ask the patient to copy the figure exactly as it is. All ten angles must be present and two must intersect to score one point. Ignore tremor and rotation.

Interpretation of the MMSE

Method	Score	Interpretation
Single Cutoff	<24	Abnormal
Range	<21	Increased odds of dementia
	>25	Decreased odds of dementia
Education	2 1	Abnormal for 8th grade education
	<23	Abnormal for high school education
	<24	Abnormal for college education
Severity	24–30	No cognitive impairment
	18–23	Mild cognitive impairment
	0–17	Severe cognitive impairment

(Folstein, Folstein & McHugh, 1975)

■ REFERENCES

Crum RM, Anthony JC, Bassett SS, Folstein MF. Population-based norms for the mini-mental state examination by age and educational level. *JAMA.* 1993;269(18):2386–2391.

Folstein MF, Folstein SE, McHugh PR. "Mini-mental state": a practical method for grading the cognitive state of patients for the clinician. *J Psychiatr Res.* 1975;12:189–198.

Rovner BW, Folstein MF. Mini-mental state exam in clinical practice. *Hosp Pract.* 1987;22(1A):99, 103, 106, 110.

Tombaugh TN, McIntyre NJ. The mini-mental state examination: a comprehensive review. *J Am Geriatr Soc.* 1992;40(9):922–935.

Appendix 14 — NIH Stroke Scale Score Sheet and Stimuli

Administer stroke scale items in the order listed. Record performance in each category after each subscale exam. Do not go back and change scores. Follow directions provided for each exam technique. Scores should reflect what the patient does, not what the clinician thinks the patient can do. The clinician should record answers while administering the exam and work quickly. Except where indicated, the patient should not be coached (i.e., repeated requests to patient to make a special effort).

Instructions	Scale Definition	Score
1a. Level of Consciousness	0 = **Alert**; keenly responsive. 1 = **Not alert**; but arousable by minor stimulation to obey, answer, or respond. 2 = **Not alert**; requires repeated stimulation to attend, obtunded and requires strong or painful stimulation. 3 = Responds only with reflex motor or autonomic effects or totally unresponsive, flaccid, and areflexic.	____
1b. LOC Questions: The patient is asked the month and his/her age.	0 = **Answers** both questions correctly. 1 = **Answers** one question correctly. 2 = **Answers** neither question correctly.	____
1c. LOC Commands: The patient is asked to open and close the eyes and then to grip and release the non-paretic hand.	0 = **Performs** both tasks correctly. 1 = **Performs** one task correctly. 2 = **Performs** neither task correctly.	____
2. Best Gaze: Only horizontal eye movements will be tested. Voluntary or reflexive (oculocephalic) eye movements will be scored.	0 = **Normal.** 1 = **Partial gaze palsy;** gaze is abnormal in one or both eyes, but forced deviation or total gaze paresis is not present. 2 = **Forced deviation,** or total gaze paresis not overcome by the oculocephalic maneuver.	____
3. Visual: Visual fields (upper and lower quadrants) are tested by confrontation, using finger counting or visual threat, as appropriate.	0 = **No visual loss.** 1 = **Partial hemianopia.** 2 = **Complete hemianopia.** 3 = **Bilateral hemianopia** (blind including cortical blindness).	____

Instructions	Scale Definition	Score
4. Facial Palsy: Ask – or use pantomime to encourage – the patient to show teeth or raise eyebrows and close eyes.	0 = **Normal** symmetrical movements. 1 = **Minor paralysis** (flattened nasolabial fold, asymmetry on smiling). 2 = **Partial paralysis** (total or near-total paralysis of lower face). 3 = **Complete paralysis** of one or both sides (absence of facial movement in the upper and lower face).	____
5. Motor Arm: The limb is placed in the appropriate position: extend the arms (palms down) 90 degrees (if sitting) or 45 degrees (if supine). Drift is scored if the arm falls before 10 seconds.	0 = **No drift;** limb holds for full 10 seconds. 1 = **Drift;** limb holds but drifts down before full 10 seconds; does not hit bed or other support. 2 = **Some effort against gravity;** limb cannot get to or maintain but has some effort against gravity. 3 = **No effort against gravity;** limb falls. 4 = **No movement.** UN = **Amputation** or joint fusion, explain: _____ **5a. Left Arm** **5b. Right Arm**	____
6. Motor Leg: The limb is placed in the appropriate position: hold the leg at 30 degrees (always tested supine). Drift is scored if the leg falls before 5 seconds.	0 = **No drift;** leg holds position for full 5 seconds. 1 = **Drift;** leg falls by the end of the 5-second period but does not hit bed. 2 = **Some effort against gravity;** leg falls to bed by 5 seconds, but has some effort against gravity. 3 = **No effort against gravity;** leg falls to bed immediately. 4 = **No movement.** UN = **Amputation** or joint fusion, explain: _____ **6a. Left Leg** **6b. Right Leg**	____

(Continued)

Instructions	Scale Definition	Score
7. Limb Ataxia: The finger-nose-finger and heel-shin tests are performed on both sides, and ataxia is scored only if present out of proportion to weakness.	0 = **Absent.** 1 = **Present in one limb.** 2 = **Present in two limbs.** UN = **Amputation** or joint fusion, explain: _____	———
8. Sensory: Sensation or grimace to pinprick when tested, or withdrawal from noxious stimulus in the obtunded or aphasic patient.	0 = **Normal;** no sensory loss. 1 = **Mild-to-moderate sensory loss;** pinprick is less sharp or is dull on the affected side; loss of superficial pain with pinprick, but patient is aware of being touched. 2 = **Severe to total sensory loss;** patient is not aware of being touched.	———
9. Best Language: A the patient is asked to describe what is happening in the attached picture, to name the items on the attached naming sheet and to read from the attached list of sentences.	0 = **No aphasia;** normal. 1 = **Mild-to-moderate aphasia.** 2 = **Severe aphasia.** 3 = **Mute, global aphasia.**	———
10. Dysarthria: An adequate sample of speech must be obtained by asking patient to read or repeat words from the attached list.	0 = **Normal.** 1 = **Mild-to-moderate dysarthria.** 2 = **Severe dysarthria.** UN = **Intubated** or other physical barrier, explain: _____	———
11. Extinction and Inattention (formerly Neglect)	0 = **No abnormality.** 1 = **Visual, tactile, auditory, spatial, or personal inattention** or extinction to bilateral simultaneous stimulation in one of the sensory modalities. 2 = **Profound hemi-inattention or extinction to more than one modality;** does not recognize own hand or orients to only one side of space.	———

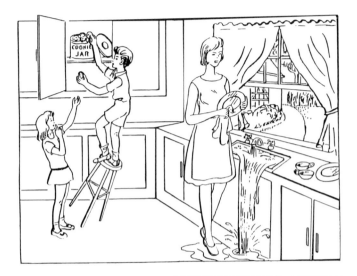

You know how.

Down to earth.

I got home from work.

Near the table in the dining room.

They heard him speak on the radio last night.

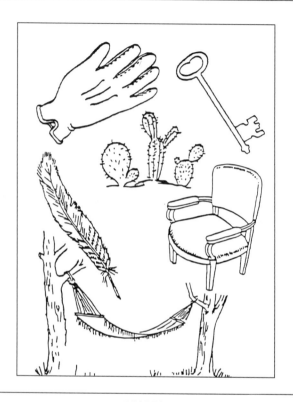

MAMA

TIP – TOP

FIFTY – FIFTY

THANKS

HUCKLEBERRY

BASEBALL PLAYER

Schematic diagram of the brachial plexus.

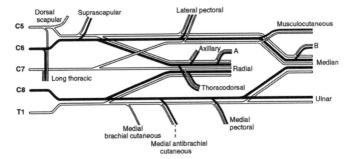

A, branch to extensor carpiradialislongus and brachioradialis; B, branch to flexor carpiradialis and pronatorteres. With permission from Fernandez HH, Eisenschenk S, Okun MS. Ultimate Review for the Neurology Boards, Second Edition. Demos Medical Publishing, New York, 2010, 458.

Lumbosacral Plexus: Schematic diagram of major nerves to the lower extremities.

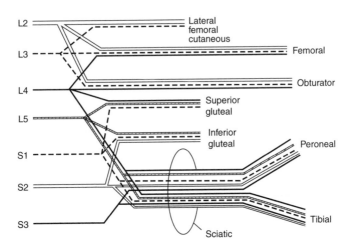

Sural nerve is a branch of both peroneal & tibal nerves

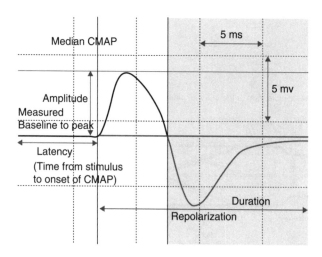

Example of compound muscle action potential (CMAP)

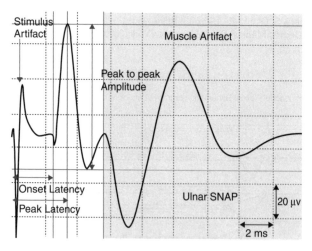

Example of Sensory nerve action potential (SNAP)

Basic Nerve Conduction Placements
Median motor to abductor pollicisbrevis (APB)

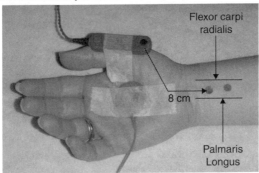

Active electrode: Abductor pollicisbrevis. Reference electrode to first metacarpophalangeal joint.

*Ground electrode should be in the dorsum of the hand, placed in the palm for visualization

Median Motor Stimulation Points

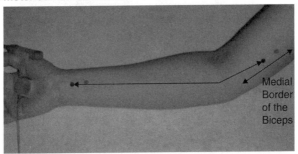

Median Sensory to First Digit

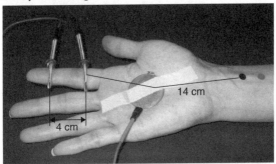

*Ground electrode should be in the dorsum of the hand, placed in the palm for visualization

Ulnarmotor to Abductor Digitiminimi (ADM)

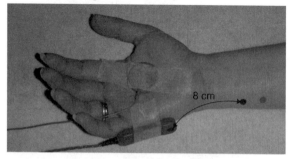

*Ground electrode should be in the dorsum of the hand, placed in the palm for visualization
Active electrode: Abductor digitiminimi (ADM)
Reference Electrode fifth metacarpophalangeal joint

Ulnar Stimulation Points

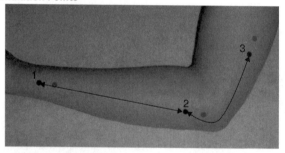

1 – 8 cm from recording site
2 – Below ulnar groove
3 – Above ulnar groove

Ulnar Sensory to Fifth Digit

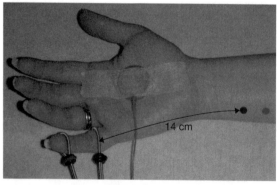

*Ground electrode should be in the dorsum of the hand, placed in the palm for visualization

Peroneal Motor to Extensor Digitorumbrevis (EDB)

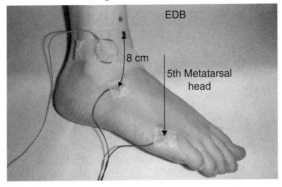

Active electrode: Extensor digitorumbrevis
Reference Electrode fifth metatarsophalangeal joint

Peroneal Stimulation Points

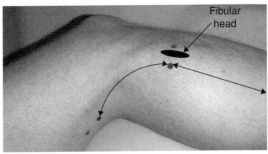

1 – (Not shown) 8 cm from recording site
2 – Straddling the fibular head
3 – Poplitealfossa

Tibial Motor to Abductor Hallucis

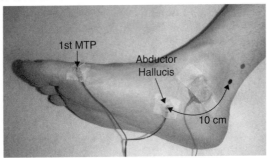

Active electrode: Abductor hallucis (medial foot)
Reference Electrode first metatarsophalangeal joint
*Second stimulation point in the poplitealfossa

Sural Sensory

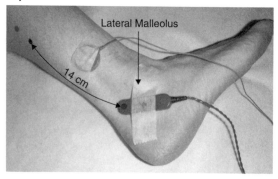

Active electrode: Posterior to lateral malleolus
Reference Electrode: 3–4 cm distal

H-Reflex

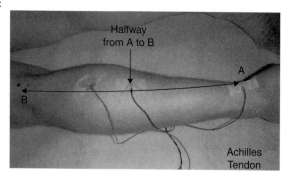

*The H-reflex is useful in S1 rediculopathy.
*Please note that the stimulation is done with the cathode proximal (stimulating up to the spinal cord and back).
*Stimulation is submaximal

■ NORMAL VALUES

EMG/Nerve Conduction Studies Adult Normal Values*

Study	Stimulation Site	Recording Site	Distance (cm)	Amplitude	Latency (msec)	Reference
				μV (peak-to-peak)	(<)	
Sensory						
Median	Mid-palm	Index finger	7	—	2.2	Felsenthal
Median	Wrist	Index finger	14	10	3.7	Melvin/Felsenthal
Median	Wrist	Middle finger	14	9	3.7	Melvin
Ulnar	Wrist	Little finger	14	10	3.7	Johnnson
	*Difference between median and ulnar should be <0.5 msec (<0.8 for workers)					Felsenthal
Ulnar DC	Forearm	Dorsum hand	8	8	2.6	Jabre
Radial	Forearm	EPL	14	13	3.3	MacKenzie/deLisa
Radial	Forearm	1st web space	10	10	2.7	Cleveland Clinic
Sural	Calf	Lateral malleolus	14	5	4.4	Izzo
Sup. Peroneal	Lateral calf	Ankle	10	6	3.2	DiBenedetto
Sup. Peroneal	Lateral calf	Lateral malleolus	12	8	3.6	Jabre
Mixed						
Median	Palm	Wrist	8	40	2.3	Med Coll Georgia
Ulnar	Palm	Wrist	8	11	2.2	Med Coll Georgia
	*Difference between median and ulnar should be <0.5 msec					Redmond/MCG
Tibial	Medial plantar		14	11	3.7	DeLisa
	Lateral plantar		14	9	3.7	Delisa
	*Absence of lateral plantar SAP after age 55 is not significant					Mayo Clinic

(*Continued*)

EMG/Nerve Conduction Studies Adult Normal Values* (Continued)

Study	Stimulation Site	Recording Site	Distance (cm)	Amplitude	Latency (msec)	Reference
Motor				mV (Base-to-peak)		
Median	Wrist	APB	8	5.0	4.3	Melvin
*median to ulnar difference should be <1.2 msec						Felsenthal
Ulnar	Wrist	ADM	8	2.5	4.2	Melvin/Checkles
*Difference to first dorsal interosseous should be <2 msec						Olney
Ulnar	SSIS	ADM	1	—	0.4	Campbell (1992)
Tibial	Medial malleolus	AH	10	3.5	5.4	Oh
Tibial	Lateral malleolus	ADQP	12	3.0	6.2	Oh
Peroneal	Ankle	EDB	8	2.6	6.2	Ma
Cranial Nerves				(mV)		
Facial	Preauric	Nasalis	—	2.5	4.1	Demeirsman/Halar
Facial	Preauric	Orb Occ	—	—	3.7	Kimura
Facial	Preauric	Orb Oris	—	—	4.2	Waylonis
CN XI	Post Trngl	Trapezius	9	3.0	3.1	Ma/Gibfried
CN XII	Submandibular	Tongue	—	1.0	3.0	Redmond/Dibene
Nerve Conduction Velocity						
Upper Extremity	48–70 m/sec					
Lower Extremity	39–55 m/sec					
*Drop in NCV of 10 or more m/sec across 2 points is significant						
Late Responses						Payan/Eisen
			R1	R2	R2' (contral)	
Blink	Preauric	Orb Occuli	12.1 msec	37.1 msec	38.1	

				Height		
			<63"	63–69"	69–74"	
Median F-wave	Wrist	APB	29	31	32	
Ulnar F-wave	Wrist	ADM	30	32	33	
Peroneal F-wave	Ankle	EDB	50	56	58	
Tibial F-wave	Ankle	AH	50	56	58	
Tibial H-reflex	Popliteal fossa	Soleus	30	32	34	

Unusual Conduction Studies

Sensory

				(µV)	(<)	
Median	Wrist	Thumb	10	7	2.9	Johnson
*Difference between radial and median should be <0.5 msec						Pease/Johnson
Radial	Wrist	Thumb	10	18	2.8	Johnson

Motor

femoral	Below inguinal ligament	Vastus medialis	~30	–	7.5	Johnson
	Above inguinal ligament	Vastus Medialis	~5	–	8.4	Johnson

Late Responses

				Height	
			<63"	63–69"	69–74"
Tibial F-wave	Popliteal Fossa	Soleus	32	34	36

*The above tables are the normal values used at the Johns Hopkins Department of Physical Medicine and Rehabilitation. The original compilation was prepared by N. Spellman, T. Dillingham, et al at Walter Reed Army medical center.

■ MUSCLES AND INNERVATION

Upper Limb

Muscle	Nerve	Root Level
Shoulder/upper trunk		
Deltoid	Axillary	**C5**, C6
Teres Minor	Axillary	**C5**, C6
Teres Major	Subscapular	**C5, C6**
Infraspinatus	Suprascapular	**C5, C6**
Supraspinatus	Suprascapular	**C5**, C6
Latissimus dorsi	Thoracodorsal	C6, **C7**, C8
Pectoralis minor	Lateral and medial pectoral	C6, C7, C8
Pectoralis major	Lateral and medial pectoral	C5, **C6, C7, C8**, T1
Levator scapulae	Dorsal scapular	**C5** (some C3, C4)
Rhomboids	Dorsal Scapular	**C5**
Serratus Anterior	Long thoracic	C5, C6, C7
Arm		
Biceps Brachii	Musculocutaneous	**C5, C6**
Brachialis	Musculocutaneous	**C5**, C6
Coracobrachialis	Musculocutaneous	**C6**, C7
Triceps Brachii	Radial	**C7, C8**, T1
Forearm		
Pronator Teres	Median	C6, **C7**
Palmaris Longus	Median	C7, **C8**, T1
Flexor Pollicis Longus	Median	C7, **C8**, T1
Flexor Carpi Radialis	Median	C6, **C7**, C8
Flexor Digitorum Superficialis	Median	C7, **C8**, T1
Pronator Quadratus	Median (Anterior Interosseus)	C7, **C8**, T1
Flexor Digitorum Profundus		
Digits 2&3	Median (Anterior Interosseus)	C7, **C8**
Digits 4&5	Ulnar	**C8**, T1
Flexor Carpi Ulnaris	Ulnar	**C8**, T1
Supinator	Radial (Posterior Interosseus)	C5, C6
Extensor Pollicis Longus	Radial (Posterior Interosseus)	**C7**, C8
Extensor Pollicis Brevis	Radial (Posterior Interosseus)	**C7**, C8
Extensor Indicis Proprius	Radial (Posterior Interosseus)	C7, **C8**

Extensor Digitorum Communis	Radial (Posterior Interosseus)	**C7**, C8
Extensor Carpi Ulnaris	Radial (Posterior Interosseus)	C6, **C7**, C8
Abductor Pollicis Longus	Radial (Posterior Interosseus)	**C7**, C8
Extensor Carpi Radialis	Radial	**C6**, C7
Brachioradialis	Radial	C5, **C6**
Anconeus	Radial	**C7**, C8

Hand

Abductor Pollicis Brevis	Median	**C8, T1**
Abductor Digiti Minimi	Ulnar	**C8, T1**
Adductor Pollicis	Ulnar	**C8, T1**
Interossei	Ulnar	C8, **T1**
Lumbricals 1st & 2nd 3rd & 4th	 Median Ulnar	 **C8**, T1 C8, **T1**
Opponens Pollicis	Median	**C8**, T1

Lower Limb

Pelvis and Hip

Gluteus maximus	Inferior gluteal	L5, **S1, S2**
Gluteus medius	Superior gluteal	L4, **L5**, S1
Gluteus minimus	Superior gluteal	L4, **L5**, S1
Tensor facsia Lata	Superior gluteal	L4, **L5**, S1
Piriformis	Nerve to Piriformis	S1, S2

Thigh

Adductor Brevis	Obturator	L2, L3, L4
Adductor Magnus	Obturator	L2, L3, L4, L5
Adductor Longus	Obturator	L2, **L3**, L4
Gracilis	Obturator	**L2, L3**, L4
Biceps Femoris Short Head Long head	 Sciatic (Peroneal Division) Sciatic (Tibial Division)	 L5, **S1, S2** L5, **S1**
Semitendinosus	Sciatic (Tibial Division)	**L5**, S1, S2
Semimembranosus	Sciatic (Tibial Division)	**L5**, S1, S2
Pectineus	Femoral	**L2, L3**, L4
Iliopsoas	Femoral	**L2, L3**, L4
Rectus Femoris	Femoral	L2, L3, L4
Sartorius	Femoral	L2, L3, L4

(Continued)

Lower Limb (*Continued*)

Muscle	Nerve	Root Level
Vastus Lateralis	Femoral	L2, **L3, L4**
Vastus Medialis	Femoral	L2, **L3, L4**
Leg		
Tibialis Anterior	Peroneal	L4, L5
Extensor Digitorum Longus	Peroneal	L4,**L5**, S1
Extensor Hallucis Longus	Peroneal	L5, **S1**
Peroneus Tertius	Peroneal	L5, S1
Peroneus Longus	Peroneal	**L5, S1**, S2
Peroneus Brevis	Peroneal	**L5, S1**, S2
Gastrocnemius	Tibial	S1, S2
Soleus	Tibial	L5, **S1, S2**
Flexor Digitorum Longus	Tibial	L5, **S1, S2**
Flexor Hallucis Longus	Tibial	**L5, S1**, S2
Tibialis Posterior	Tibial	**L5**, S1
Foot		
Extensor Digitorum Brevis	Peroneal	L5, S1
Abductor Hallucis	Tibial (Medial Plantar)	S1, S2

Adapted from Perotto AO. *Anatomical Guide for the Electromyographer.* 3rd ed. Springfield, IL: Thomas Publishers; 1994. Preston DC, Shapiro BE. *Electromyography and Neuromuscular Disorders.* 2nd ed. Philadelphia, PA: Elsevier; 2005.

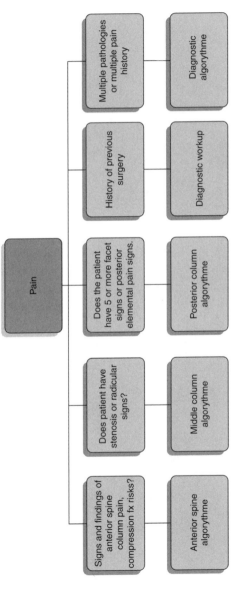

Initial pain algorithm.

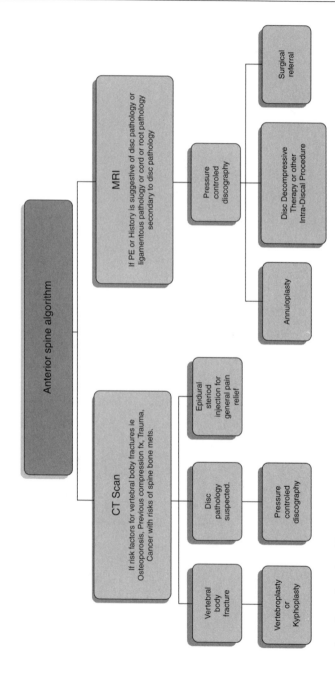

Anterior spine algorithm.

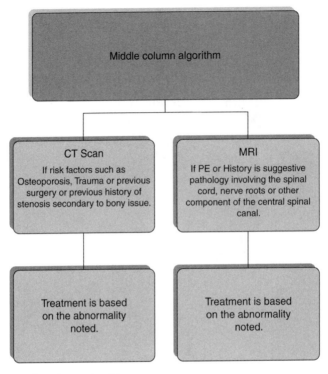

Middle column algorithm.

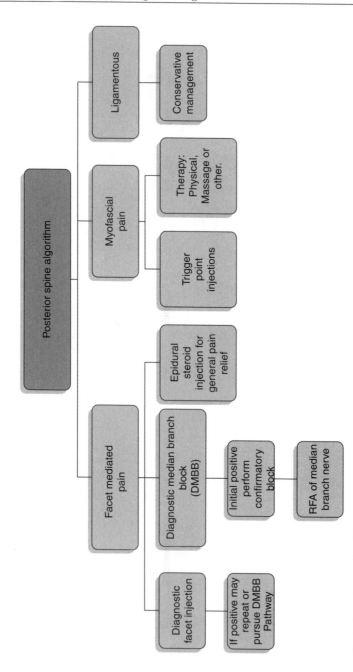

Posterior column algorithm.

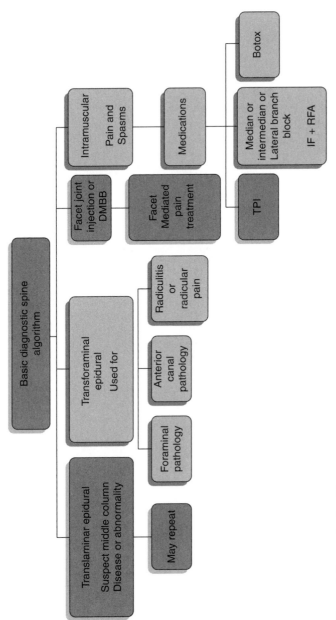

General diagnostic algorithm.

Level I:	**No Response** to pain, touch, sound, or sight.
Level II:	**Generalized Reflex Response** to pain.
Level III:	**Localized Response.**
Level IV:	**Confused—Agitated.** Alert, very active, aggressive or bizarre behaviors; performs motor activities but behavior is nonpurposeful, and extremely short attention span.
Level V:	**Confused—Nonagitated.** Gross attention to environment, highly distractible, requires continual redirection, difficulty learning new tasks, and agitated by too much stimulation. May engage in social conversation but with inappropriate verbalizations.
Level VI:	**Confused—Appropriate.** Inconsistent orientation to time and place, retention span/recent memory impaired, begins to recall past, consistently follows simple directions, and goal-directed behavior with assistance.
Level VII:	**Automatic—Appropriate.** Performs daily routine in highly familiar environment in a nonconfused but automatic robot-like manner. Skills notably deteriorate in unfamiliar environment. Lacks realistic planning for own future.
Level VIII:	**Purposeful—Appropriate.**

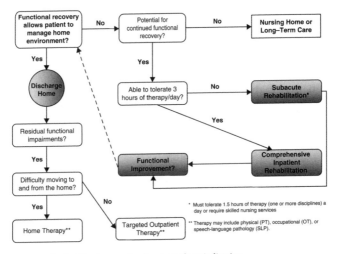

Determination of rehabilitation needs after acute hospitalization.

From González-Fernández M, Feldman D. Rehabilitation of the Stroke Patient. In Conn's Current Therapy 2010. Bope ET, Rakel RE, Kellerman RD, eds. Elsevier, with permission.

SBAR Communication Tool for Rehabilitation

S Describe **SITUATION**	My name is ...... and I work ...... (*your service*) I need to talk to you about: ❑ an urgent safety issue regarding ...... (*name of client*) ❑ a quality of care issue regarding ...... (*name of client*) I need about ...... (*minutes*) to talk to you, if not now, when can we talk? I need you to know about: ❑ changes to a patient status ❑ changes to treatment plan, procedures or protocols ❑ environmental/organizational issues related to patient care
B Provide **BACKGROUND**	Are you aware of ...... (*specific problem*) The patient is ...... (*age*) and has a diagnosis of ..... (*diagnosis*) as well as ..... (*diagnosis*) He/She was admitted on ...... (*date*) and is scheduled for discharge on ...... (*date*) His/Her treatment plans related to this issue to date include ..... (*treatment*) He/She is being monitored by ...... (*specialist*) and has appointments for ...... (*procedures*) This patient/family/staff is requesting that ...... (*requests*)
A Provide client **ASSESSMENT**	I think the key underlying problem/concern is ...... (*describe*) The key changes since the last assessment related to the specific concern are: **Person Level Changes** ❑ Vital Signs/GI/Cardio-Respiratory ❑ Neurological ❑ Musculoskeletal/Skin ❑ Pain ❑ Medications ❑ Psychosocial/Spiritual ❑ Sleep ❑ Cognitive/Mental Status/Behavioural ❑ Nutrition/Hydration **Activity/Participation/Functional Changes** ❑ ADL ❑ Transfers ❑ Home/Community Safety **Environmental Changes** ❑ Organizational/Unit Protocols/Processes ❑ Discharge Destination ❑ Social/Family Supports
R Make **RECOMMENDATION**	Based on this assessment, I request that: ❑ we discontinue/continue with ...... ❑ we prepare for discharge OR extend discharge date ❑ you approve recommended changes to treatment plan/goals including ...... ❑ you reassess the patient's ...... ❑ the following tests/assessments be completed by ...... ❑ the patient be transferred out to.../be moved to ...... ❑ you inform other team members/family/patients about change in plans ❑ I recommend that we modify team protocols in the following ways ...... To be clear, we have agreed to... Are you ok with this plan? ❑ I would like to hear back from you by ...... ❑ I will be in contact with you about this issue by ......

Adapted SBAR Tool.

Spasticity Medications

Oral Spasticity Medications

Drug	Half Life	Starting Dose	Maximum Dose	Common/Serious Side Effects	Mechanism of Action
Baclofen (Lioresal®)	3.5 h	5 mg TID	Max dose 80 mg (20 mg QID) (Higher doses up to 200 mg have been used but are not approved by the FDA)	Vertigo, urinary frequency, muscle weakness, drowsiness, confusion, headache, nausea, seizures, constipation, dyspnea, impaired vision, severe fatigue, urticaria, edema **Hepatotoxicity** **May lower seizure threshold hallucinations**	Analog of GABA decreases release of excitatory neurotransmitters from afferent terminals
Tizanidine (Zanaflex®)	2 h	1–2 mg daily	Max dose 36 mg/d	Sedation, orthostatic hypotension, dry mouth, dizziness, renal impairment, psychosis **Hepatotoxicity**	α2-adrenergic receptor agonist reduces spasticity by increasing presynaptic inhibition
Dantrolene (Dantrium®)	8.7 h	25 mg daily	Max dose 400 mg/d (divided TID or QID) Doses above 400 mg have been used but may increase risk of hepatotoxicity	Drowsiness, dizziness, weakness, malaise, fatigue, and diarrhea **Hepatotoxicity**	Reduces the release of calcium (sarcoplasmic reticulum)
Diazepam (Valium®)	27–37 h	2–2.5 mg daily	10 mg TID or QID	Sedation, ataxia, and fatigue	GABA postsynaptic facilitation
Clonazepam (Klonopin®)	30–40 h	0.5–1 mg at bedtime	20 mg	Weakness, hypotension, ataxia, dyscoordination, sedation, depression, and memory impairment **High risk for addiction**	GABA postsynaptic facilitation
Clonidine (Catapres®)	12–16 h	0.1 mg twice a day	Max dose 2.4 mg/d	**Hypotension**	Selective α2-receptor agonist may increase presynaptic inhibition

■ **REFERENCES**

Micromedex Heathcare series 1.0, Drugdex.

Movement Disorders Virtual University. *http://www.mdvu.org/library/disease/spasticity/spa_mtop.asp*. Accessed September 1, 2010.

Rossi R, Alexander M, Cuccurullo S. Pediatric rehabilitation. In: Cuccurullo S, ed. *Physical Medicine and Rehabilitation Board Review*. Demos, NY. Table 10–27.

Spasm Frequency Scale

How many spasms has the patient had in the last 24 hours in affected muscles or extremity?

Definitions of spasms:

■ Spasm is a jumping or twitching of the muscle or limb without control

■ A spasm can be a "shooting" of the body part into a position without control

■ A rapid series of "spasms" without significant pausing/resting is defined as one spasm.

Level	Definition	Level	Definition
0	No spasms	3	5–9 spasms/d
1	1 spasm or fewer/d	4	10 or more spasms/d
2	1–5 spasms/d		

Snow BJ, Tsui JKC, Bhart MH, Varelas M, Hashimoto SA, Calne DB. Treatment of spasticity with botulinum toxin: a double-blind study. *Ann Neurol.* 1990;28:512–515.

Modified Ashworth Scale[3]

Score	Description
0	No increase in muscle tone
1	Slight increase in muscle tone, manifested by a catch and release or by minimal resistance at the end of the range of motion when the affected part(s) is moved in flexion or extension.
1+	Slight increase in muscle tone, manifested by a catch, followed by minimal resistance throughout the reminder (<50%) of the range of motion.
2	More marked increase in muscle tone through most of the ROM (>50%), but affected part(s) easily moved.
3	Considerable increase in muscle tone passive, movement difficult.
4	Affected part(s) rigid in flexion or extension.

Bohannon RW, Smith MB. Interrater reliability of a modified Ashworth scale of muscle spasticity. *Phys Ther* 1987;67:206–207.

Snow BJ, Tsui JKC, Bhart MH, Varelas M, Hashimoto SA, Calne DB. Treatment of spasticity with botulinum toxin: a double-blind study. *Ann Neurol.* 1990;28:512–515.

Appendix 22 — *Swallowing Screening*

Rosemary Martino

■ THE TORONTO BEDSIDE SWALLOWING SCREENING (TOR-BSST(C)): AN EXAMPLE FOR SWALLOWING SCREENING AFTER STROKE

The Toronto Bedside Swallowing Screening Test (TOR-BSST©) was developed with a large stroke population across the continuum of care. It aims to predict the presence of dysphagia defined by aspiration and/ or any physiological abnormality. The TOR-BSST© was conceptualized and developed on the premise that earlier detection of dysphagia by screening shortens recovery and also improves overall patient health. The TOR-BSST© items were generated using the best available evidence derived from an extensive systematic review (1). A standardized didactic workshop is available to train screeners on administration and interpretation of the test. The TOR-BSST© was assessed for reliability and validity with trained screeners using a sample of over 300 stroke patients across acute and rehabilitation settings (2). The TOR-BSST© can be administered, scored, and placed on the medical chart in approximately 10 minutes. Because administration continues only until the first TOR-BSST© item is failed, patients with severe dysphagia typically fail an early item thereby reducing administration to less than 10 minutes.

The TOR-BSST© is intended for use by any health care professional trained by a speech-language pathologist on its administration and interpretation. This training is critical to maintain its proven accuracy in detecting the presence of dysphagia. The TOR-BSST© is designed so that it can be administered to patients across all settings, including acute, rehabilitative, and chronic facilities.

More information about the TOR-BSST© and its training can be obtained at http://swallowinglab.uhnres.utoronto.ca/torbsst.html.

■ REFERENCES

1. Martino R, Pron G, Diamant N. Screening for oropharyngeal dysphagia in stroke: insufficient evidence for guidelines. *Dysphagia*. 2000;15:19–30.
2. Martino R, Silver F, Teasell R. The Toronto Bedside Swallowing Screening Test (TOR-BSST©): development and validation of a dysphagia screening tool for patients with stroke. *Stroke*. 2009;40(2):555–561.

TOR-BSST©
The Toronto Bedside Swallowing
Screening Test©

(addressograph)

DATE: _____*(mm/dd/yyyy)*   TIME: _____ *(hh/mm)*

A) Before water intake:

(Mark either abnormal or normal for each task.)

1. Have patient say 'ah' and judge voice quality

Abnormal	Normal
☐	☐

2. Ask patient to stick their tongue out and then move it from side to side.

Abnormal	Normal
☐	☐

B) Water intake: Have the patient **sit upright** and give water. Ask patient to **say "ah"** after each intake. Mark as abnormal if you note any of the following signs: **coughing, change in voice quality** *or* **drooling.** If abnormal, stop water intake and advance to 'D'.

1) One Tsp Swallows	Cough during/after swallow	Voice change after swallow	Drooling during/after swallow	Normal
Swallow 1	☐	☐	☐	☐
Swallow 2	☐	☐	☐	☐
Swallow 3	☐	☐	☐	☐
Swallow 4	☐	☐	☐	☐
Swallow 5	☐	☐	☐	☐
Swallow 6	☐	☐	☐	☐
Swallow 7	☐	☐	☐	☐
Swallow 8	☐	☐	☐	☐
Swallow 9	☐	☐	☐	☐
Swallow 10	☐	☐	☐	☐
2) Cup drinking	☐	☐	☐	☐

C) After water intake:

(Administer at least a minute after you finish Section B.)

1. Have patient say 'ah' again and judge voice quality.

Abnormal	Normal
☐	☐

D) Results: ☐ **Passed**   ☐ **Failed → Initiate referral to SLP**
                  (no abnormal signs)   (1 or more abnormal signs)

TOR-BSST© Screener's Signature: _____

Some Guidelines and Tips for the TOR-BSST©

Before the start of screening, remember to: a) have a cup of water and a teaspoon; b) ensure patient's mouth is clean; and c) ensure patient is sitting upright at 90°.

A. Before water intake:

1. *"I want you to say "ah" for 5 seconds using your speaking voice."*
- o Model a clear "ah" for the patient.
- o Remind them not to sing "ah" or use a quiet voice.
- o You can ask them to stretch the last syllable of the word *Ottawa*.
- o Remember to take note of the patient's voice when speaking. If his/her voice sounds different when saying "ah" re-instruct the patient to use a normal voice using any of the suggestions above.
- O **You are looking for any breathiness, gurgles, hoarseness, or whisper quality to the voice. If you perceive any of these, even to a mild degree, mark as abnormal.**

2. *"Open your mouth. Now stick out your tongue as far as it will go. Now move it back and forth across your mouth."*
- o Stick your tongue straight out. If no deviation, model a consistent back and forth motion for the patient.
- o **You are looking for any deviation of the tongue towards one side on protrusion, or any difficulty in moving the tongue to one side. Mark as abnormal if you perceive any of these features.**
- o If the patient is unable to protrude his/her tongue at all, mark as abnormal.

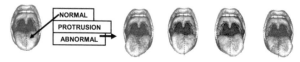

NORMAL PROTRUSION
ABNORMAL

B. Water Swallows:

Give the patient 10 X 1 tsp of water. Remind the patient to say "ah" after every teaspoon swallow. If normal, give cup to patient for drinking.
- o The patient should always be fed the teaspoon of water.
- o Ensure that full teaspoon amounts are given.
- o Lightly palpate the throat to monitor for movement of the larynx on the first few swallows.
- o **You are looking for any coughing, drooling or change in the patient's voice suggesting wetness, hoarseness, etc. If you perceive this, mark accordingly and stop the water swallows.**
- o **If you see what looks like a stifled or suppressed cough, mark this as a cough.**
- o **If there is no coughing, drooling, wet voice or hoarseness mark as normal.**

C. Voice after Water Swallows:
- o Wait one minute after the end of the water swallows.(You can use this time to clear away the cup etc. and mark the form)
- o Ask the patient to say "ah" as in the first part of the screen.

D. Final Scoring:
If you have marked *any* of the *items* as *abnormal*, score the patient as *Failed.*

Normal Wound Healing

Stage	Time	Factors
Inflammatory	0–4 d	Macrophages
Proliferative	3 d–4 wk	Fibroblasts
Reodelig	3 wk–1 y	

Factors in Wound Healing

Oxygen	PO2 >40 mmHg	
Anemia	Questionable	Controversial
Vitamin C	Co-factor for Collagen	
Vitamin E	Possible role in irradiated tissue	Large doses can inhibit healing
Zinc	Essential for epithelial and fibroblast proliferation	Deficiency impairs epithelial and fibroblast proliferation
Steroids	Reversed by vitamin A	Impairs healing

Additional Factors in Wound Healing

NSAIDs	Decrease collagen synthesis 45% at NL dose
Smoking	Impairs oxygen, blood flow, healing
Age	Older lose of tensil strength and slower closure rate
Nutrition	Protein <2 g associated with prolonged inflammatory phase
Environment	Temp 30°C
Impairments	Infection, chemotherapy, radiation(damages fibroblasts), DM, neuropathy

Pathophysiology

Extrinsic	Intrinsic
Pressure	Fibrosis/local ischemia
Shear (Damages blood vessels)	Loss of autonomic control
Friction (Damages epidermis)	Infection
	Impaired mobility
	Incontinence(fecal and urinary)
	Poor nutritional status

PREVENTION

1. Minimize skin moisture/control to minimize risk of skin maceration and increased friction coefficient

2. Control spasticity

3. Pressure relief:

- Low air loss mattress (25 mm Hg pressure)

- Air-Fluided beds (20 mm Hg pressure)

- HOB >45 degrees

- Turn every 2 hours

- Pressure lift 10 second lift every 10 minutes when sitting

■ TYPICAL WOUND CARE SUPPLIES BY CLASS

Alginates
Algisite M (Smith & Nephew)

Kaltostat (ConvaTec)

Maxorb (Medline)

Hydrogels
Duoderm (Convatec)

Hypergel (Molnlycke Health Care)

IntraSite (Smith & Nephew)

Hydrofiber
Aquacel (ConvaTec)

Silver Impregnated Dressings
Aquacel Ag (Convatec)

Acticoat (Smith & Nephew)

Maxorb Ag (Medline)

Antimicrobial gels and creams
Bactroban Ointment

Bacitracin Ointment

Gentamicin cream

Silver sulfadiazine cream

Compression Wraps
Dyna-Flex (Johnson & Johnson)

Profore (Smith & Nephew)

Sub-atmospheric Dressings
V.A.C. (KCI)

Versatile 1 (Smith & Nephew)

Skin Substitutes (Cellular)
Apligraf (Organogenesis)

Dermagraft (Advanced Biohealing)

Skin Substitutes (Acellular)
Oasis (Healthpoint)

Integra (Integra LifeSciences)

Appendix 24   *Websites*

General Rehabilitation Professional Organizations

American Academy of Physical Medicine and rehabilitation (AAPMR)
    http://www.aapmr.org

American Association of Neuromuscular and Electrodiagnostic (AANEM)
    http://www.aanem.org/

American Association of People with Disabilities (AAPD)
    http://www.aapd.com

American Board of Physical Medicine and Rehabilitation
    http://www.abpmr.org

American Congress of Rehabilitation Medicine
    http://www.acrm.org

Association of Academic Physiatrists (AAP)
    http://www.physiatry.org

Foundation for PM&R
    http://www.foundationforpmr.org/

International Society of Physical and Rehabilitation Medicine (ISPRM)
    http://www.isprm.org/

Rehabilitation Engineering and Assistive Technology Society
    of North America (RESNA)
    http://www.resna.org

The National Rehabilitation Association (NRA)
    http://www.nationalrehab.org

Special Interest

Alzheimer's Association
    http://www.alz.org/index.asp

American Academy of Orthotists and Prosthetists
    http://www.oandp.com/

American occupational Therapy Association
    http://www.aota.org

American Physical Therapy Association
    http://www.apta.org

American Psychological Association—Division 22 Rehabilitation Psychology
    http://www.apa.org/about/division/div22.aspx

American Speech language and Hearing Association
    http://www.asha.org

American Stroke Association
    http://www.strokeassociation.org

American Therapeutic Recreation Association
    http://www.atra-online.com

Amputee Coalition of America
    http://www.amputee-coalition.org

Arthritis Foundation
    http://www.arthritis.org

Muscular Dystrophy Association
http://www.mda.org
National Brain Injury Association
http://www.biausa.org
National Institute on Disability and Rehabilitation Research (NIDRR)
http://www.ed.gov/offices/OSERS/NIDRR
National Multiple Sclerosis Society
http://www.nmss.org
National Spinal Cord Injury Association
http://www.spinalcord.org/
National Stroke Association
http://www.stroke.org
Needle EMG Anatomy Atlas
http://www.teleemg.com/new/atlas.htm
Office of Disability Employment Policy (ODEP)
http://www.dol.gov/odep/welcome.html
Paralyzed Veterans of America
http://www.pva.org
The Orthotics & Prosthetics Virtual Library
http://www.oandplibrary.org/
Visible Human Project
http://www.nlm.nih.gov/research/visible/visible_human.html
Worldwide Education and Awareness for Movement Disorders (WE MOVE)
http://www.wemove.org

Rehabilitation Journals

American Journal of Physical Medicine & Rehabilitation
http://www.amjphysmedrehab.com
Archives of Physical Medicine and Rehabilitation
http://www.archives-pmr.org
Journal of Rehabilitation Medicine
http://jrm.medicaljournals.se
PM&R
http://www.pmrjournal.org